Frontiers in Celiac Disease

Pediatric and Adolescent Medicine

Vol. 12

Frontiers in Celiac Disease

Volume Editors

Alessio Fasano Baltimore, Md.
Riccardo Troncone Naples
David Branski Jerusalem

52 figures, 19 in color, and 25 tables, 2008

KARGER

Basel · Freiburg · Paris · London · New York · Bangalore · Bangkok · Shanghai · Singapore · Tokyo · Sydney

Prof. Alessio Fasano, MD
Center for Celiac Research and
Mucosal Biology Research Center
University of Maryland School of Medicine
Baltimore, Md., USA

Prof. Riccardo Troncone, MD
Department of Pediatrics and European Laboratory for
the Investigation of Food-Induced Diseases
University Federico II
Naples, Italy

Prof. David Branski, MD
Division of Pediatrics
Hadassah University Hospitals
Jerusalem, Israel

Library of Congress Cataloging-in-Publication Data

Frontiers in celiac disease / volume editor, Alessio Fasano, Riccardo
Troncone, David Branski.
p. ; cm. – (Pediatric and adolescent medicine, ISSN 1017–5989; v. 12)
Includes bibliographical references and indexes.
ISBN 978-3-8055-8526-2 (hard cover: alk. paper)
1. Celiac disease. I. Fasano, Alessio. II. Troncone, R. (Riccardo) III. Branski, D.
IV. Series.
[DNLM: 1. Celiac disease—immunology. 2. Celiac Disease. W1 PE163HL
v.12 2008 / WD 175 F935 2008]
RC862.C44F76 2008]
616.3′99–dc22 2008007963

Bibliographic Indices. This publication is listed in bibliographic services, including Current Contents®.

Disclaimer. The statements, options and data contained in this publication are solely those of the individual authors and contributors and not of the publisher and the editor(s). The appearance of advertisements in the book is not a warranty, endorsement, or approval of the products or services advertised or of their effectiveness, quality or safety. The publisher and the editor(s) disclaim responsibility for any injury to persons or property resulting from any ideas, methods, instructions or products referred to in the content or advertisements.

Drug Dosage. The authors and the publisher have exerted every effort to ensure that drug selection and dosage set forth in this text are in accord with current recommendations and practice at the time of publication. However, in view of ongoing research, changes in government regulations, and the constant flow of information relating to drug therapy and drug reactions, the reader is urged to check the package insert for each drug for any change in indications and dosage and for added warnings and precautions. This is particularly important when the recommended agent is a new and/or infrequently employed drug.

www.karger.com
Printed in Switzerland on acid-free and non-aging paper (ISO 9706) by Reinhardt Druck, Basel
ISSN 1017–5989
ISBN 978–3–8055–8526–2

Contents

Preface

Celiac disease (CD) is an immune-mediated enteropathy triggered by the ingestion of gluten-containing grains (including wheat, rye and barley) in genetically susceptible individuals. Epidemiological studies conducted during the past decade revealed that CD is one of the most common lifelong disorders worldwide. CD can manifest itself with a previously unappreciated range of clinical presentations, including the typical malabsorption syndrome and a spectrum of symptoms potentially affecting any organ system. Since CD often presents in an atypical or even silent manner, many cases remain undiagnosed and carry the risk of long-term complications, including anemia, osteoporosis, infertility or cancer. The high prevalence of the disease and its variety of clinical outcomes raise several interesting questions. Why is a disease that, if not treated, is associated with a high rate of morbidity and increased mortality yet not segregated by genetic evolution, and why does it remain one of the most frequent genetically based disorders of humankind? One possible explanation is that gluten, a protein introduced in large quantities in the human diet only after the advent of agriculture, activates 'by mistake of evolution' mechanisms of innate and adaptive immunity that are too important for human survival to be eliminated. Another unresolved issue concerns the variable(s) that dictates the length of clinical latency and the type of symptoms experienced by CD patients when the disease becomes clinically apparent. In recent years, there have been noticeable shifts in the age of onset of symptoms and in the clinical presentation of CD, changes that seem to be associated with a delayed introduction of gluten coupled with its reduced amount in the diet. Another controversial topic concerns the complications of untreated CD. Multiple studies that have focused on the biochemistry and toxicity of gluten-containing grains and the immune response to these grains suggest that individuals affected by CD should be treated, irrespective of the presence or absence of symptoms and/or associated conditions. However, well-designed prospective clinical studies to address this point have not been performed, nor can they be conceived, given the ethical implications of such studies. Nevertheless, there is general agreement that the persistence of mucosal injury, with or without typical symptoms, can lead to severe complications in CD patients who do not strictly comply with a gluten-free diet. Another controversial issue is related to screening policies in terms of who should be screened for CD. The prevalence of the disease and the burden of illness related to this condition, particularly if not treated, are so high as to possibly support a policy of general population screening. However, cost-effective analyses and 'return on investment' for patients, healthcare providers and policy makers keep the debate open.

This book covers most of the aforementioned controversial and yet unresolved topics by capitalizing on the contribution of opinion leaders expert in CD and of its multidisciplinary ramifications. What the reader will surely find stimulating about this book is not only its exhaustive coverage of our current knowledge of CD, but also of provocative new concepts in disease pathogenesis, treatment and prevention that can be extrapolated to other immune-mediated pathologies. Indeed, given the undisputable role of gluten in causing inflammation and immune-mediated tissue damage, CD represents a unique model of autoimmunity in which, in contrast to most other autoimmune diseases, a close genetic association with HLA genes (DQ2 and/or DQ8), a highly specific humoral autoimmune response (autoantibodies to tissue transglutaminase) and, most importantly, the triggering environmental factor (gluten) are known. This information provides the rationale for the treatment of the disease based on complete avoidance of gluten-containing grains from the patients' diet. Therefore, CD represents the only autoimmune disorder for which a treatment is available, since the trigger(s) involved in the pathogenesis of other autoimmune diseases remain elusive at best. This also implies that CD could represent the best model to study autoimmune pathogenesis and, eventually, to develop novel therapeutic strategies for the treatment of conditions still orphan of any possible solution.

We want to take the opportunity to thank all the contributors of this book who took time from their busy schedule to realize this project. This book would not have been possible without the expertise and invaluable contribution and technical support of Mrs. Donna Bethke and of the Karger editorial team.

Alessio Fasano, Baltimore, Md.
Riccardo Troncone, Naples
David Branski, Jerusalem

Fasano A, Troncone R, Branski D (eds): Frontiers in Celiac Disease.
Pediatr Adolesc Med. Basel, Karger, 2008, vol 12, pp 1–11

Historical Perspective of Celiac Disease

Stefano Guandalini

Division of Pediatric Gastroenterology, Hepatology and Nutrition, University of Chicago, Chicago, Ill., USA

Abstract

Ten thousand years ago, celiac disease (CD) appears on the face of the Earth with the most dramatic change in human history: the agricultural revolution that brought to man's table foods that he had never experienced in his previous 2.5 million years. Among them eventually wheat was domesticated, selected mostly for the appearance of mutants with large grains and with ears resistant to harvesting. Not all humans adapted and, among those who had a genetic predisposition to develop an abnormal immune response rather than tolerance, CD emerged, becoming soon a major killer of infants for many generations. Little less than 2,000 years ago, a clever Greek physician named Aretaeus of Cappadocia wrote a total of 8 books on medicine, providing the first known description of adult patients with CD. He had quite a grasp on this condition, that he named 'koiliakos' after the Greek word 'koelia' (abdomen), to imply that these patients were 'suffering in their abdomen'. Seventeen centuries went by. On October 5, 1887, at Great Ormond Street in London, Dr. Samuel Gee, a Lecturer in Medicine at St. Bartholomew's Hospital as well as Physician in the Hospital for Sick Children at Great Ormond Street, gave to medical students a lecture on the 'celiac affection' that was published the following year: this constitutes the modern 'rediscovery' of CD. Also Dr. Gee had good insights into CD, as he wrote: 'If the patient can be cured at all, it must be by means of diet', adding: 'The allowance of farinaceous food must be small'. In 1924 Sidney Haas described his successful treatment of 8 children whom he had diagnosed as having CD, by using a diet based mostly on bananas. The banana diet, of which he became soon a fervent, strenuous advocate, ruled the world as the only treatment for CD for decades, even years after Dicke, Weijers and van de Kamer had produced their famous series of seminal papers documenting for the first time the role of gluten from wheat and rye in causing the harm of CD. Soon after the role of gluten in causing the flat lesion of CD had been ascertained, theories began to be put forward as to why gluten would be causing that intestinal damage and its subsequent symptoms. The first was an enzymatic one: an enzyme ought to be either missing or malfunctioning, thus leading to an inability to properly digest gluten, generating toxic fragments. This theory persisted for many years without any solid evidence but was put to rest when it became finally clear that CD had an immunological basis, and its autoimmune nature was convincingly demonstrated by the identification, in 1997, by a German group led by Dietrich, of the autoantigen: the ubiquitous enzyme tissue transglutaminase. Along with the progress in the clinical description of CD and in its diagnosis (something that flourished after the availability in the early 60s of the peroral biopsy capsule), efforts were made especially by the European Society for Pediatric Gastroenterology (today the European Society for Pediatric Gastroenterology, Hepatology and Nutrition) to define precise diagnostic criteria. Such criteria were put forward in 1970, revised in 1990 and accepted basically worldwide until now. Currently in fact, the fast advancing knowledge on CD pathophysiology, its many forms and its natural history is knocking at the door for their further revision.

Celiac Disease Appears in the World's Scenario

A long, long time ago there was no celiac disease (CD) on the planet Earth. This was not the result of lack of awareness, poor diagnostic techniques or the fact that humankind had different gene pools. It was the result of the fact that simply there *was* no gluten. Man was a (happy?) gatherer and hunter, and his diet consisted of fruits, nuts and perhaps tubers, dug up with simple tools. He also had occasional feasts on meats obtained by actively hunting particularly large-bodied prey, and possibly also on scavenging carcasses. These dietetic habits went on for an extremely long period of time, roughly since inception of humans as we know them (about 2.5 million years ago), and remained unchanged until about only 10,000 years ago.

But what happened then was going to change our way of life forever: the Neolithic era agricultural revolution. It is thought that it might have been an incidental observation (most likely by women, who – besides being notoriously cleverer than men – were more likely to stay 'home' while the men were out hunting) that a seed fallen from a wild plant had later sprung into another similar plant that led to the intuition that 'food'-bearing plants could actually be cultivated. This soon was to transform society: the hunter-gatherer way of life was in fact replaced by domestication of crops and animals, enabling people to live sedentary lives next to their sources of food, instead of having to constantly move from one location to another in perpetual search of food sources. Thus, permanent settlements arose, beginning in an area of the Middle East called the 'Fertile Crescent' (a term coined by the University of Chicago archaeologist James H. Breasted), creating previously unforeseen forms of social, cultural, economic and political institutions. The modern times had begun!

Wheat and barley were the first cereals to have been domesticated. Specifically, wheat, in all its subspecies, originated in the Fertile Crescent. Ten thousand years ago, wild einkorn *(Triticum monococcum)* and emmer wheat (*Triticum dicoccoides*, in Europe and especially Italy still known as 'farro') were domesticated as part of the early agriculture in the Fertile Crescent, although both are now considered 'relic' crops [1]. Parenthetically, it is of interest that recently it has been shown that the gliadin of the original wheat *T. monococcum* lacks toxicity for celiac patients in an in vitro organ culture system [2]. Cultivation and repeated harvesting and sowing of the grains of wild grasses led to the domestication of wheat by selection of mutant forms with lager grains and with ears resistant to harvesting [3].

Next, the cultivation of wheat began to spread beyond the Fertile Crescent during the Neolithic period. Of interest, this massive westward spreading of wheat cultivation (and more in general of the agricultural revolution) should not be seen simply as the spreading of the new technology, but actually as a true migration of masses of populations that progressively moved westward, perhaps because the original settlements were becoming overcrowded, and because that was the time of melting of the last ice Age, making new and more northerly destinations attractive again [4, 5]. This massive migration is considered one of the major events in the whole of human history, and recently obtained evidence has conclusively shown its occurrence, further identifying the speed of its progression at about 1 km/year [6]. Of note, this massive population migration also coincided with the spreading of the Indo-European languages, a language family linked to the domestication of wheat, and particularly to its 'Centum' subbranch, whose geographical extension strikingly overlaps with the extension of the agricultural spreading, with the exception of the Basque region [7] (fig. 1).

By 5,000 years ago, wheat had reached Ireland and Spain. A millennium later it reached also China [3]. Today, the annual world's production of wheat amounts to approximately 630 millions of tons!

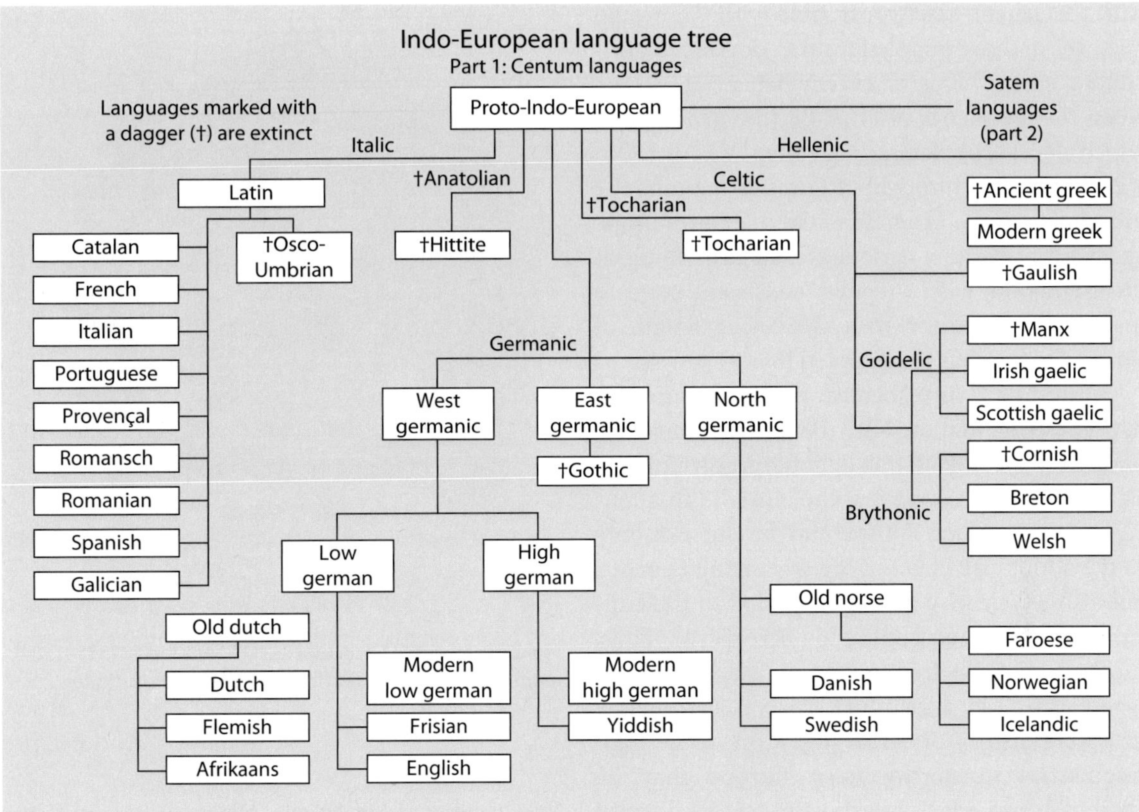

Fig. 1. The Indo-European language (Centum branch) overlaps completely with the geographical distribution of the Neolithic agricultural spreading (from http://www.danshort.com/ie/iecentum_c.shtml; used with permission).

In contrast to the many positive consequences of this revolution however, some unanticipated problems also arose. In fact, our gut had progressively developed, over more than 2 million years, into a sophisticated organ happily interacting with billions of bacteria and capable of selectively distinguishing, among the constant load of antigens presented to it day after day, those that were to be fought as strangers and potentially dangerous from those that could be accepted as innocuous. In other words, the evolution had provided us with the ability to show immunological tolerance to food antigens that have been the staple of our diet over many hundreds of thousands of years; but how to react to completely new antigens, suddenly appearing in the diet? The agricultural revolution of the Neolithic, with its domestication of cattle *(Bos taurus* and *Bos indicus)* from wild aurochsen *(Bos primigenius)*, various species of birds and the production of cereals, generated in fact a whole battery of food antigens previously unknown to men: protein from cow, goat, donkey milks, as well as birds' eggs, and cereals such as wheat and barley became all of a sudden totally new and major components of man's diet.

Not everybody adapted, food intolerances appeared and CD was born.

It can be assumed that most of the individuals who developed CD succumbed to this condition, and thus the overall prevalence of adult individuals with the genetic asset compatible with CD would be lower in those populations that developed agriculture earlier. This is exactly what was found when the prevalence of HLA-B8 (the genotype to which all celiacs belong being either DQ2 or DQ8) was investigated throughout Europe: mapping the prevalence of the HLA-B8 antigen across Europe against the spread of agriculture, an east-west gradient is found, with a regular, consistent increase in antigen frequency with decreasing length of time since farming was adopted [8].

Simoons [9] investigated this phenomenon, hypothesizing that the HLA-B8 antigen may once have been prevalent throughout preagricultural Europe and suggesting that the HLA-B8 frequencies across modern Europe may be due not only to the admixture effect of the advancing farmers, but also to selective pressures related to the consumption of gluten-containing cereals [9]. Thus, the low HLA-B8 frequencies in the Near East, where as we saw agriculture arose, is attributable to a long history of cereal ingestion, while high frequencies in northwestern Europe may be attributable to a lack of exposure to cereals until relatively recently. Possession of CD genes would confer a disadvantage to those living in areas of high cereal consumption, accounting for the well-documented inverse relationship between the frequency of CD in an area and the length of time since the introduction of agriculture.

Celiac Disease Is Recognized and Described

Now, fast-forward several millennia: more or less 8,000 years after its onset, and probably for a long time undetected amidst the large number of infant and childhood deaths due to infectious diarrheal diseases, CD was identified and received its name. A clever Greek physician named Aretaeus of Cappadocia (fig. 2), living about a century before the more famous ancient Roman physician Galen, wrote in the first century AD a total of 8 books on medicine, arriving to us in their Latin version and

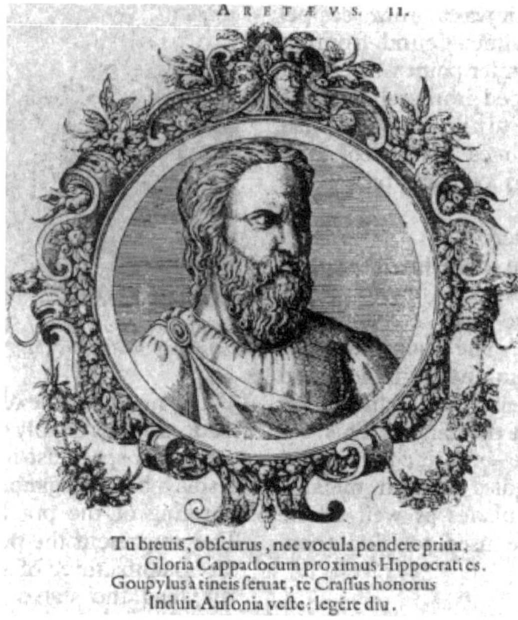
ARETÆVS. II.
Tu breuis, obſcurus, nec vocula pendere priua,
Gloria Cappadocum proximus Hippocrati es.
Goupylus à tineis ſeruat, te Craſſus honorus
Induit Auſonia veſte: legére diu.

WELLCOME INSTITUTE LIBRARY, LONDON

Fig. 2. Aretaeus of Cappadocia (by J. Sambucus, 1531–1584); reprinted with permission from the Wellcome Institute Library, London.

later translated by Francis Adams and printed for the Sydenham Society in 1856 [10]: two *De causis et signis acutorum morborum*, two *De causis et signis diuturnorum morborum*, two *De curatione acutorum morborum* and two *De curatione diuturnorum morborum*. In one word: all you need to know about acute and chronic illnesses! In his treaties, Aretaeus had a section on 'the coeliac affection' considered the very first description of CD (the classical, gastrointestinal form, to be clear), proving that he had quite a grasp on this condition, that he named 'koiliakos' after the Greek word 'koelia' (abdomen), to imply that these patients were 'suffering in their abdomen'. Here – in the 19th-century English translation mentioned – is what he had to say when describing celiac patients: 'If the stomach be irretentive of the food and if it pass through undigested and crude, and nothing ascends into the body, we call such persons coeliacs.' He must even be credited with the astute observation that the disease is more prevalent in women!

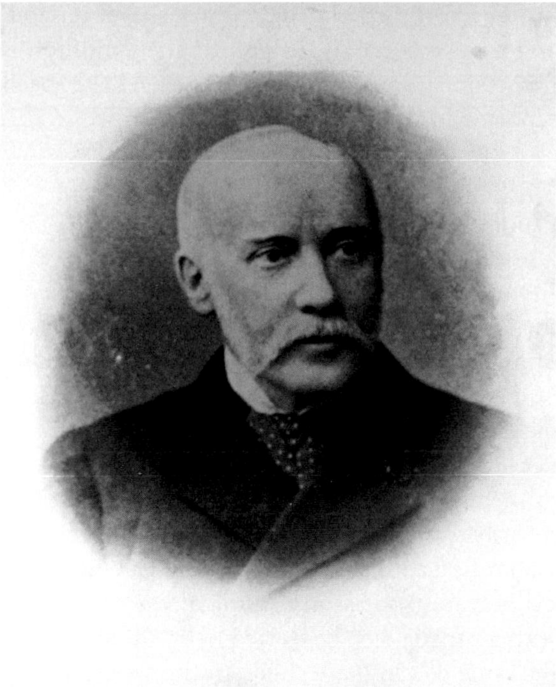

Fig. 3. Samuel Gee. Reprinted with permission from the Wellcome Institute Library, London.

Another 17 centuries went by, and in the early 19th century a Dr. Mathew Baillie, probably unaware of Aretaeus, published his observations on a chronic diarrheal disorder of adults causing malnutrition and characterized by a gas-distended abdomen. He even went on to suggest dietetic treatment, writing [11]: 'Some patients have appeared to derive considerable advantage from living almost entirely upon rice.' Baillie's observations however got practically unnoticed, as pointed out by Lewkonia [12], and it was for the English doctor Samuel Gee (fig. 3) to take full credit for the modern-times description of CD.

At the time of his description of CD, Dr. Gee was Lecturer in Medicine at St. Bartholomew's Hospital as well as Physician in the Hospital for Sick Children at Great Ormond Street, London, where he was a leading authority in pediatric diseases. On October 5, 1887, at Great Ormond Street he gave to medical students a lecture on the 'celiac affection' that was published the following year [13] and remains to this date the milestone description of this disorder in modern times.

Let's look at some of his writings, as they represent an elegant and amazingly detailed description of what is today called 'classical' CD: 'There is a kind of chronic indigestion which is met with in persons of all ages, yet is especially apt to affect children between one and five years old. Signs of the disease are yielded by the faeces; being loose, not formed, but not watery; more bulky than the food taken would seem to account for; pale in colour, as if devoid of bile; yeasty, frothy, an appearance probably due to fermentation; stinking, stench often very great, the food having undergone putrefaction rather than concoction... The onset is generally gradual, so that its time is hard to fix: sometimes the complaint sets in suddenly, like an accidental diarrhea; ... The patient wastes more in the limbs than in the face ... The belly is mostly soft, doughy and inelastic; sometimes distended and rather tight ...'. He noted that 'because of the wasting, weakness, and pallor of the patient, the bowel complaint might be easily overlooked... The course of the disease is always slow, whatever be its end; whether the patient live or die, he lingers ill for months or years. Death is a common end ...'.

As for a treatment, he had the intuition, like Baillie before him, that 'if the patient can be cured at all, it must be by means of diet.' And he adds that 'the allowance of farinaceous food must be small' and also describes 'a child who was fed upon a quart of the best Dutch mussels daily, throve wonderfully, but relapsed when the season for mussels was over; next season he could not be prevailed upon to take them. This is an experiment which I have not yet been able to repeat.' Samuel Gee therefore concurs, unknowingly, with Mathew Baillie in documenting the improvement following the introduction of a gluten-free diet, and he even shows for the first time the relapse after reintroduction of gluten!

Years later CD began to be increasingly recognized and reported, although certainly still vaguely, if at all, differentiated from other conditions causing malabsorption. The landmark of malabsorption, steatorrhea, was identified as typical of CD children already more than a century ago, when it was noticed and quantitatively demonstrated by Cheadle [14], who however thought that the main pathophysiological problem was the lack of bile in stools, and hence called the disease 'acholia' and concluded that the cause of the disease was 'most obscure'.

In fact, for many decades there was no clue as to what could be causing CD and no hint (in spite of autopsies frequently performed given the high mortality rate) of the damage to the intestinal mucosa. Still in the mid 1950s CD was in fact thought to have 'no anatomic abnormality of the digestive tract' [15].

Yet, it is remarkable that some of the present-day findings, which we tend to consider as recent advances, were indeed well known a long time ago.

For instance, it was already in the early 1920s that Miller and Perkins [16] recognized that CD could be present without diarrhea, as they wrote differentiating 'the diarrheic or classical type and the non-diarrheic type'. Moreover, the protective role of breastfeeding in the development and severity of CD, recently documented by a rigorous evidence-based approach [17], was already postulated with great confidence by several authors [18–20] 60 years ago. Furthermore, although nothing was known on predisposing genes, the celebrated Swiss pediatrician Guido Fanconi had recognized already in 1938 an increased familial incidence and its occurrence in twins [21].

As for what was thought in terms of its worldwide prevalence, the modern reader will be surprised to learn what Doris Anderson writes in the USA in 1959 [22]: 'The geographic distribution now appears to be associated largely with the use of wheat or rye ... Most of the cases have been observed in England and America (sic!); next in order come Germany and Austria, while others have been recorded in Scandinavia, Switzerland, and the Netherlands. In France, the condition is rare (sic!), and only a few cases have been reported from Italy (double sic!).'

Progress in Treatment

In the face of a prolonged lack of knowledge about the etiology and pathogenesis of CD, and after the original astute observations about the importance of diet in obtaining remission, in the 1920s a new dietetic treatment irrupted in the scene and for decades established itself as the main cornerstone of therapy: the banana diet. In 1924 Sidney Haas described his successful treatment of 8 children whom he had diagnosed as having CD. Based on his previous success in treating a case of anorexia with a banana diet, he elected to try to experiment the same diet in these children who were too very anorectic. He published [23] 10 cases, 8 of them treated ('clinically cured') with the banana diet, whilst the 2 untreated ones died. This paper encountered enormous success and for decades the banana diet enjoyed wide popularity, indeed benefiting a large number of celiac children and probably preventing many deaths. The diet – aimed at avoiding all complex carbohydrates – specifically excluded bread, crackers, potatoes and all cereals, and it's easy now to argue that its success was based on the elimination of gluten-containing grains.

Haas was very proud of his insight that carbohydrates were the culprit and had to be eliminated and he was very resistant to accept different views, no matter how well documented they might be. Indeed, even as late as 40 years later [24], well after Dicke et al. [25] had convincingly shown that wheat protein, and not starch, was the only culprit, Haas still insisted that with his banana diet 'all patients are cured by the specific carbohydrate diet, a cure which is permanent without relapse'. He even went on to say (a quote from the same paper) that 'Dicke's demonstration was an excellent achievement scientifically ... but clinically it was a possible disservice, since it ignored other carbohydrates as aetiological factors'. So much for 'expert opinion'!

Progress in Understanding the Pathogenesis

The breakthrough that Haas chose to deliberately downplay was however to change forever our view of CD. Dicke, a Dutch pediatrician, had in fact noticed that during the shortage of bread caused by World War II in the Netherlands, children with CD improved. Additionally, he also noticed that when planes from the Allies dropped bread into the Netherlands, celiac children quickly deteriorated. A few years later, working with Weijers and van de Kamer, they produced a series of seminal papers [25, 26] documenting for the first time the role of gluten from wheat and rye in causing the harm of CD.

Thus, soon after the role of gluten in causing the flat lesion of CD was ascertained, theories began to be put forward as to why gluten would be causing that intestinal damage and its subsequent symptoms.

The first was an enzymatic one: an enzyme ought to be either missing or malfunctioning, thus leading to an inability to properly digest gluten, generating toxic fragments. Although the search for a missing or defective enzyme was destined to be unsuccessful [27–29], as all the deficiencies in the hydrolysis or transport of peptides found in celiacs were invariably shown to be simply secondary to the reduced absorptive surface, it was nevertheless instrumental in the acquisition of a formidable wealth of new information on the pathophysiology of intestinal digestion and absorption of protein.

In the 70s and well into the 80s, a new theory became fashionable: the 'lectin theory' [30]. The theory surmised the presence in gluten of a toxic lectin (lectins are vegetable proteins that recognize carbohydrate moieties of glycoprotein and glycolipids and bind to them, eliciting subsequent biological effects). In CD, it was hypothesized that this binding to the brush border would initiate a series of toxic events, which indeed some investigators were able to show in vitro [31, 32]. This hypothesis persisted throughout the 80s and only in the early 90s was it challenged and definitively put to rest [33] in the face of the rising fortune of the 'immunological theory' that was quickly gaining ground.

After 1990, CD was increasingly accepted as an example of an autoimmune disease, associated with a specific HLA haplotype (either DQ2 or DQ8). The missing autoantigen was finally identified in 1997 by Dieterich et al. [34], in Germany, as the ubiquitous enzyme tissue transglutaminase. These authors recognized tissue transglutaminase as the unknown endomysial autoantigen, and in that seminal paper even showed that 'gliadin is a preferred substrate for this enzyme, giving rise to novel antigenic epitopes'. Thus, the mystery was finally broken and the long sequence of theories and conjectures was once and forever over, with the universal acceptance that CD is an autoimmune condition whose trigger (gluten) and autoantigen (tissue transglutaminase) are known.

Progress in Delineating the Clinical Spectrum

Another interesting phenomenon pertaining to the perceived clinical expression of CD began to appear in the 80s: on one side it became increasingly clear that CD may be associated with other conditions, mostly autoimmune disorders such as type 1 diabetes, but also some syndromes such as Down [35–39]; on the other side, it was obvious that CD was changing patterns of presentation, becoming less and less an intestinal disorder, and more and more a variety of extraintestinal symptoms and signs [40]. These facts, today well known, were described and immediately appreciated mostly in Europe, while in North America no one seemed to pay attention to them. This phenomenon probably greatly contributed to make CD the

Cinderella of pediatric disorders in North America, where the classical, gastrointestinal presentation (that decades earlier was considered common, as we have seen) was considered rare and not worth of much attention, thus generating the progressive lag of attention to CD in that part of the world. In fact, a recent observation by Rampertab et al. [41] confirms that in a population of celiac patients in the USA, with time the pattern of clinical presentation has significantly shifted toward later presentation and more extraintestinal manifestations.

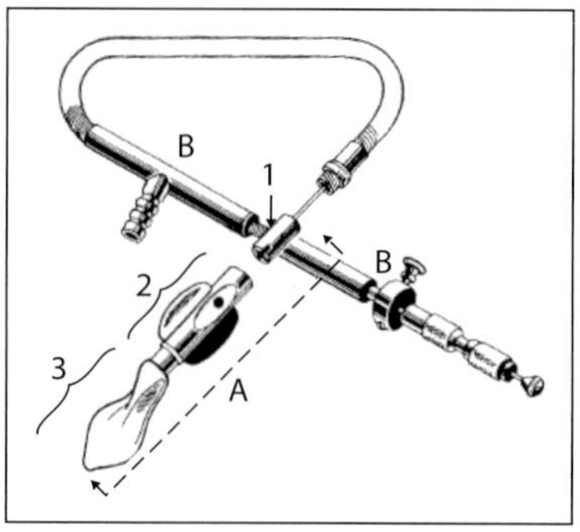

Fig. 4. Margot Shiner's jejunal biopsy tube; reprinted from Shiner [42], with permission.

Progress in Diagnosis

As mentioned, for a very long time there was no clue as to what was the reason for the chronic diarrhea and subsequent wasting. Although Fanconi had the intuition that the condition was due to a dysfunction of the small intestine [21], it was not until Margot Shiner provided gastroenterologists the world over with the chance of doing intestinal biopsies in children that the duodenojejunal damage typical of CD was recognized. Shiner conducted important studies on the ultrastructure and cytopathology of the human small intestine at the Central Middlesex Hospital. In January of 1956, in a two-paper series published in the *Lancet* [42, 43], she described a new jejunal biopsy tube (fig. 4) based on a modification of the gastric mucosal biopsy instrument introduced a few years earlier by Ian Wood in Australia [44], with which she successfully reached and biopsied the distal duodenum. This – and the development of the less cumbersome, more user-friendly capsule developed shortly after by the American Lieutenant Colonel Crosby [45] – was a huge milestone development in the history of celiac disease, as it allowed for the first time to link the disease with a specific, recognizable pattern of damage to the proximal small-intestinal mucosa.

Thus, at the dawn of the 60s we had these 3 important elements: (1) the knowledge of gluten being the triggering agent for CD; (2) the notion that there was a remarkable and easily identifiable mucosal lesion, and finally (3) the availability of an instrument to obtain biopsies and thus beginning to unravel the mystery of CD pathogenesis (see below).

But perhaps more importantly the medical community could now begin to differentiate CD from other causes of chronic diarrhea and wasting, and could fund diagnostic practices on firmer grounds. This is the point where we see a new, emerging field quickly take the lead in this process: the field of pediatric gastroenterology. Essentially born in Europe with mostly biochemical research around the description of several new congenital disorders of digestion and absorption, pediatric gastroenterology soon emerged and became a powerful force in defining CD and in indicating how to properly diagnose it. In the mid to late 60s, it had become clear that CD could be diagnosed with the peroral jejunal biopsy showing atrophy of the villi, but since many were the causes of that lesion (and at that time especially chronic intestinal infections and milk protein allergy), a strong word of caution was exerted by the medical community not to diagnose CD until it could be proven that gluten was indeed the cause of the mucosal atrophy. Thus, not only was a clinical complete remission on a gluten-free diet considered necessary, but this had to be followed by the documentation of the normalization of the lesion, and finally by its recurrence

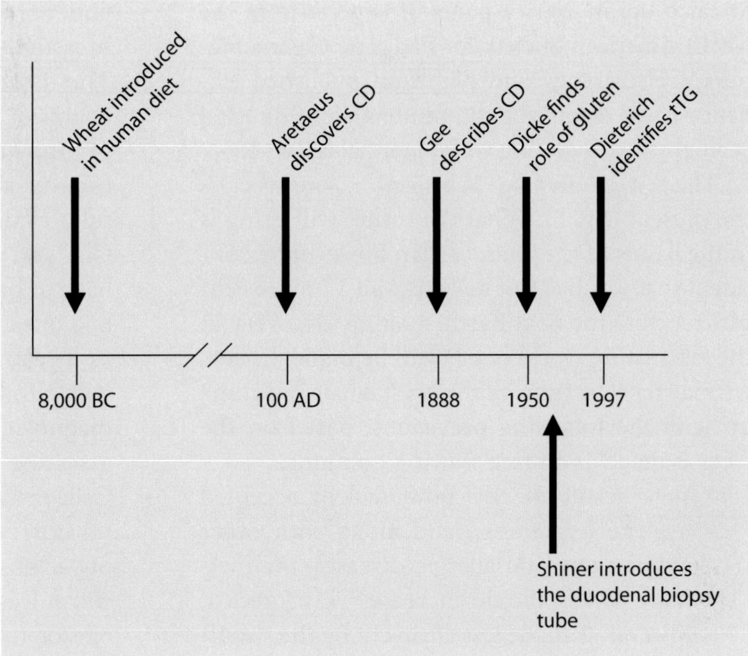

Fig. 5. A diagrammatic summary of the history of CD. tTG = Tissue transglutaminase.

once gluten was reintroduced into the diet. These criteria were formalized in 1969 by a panel of experts in the then newly born European Society for Pediatric Gastroenterology (today ESPGHAN – European Society for Pediatric Gastroenterology, Hepatology and Nutrition) in the so-called 'Interlaken criteria' [46] which for over 20 years served worldwide as the accepted diagnostic standard.

The Interlaken criteria did however not take into account another important discovery that had been made just a few years earlier: CD children presented in their blood antibodies caused by the ingestion of gluten. The first category to be discovered were the antigliadin antibodies, detected and reported by Berger et al. [47] in 1964. Seven years later, Seah et al. [48] identified for the first time not an antifood protein, but an actual autoantibody in the serum of celiac children: the antireticulins. It took however several years before their diagnostic utility was fully appreciated, and the real leap forward occurred in 1984 when the antiendomysium antibodies were described [49], which soon dominated the scene for their high specificity.

In the late 80s, a large multicenter Italian study could demonstrate that by relying on strict clinical and laboratory criteria, and now also supported by the antiendomysium antibodies, a correct diagnosis of CD could be reached in 95% of cases by limiting intervention to the one initial biopsy [50]. This plea for a change was soon followed by new diagnostic guidelines published the following year by the ESPGHAN [51]. These guidelines have been widely followed worldwide, not only in pediatric, but also in adult gastroenterology. Even though they were not 'evidence based' in the strictest sense of the word as used today [52], such recommendations still stemmed largely from the cited experience [50] and proved very useful not only in clinical practice, but also as a reference for research.

North America, that as mentioned in spite of an early start was markedly lagging behind as for the rate of diagnosis and diagnostic delay (at some point estimated to be higher than 10 years), began to catch up: in 2005 a panel of experts from the North American Society for Pediatric Gastroenterology, Hepatology and Nutrition published evidence-based diagnostic recommendations directed at all physicians dealing with potential celiacs [53].

The rest, as they say, is history … or rather, is the present (fig. 5). What the future will bring is in the hands of the gods: we can however be confident that we shall not have to wait 17 more centuries before the next Earth-shaking discovery in the fascinating world of CD will be made. In fact, we may try to scrutinize the crystal ball and come up with the following previsions, based on the facts as much as on free-flowing opinions.

(1) As a result of the now widely accepted 'hygiene hypothesis', and along with other autoimmune and allergic diseases, the incidence of CD should increase. This forecast, however, is made less clear-cut by the simultaneous emergence of possible preventative measures, such as; anti-Rotavirus vaccination (CD prevalence is higher in children who as infants had 2 or more Rotavirus infections [54]), prolonged breastfeeding, and especially introducing small amounts of gluten [55] to infants who are still being breastfed [17].

(2) The diagnostic criteria of CD will again be changed: once the issues of properly interpreting *mucosal* autoimmunity and minimal (or even absent!) histologic changes have been fully evaluated [56], the definition itself of CD, and hence its diagnostic criteria, will have to be rewritten in much broader terms, and our limited and limiting thinking of CD as a gastrointestinal malabsorptive disorder will be obsolete. Also, we may end up by diagnosing CD with a simple blood test assessing gluten-specific T cells [57].

(3) Celiac patients will likely enjoy better peace of mind by being able to occasionally eat out without an obsessive attention to the menu, as they will at least partially be protected by ingesting one or the other preparations that are being developed [58, 59] to attenuate the harmful effects of low amounts of ingested gluten. Also, they may be able to enjoy a broader selection of foods increasingly more similar to bread, by the availability of pretreated wheat [60].

All in all, the future does look bright and exciting!

References

1 Heun M, et al: Site of einkorn wheat domestication identified by DNA fingerprinting. Science 1997;278:1312–1314.

2 Pizzuti D, et al: Lack of intestinal mucosal toxicity of *Triticum monococcum* in celiac disease patients. Scand J Gastroenterol 2006;41:1305–1311.

3 Smith C: Crop Production: Evolution, History and Technology. Hoboken, Wiley & Sons, 1995, pp 60–62.

4 Colledge S, Conolly J, Shennan S: Archaeobotanical evidence for the spread of farming in the eastern Mediterranean. Curr Anthropol 2004;45:S35–S59.

5 Diamond J, Bellwood P: Farmers and their languages: the first expansions. Science 2003;300:597–603.

6 Pinhasi R, Fort J, Ammerman AJ: Tracing the origin and spread of agriculture in Europe. PLoS Biol 2005;3:e410.

7 Fortson B: Indo-European Language and Culture: An Introduction. Oxford, Blackwell Synergy, 2004.

8 Ryder LP, Andersen E, Svejgaard A: An HLA map of Europe. Hum Hered 1978; 28:171–200.

9 Simoons FJ: Celiac disease as a geographic problem; in Kretchmer DNWaN (ed): Food, Nutrition and Evolution. New York, Masson, 1981, pp 179–199.

10 Adams F: The Extant Works of Aretaeus the Cappadocian. London, The Sydenham Society, 1856.

11 Baillie M: Observations on a Particular Species of Purging. Med Trans the R Coll Phys 1815;5:166–169.

12 Lewkonia RM: Samuel Gee, Aretaeus, and the coeliac affection. Br Med J 1974;iii:442.

13 Gee SJ: On the celiac affection. St. Bartholomew's Hosp Rep 1888;24: 17–20.

14 Cheadle WB: A clinical lecture on acholia. Lancet 1903;i:1497.

15 Andersen DH, Mike EM: Diet therapy in the celiac syndrome. J Am Diet Assoc 1955;31:340–346.

16 Miller R, Perkins H: The non-diarrhoeic type of coeliac disease: a form of chronic fat indigestion in children. Lancet 1923;ii:72–76.

17 Akobeng AK, et al: Effect of breast feeding on risk of coeliac disease: a systematic review and meta-analysis of observational studies. Arch Dis Child 2006;91:39–43.

18 Brown A: Some etiological factors in the coeliac syndrome. Arch Dis Child 1949;24:99.

19 Jeans PC, Marriott WM: Infant Nutrition: A Textbook of Infant Feeding for Students and Practitioners of Medicine, ed 4. St Louis, Mosby, 1947.

20 Parsons LG: Celiac disease. Am J Dis Child 1932;43:1293.
21 Fanconi G: Zöliakie. Dtsch Med Wochenschr 1938;64:1607.
22 Anderson DM: History of celiac disease. J Am Diet Assoc 1959;35:1158–1162.
23 Haas S: The value of the banana in the treatment of coeliac disease. Am J Dis Child 1924;24:421–437.
24 Haas SV: Coeliac disease. NY State J Med 1963;1:1346–1350.
25 Dicke WK, Weijers HA, van de Kamer JH: Coeliac disease. 2. The presence in wheat of a factor having a deleterious effect in cases of coeliac disease. Acta Paediatr 1953;42:34–42.
26 van de Kamer JH, Weijers HA, Dicke WK: Coeliac disease. 4. An investigation into the injurious constituents of wheat in connection with their action on patients with coeliac disease. Acta Paediatr 1953;42:223–231.
27 Cornell HJ, Townley RR: Investigation of possible intestinal peptidase deficiency in coeliac disease. Clin Chim Acta 1973;43:113–125.
28 Lindberg T, Norden A, Josefsson L: Intestinal dipeptidases: dipeptidase activities in small intestinal biopsy specimens from a clinical material. Scand J Gastroenterol 1968;3:177–182.
29 Townley RR: Celiac disease – an inborn error of metabolism. Am J Dig Dis 1973; 18:797–800.
30 Weiser MM, Douglas AP: An alternative mechanism for gluten toxicity in coeliac disease. Lancet 1976;i:567–569.
31 Auricchio S, et al: Agglutinating activity of gliadin-derived peptides from bread wheat: implications for coeliac disease pathogenesis. Biochem Biophys Res Commun 1984;121:428–433.
32 Kottgen E, et al: Gluten, a lectin with oligomannosyl specificity and the causative agent of gluten-sensitive enteropathy. Biochem Biophys Res Commun 1982;109:168–173.
33 Ruhlmann J, et al: Studies on the aetiology of coeliac disease: no evidence for lectin-like components in wheat gluten. Biochim Biophys Acta 1993;1181:249–256.
34 Dieterich W, et al: Identification of tissue transglutaminase as the autoantigen of celiac disease. Nat Med 1997;3:797–801.
35 Dias JA, Walker-Smith J: Down's syndrome and coeliac disease. J Pediatr Gastroenterol Nutr 1990;10:41–43.
36 Green FH, Carty JE: Letter: coeliac disease and autoimmunity. Lancet 1976;i: 964.
37 Mulder CJ, Tytgat GN: Coeliac disease and related disorders. Neth J Med 1987; 31:286–299.
38 Scott BB, Losowsky MS: Coeliac disease: a cause of various associated diseases? Lancet 1975;ii:956–957.
39 Shiner M: Present trends in coeliac disease. Postgrad Med J 1984;60:773–778.
40 Rosenthal E, et al: Immunofluorescent antigluten antibody test: titer and profile of gluten antibodies in celiac disease. Am J Dis Child 1984;138:659–662.
41 Rampertab SD, et al: Trends in the presentation of celiac disease. Am J Med 2006;119:e9–14.
42 Shiner M: Jejunal-biopsy tube. Lancet 1956;i:85.
43 Shiner M: Duodenal biopsy. Lancet 1956; i:17–19.
44 Haubrich WS: Shiner of the Shiner mucosal biopsy tube. Gastroenterology 2004;127:740.
45 Crosby WH, Kugler HW: Intraluminal biopsy of the small intestine. Am J Dig Dis 1957;2:236–241.
46 Meeuwisse G: Round table discussion: diagnostic criteria in coeliac disease. Acta Paediatr Scand 1970;59:461–463.
47 Berger E, Buergin-Wolff A, Freudenberg E: Diagnostic value of the demonstration of gliadin antibodies in celiac disease. Klin Wochenschr 1964;42:788–790.
48 Seah PP, et al: Anti-reticulin antibodies in childhood coeliac disease. Lancet 1971; ii:681–682.
49 Chorzelski TP, et al: IgA anti-endomysium antibody: a new immunological marker of dermatitis herpetiformis and coeliac disease. Br J Dermatol 1984;111: 395–402.
50 Guandalini S, et al: Diagnosis of coeliac disease: time for a change? Arch Dis Child 1989;64: 1320–1324, discussion 1324–1325.
51 Walker-Smith J, et al: Revised criteria for diagnosis of coeliac disease: report of a working group of ESPGAN. Arch Dis Child 1990;65:909–911.
52 Schoenfeld P, et al: An evidence-based approach to gastroenterology diagnosis. Gastroenterology 1999;116:1230–1237.
53 Hill ID, et al: Guideline for the diagnosis and treatment of celiac disease in children: recommendations of the North American Society for Pediatric Gastroenterology, Hepatology and Nutrition. J Pediatr Gastroenterol Nutr 2005;40:1–19.
54 Stene LC, Honeyman MC, Hoffenberg EJ, et al: Rotavirus infection frequency and risk of celiac disease autoimmunity in early childhood: a longitudinal study. Am J Gastroenterol 2006;101:2333–2340.
55 Hernell O, Forsberg G, Hammarström M-L, et al: Celiac disease: effect of weaning on disease risk; in Hernell O, Schmitz J (eds): Feeding during Late Infancy and Early Childhood: Impact on Health. Nestlé Nutr Workshop Ser Pediatr Program. Vevey, Nestec/Basel, Karger, 2005, vol 56, pp 27–42.
56 Kaukinen K, Peraaho M, Collin P, et al: Small-bowel mucosal transglutaminase 2-specific IgA deposits in coeliac disease without villous atrophy: a prospective and randomized clinical study. Scand J Gastroenterol 2005;40:564–572.
57 Raki M, Fallang LE, Brottveit M, et al: Tetramer visualization of gut-homing gluten-specific T cells in the peripheral blood of celiac disease patients. Proc Natl Acad Sci USA 2007;104:2831–2836.
58 Gass J, Bethune MT, Siegel M, et al: Combination enzyme therapy for gastric digestion of dietary gluten in patients with celiac sprue. Gastroenterology 2007;133:472–480.
59 Paterson BM, Lammers KM, Arrieta MC, et al: The safety, tolerance, pharmacokinetic and pharmacodynamic effects of single doses of AT-1001 in coeliac disease subjects: a proof of concept study. Aliment Pharmacol Ther 2007;26:757–766.
60 Rizzello CG, De Angelis M, Di Cagno R, et al: Highly efficient gluten degradation by lactobacilli and fungal proteases during food processing: new perspectives for celiac disease. Appl Environ Microbiol 2007;73:4499–4507.

Prof. Stefano Guandalini, MD
Division of Pediatric Gastroenterology, Hepatology and Nutrition, University of Chicago
5839 S. Maryland Avenue, MC 4065
Chicago, IL 60637 (USA)
Tel. +1 773 702 6418, Fax +1 773 702 0666, E-Mail sguandalini@peds.bsd.uchicago.edu

Fasano A, Troncone R, Branski D (eds): Frontiers in Celiac Disease.
Pediatr Adolesc Med. Basel, Karger, 2008, vol 12, pp 12–17

Natural History of Celiac Disease

Katri Kaukinen[a,b] · Pekka Collin[a,b] · Markku Mäki[a,c]

[a]Medical School, University of Tampere, and Departments of [b]Gastroenterology and Alimentary Tract Surgery and [c]Pediatrics, Tampere University Hospital, Tampere, Finland

Abstract
In celiac disease a gluten-induced small-bowel mucosal lesion develops gradually in genetically susceptible persons. Evidence shows that clinically pertinent celiac disease exists despite a normal small-bowel villous architecture. The characteristic villous atrophy with crypt hyperplasia, a flat lesion, may become evident only after decades of gluten ingestion, representing the end stage of the mucosal response to the environmental trigger, gluten. Positive serum celiac autoantibodies in individuals with normal histology indicate early developing celiac disease. When these autoantibodies are demonstrated in vivo in small-intestinal mucosa – where they are in fact produced – it is possible to find even more reliably patients having celiac disease in its early stages. It is foreseen that the demonstration of enteropathy will no longer be the gold standard in the diagnosis of celiac disease, and the diagnostic criteria are extended to include 'genetic gluten intolerance'.

Markers of Early Developing Celiac Disease

Celiac disease is an autoimmune-mediated enteropathy triggered by the ingestion of a single dietary factor – wheat-, rye- and barley-derived gluten – in genetically susceptible persons. Of the genetic factors that contribute to celiac disease susceptibility, the strongest recognized association is with HLA-DQ2 and -DQ8 – one or other of which is to be found in 95–100% of the patients [1]. The use of HLA in the diagnosis remains limited, since 30–40% of the general population also carry the HLA-DQ2 or -DQ8 molecules, and the twin and family studies strongly indicate the presence of additional genetic risk factors [1]. Small-bowel villous atrophy with crypt hyperplasia and recovery of the lesion on a gluten-free diet are currently required for the diagnosis of the disease [2]. There is much evidence to suggest that villous atrophy comprises only the end stage of the clinical course of the disease, and celiac disease clearly develops gradually from mucosal inflammation (infiltrative lesion, Marsh 1), to crypt hyperplasia (hypertrophic lesion, Marsh 2) and finally to overt villous atrophy (atrophic lesion, Marsh 3) [3]. The concept of latent celiac disease is well recognized: a patient having a normal small-bowel mucosal structure while on a gluten-containing diet later develops typical mucosal villous atrophy with crypt hyperplasia [4–8]. The late concordance in the appearance of celiac disease in monozygotic twins also suggests that the disorder may remain in the latent stage for long periods [9, 10]. In today's literature, potential celiac disease is again attributed to cases with markers of early developing celiac disease but where a diagnostic biopsy finding is lacking. Altogether this means that the normal

Table 1. Sensitivities and specificities (%) of different markers in detecting celiac disease in its early stages before the development of villous atrophy

	Sensitivity	Specificity
Intestinal mucosal TG2-specific IgA deposits present	93	93
Serum IgA class celiac autoantibodies present	76	83
Increased density of villous-tip IELs in intestinal mucosa	88	71
Increased density of $\gamma\delta+$ IELs in intestinal mucosa	76	60
Intestinal mucosal Marsh 1 lesion (lymphocytosis)	59	57
HLA-DQ2/DQ8 present	100	66

TG2 = Transglutaminase 2; IELs = intraepithelial lymphocytes. Data modified from Salmi et al. [7].

small-bowel mucosal architecture does not necessarily exclude celiac disease in the long term.

It is often difficult to interpret whether minor small-bowel mucosal changes are due to celiac disease in its early stages. A mucosal Marsh 1 lesion (lymphocytosis) may indicate early developing celiac disease (sometimes referred to as mild enteropathy celiac disease) but this finding is also associated with other disorders since, according to the literature, only 2–43% of patients are eventually shown to suffer from genetic gluten intolerance [7, 11, 12]. An increased density of $\gamma\delta+$ or villous-tip intraepithelial lymphocytes has been shown to be predicting forthcoming celiac disease better than intraepithelial lymphocytes in general [7]. Nevertheless, the specificity of $\gamma\delta+$ and villous-tip intraepithelial lymphocytes in the diagnosis of early developing celiac disease has remained rather low – 60 and 71%, respectively (table 1).

A typical feature for celiac disease, in addition to the mucosal changes, is gluten-dependent serum IgA class autoantibodies against transglutaminase 2 (TG2). These serum autoantibodies – endomysial and TG2 antibodies – are powerful tools in disclosing celiac disease with overt villous atrophy [13]. Furthermore, positive serum celiac autoantibodies have predicted impending celiac disease in many patients evincing normal small-bowel mucosal villous architecture [4, 5, 7, 8, 14, 15]. Hence, patients having 'false-positive' celiac autoantibodies in serum are in fact at risk of developing overt celiac disease later. In a recent study by Salmi et al. [7] the specificity of IgA class celiac autoantibodies proved to be high in early developing celiac disease (table 1). Some patients with positive serum endomysial or tissue transglutaminase antibodies may still seroconvert negatively during the follow-up. On the other hand, it is well recognized that in some cases serum celiac autoantibodies fluctuate before the patients eventually develop overt celiac disease after a longer follow-up period (fig. 1) [16]; the reason for this has remained obscure.

Studies on phage display library and organ culture methods have shown that TG2-targetted celiac disease autoantibodies are produced in small-intestinal mucosa and not peripherally [17, 18]. In untreated celiac disease the autoantibodies can also be found deposited in vivo in situ in small-bowel mucosa alongside extracellular TG2, even in cases who have no measurable autoantibodies in their sera [19, 20]. Recent data indicate that by looking at celiac autoantibodies on site where they are produced (that is intestinal TG2-specific IgA deposits), it is possible to detect reliably early developing celiac disease without villous atrophy (table 1) [7, 19, 21]. Future studies will show whether the detection of intestinal mucosal TG2-specific IgA deposits works also well in the diagnostic workup of celiac disease in larger series, and whether there are variations in different laboratories.

Latent Celiac Disease in Gluten Challenge Studies

The permanency of gluten intolerance in celiac disease was suggested in early studies, which

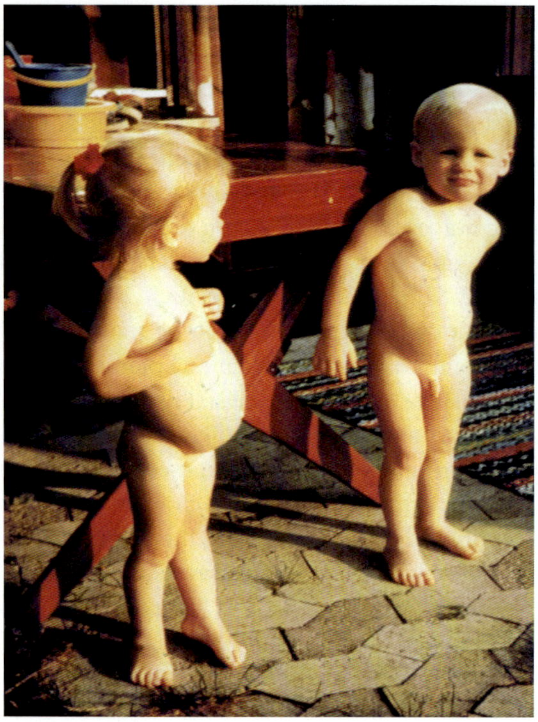

Fig. 1. Two-year-old twins: the girl having a protruding abdomen was diagnosed to have celiac disease; her brother had positive serum endomysial antibodies but a normal small-bowel mucosal villous architecture. He continued on a gluten-containing diet and serocoverted negatively during the follow-up. Seventeen years later, he developed symptoms suggestive of celiac disease; serum autoantibodies were positive again, and the small-bowel mucosa showed villous atrophy with crypt hyperplasia; the diagnosis of celiac disease was eventually established. Copyright Raili Oinonen, with permission.

showed that symptoms and intestinal lesion occurred usually within 2 years when gluten was reintroduced to the diet [2]. Later it was recognized that the process of gluten-induced mucosal deterioration may take years or even decades in some individual cases [22]. In our postpubertal gluten challenge study, 4 out of 29 celiac disease children did not relapse within 2 years [23]; a longer follow-up has revealed that 1 additional case relapsed 6 years later and 1 developed dermatitis herpetiformis with mild enteropathy at the age of 33 years, being then also endomysial antibody positive [M. Mäki, pers. commun.]. In individual cases the clinical presentation of celiac disease may thus change from classical malabsorption syndrome to extraintestinal manifestation at different time points.

Recently, a French group elucidated the clinical course of a less common form of latent celiac disease: 13 patients with celiac disease did not show clinical or histological relapse on a long-term gluten challenge up to 21 years [24]. Interestingly, 2 out of the 13 evinced small-bowel mucosal atrophy shortly after the beginning of the gluten challenge, but their mucosa normalized when the gluten ingestion continued. The authors concluded that some celiac disease patients may develop true latency or tolerance against dietary gluten. However, many of these latent cases suffered from mild symptoms and had mild anemia or other nutritional deficiencies, showing positive celiac autoantibodies and minor small-bowel mucosal inflammatory changes at the same time. Furthermore, during the longer follow-up 2 of the patients relapsed clinically and histologically [24]. Altogether these findings suggest that the patients had not developed tolerance against gluten, but were still suffering from celiac disease without villous atrophy.

Treatment with a Gluten-Free Diet before the Development of Villous Atrophy

Celiac disease is clearly not restricted to small-bowel mucosal villous atrophy. Therefore, the next inevitable question is whether patients having evidence of early developing celiac disease should be treated with a gluten-free diet even in the absence of intestinal mucosal villous atrophy. In dermatitis herpetiformis the spectrum of enteropathy varies, and approximately 20% of the patients show an apparently normal small-bowel mucosal villous architecture; however, there are virtually always inflammatory changes consistent with latent celiac disease [25, 26]. Thus, dermatitis herpetiformis constitutes a model for early-stage celiac disease,

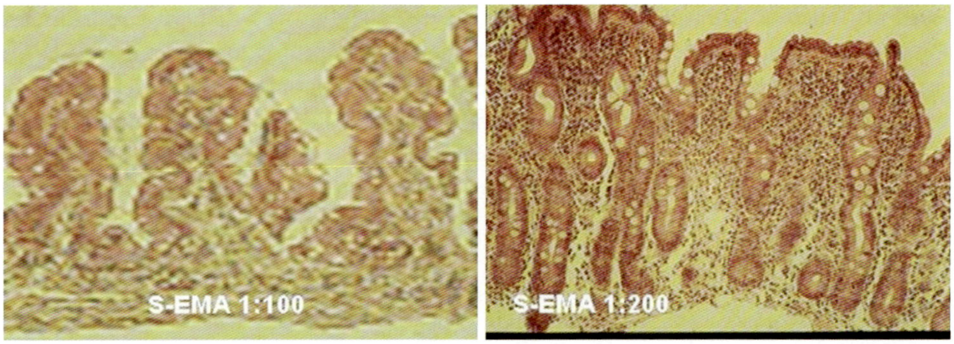

a b

Fig. 2. An asymptomatic 15-year-old boy suffering from type I diabetes mellitus was found to have positive serum endomysial antibodies (S-EMA) upon risk group screening; small-bowel mucosal biopsies were interpreted not to represent overt celiac disease, and based on the current diagnostic criteria he was not prescribed a gluten-free diet (**a**). Twelve years later, he was diagnosed to have dementia and brain atrophy, no abdominal symptoms occurred. Serum endomysial antibodies were still positive, and this time the small-bowel mucosa was compatible with celiac disease (**b**). No other definite explanation than celiac disease was shown to be related to these severe neurological findings.

where treatment of gluten intolerance is indicated irrespectively of small-bowel mucosal damage.

Interestingly, many patients diagnosed to have dermatitis herpetiformis during adulthood evince celiac-type dental enamel defects suggesting that they have suffered from a gluten-induced condition already in early childhood [27]. Similarly, many patients having latent celiac disease in fact have suffered from gluten-dependent symptoms already before the development of small-bowel mucosal villous atrophy; some had had osteopenia or osteoporosis, definitely warranting the early treatment [14, 21, 28]. It is not known whether untreated patients having early developing celiac disease carry an increased risk of malignancies; so far there is only one case report indicating that intestinal lymphoma may appear in the latent stage of celiac disease [29]. Recently, it has been suggested that in celiac disease gluten may affect also both the peripheral and central nervous system, and celiac disease may present with peripheral neuropathy, ataxia, epilepsy or even with brain atrophy [30–32]. In gluten ataxia patients, severe neurological symptoms develop but only some of the patients show gluten-dependent small-bowel mucosal atrophy with crypt hyperplasia or gastrointestinal complaints. In a recent study all gluten ataxia patients with or without villous atrophy were found to have celiac-type TG2-specific autoantibody deposits in their intestinal mucosa – interestingly, one of the patients was shown to have similar TG2-targetted IgA deposits in the small vessels of the brain [32]. Nervous tissue, in general, owns a poor regenerative capacity. Therefore, it has been suggested that only early treatment with a gluten-free diet might be beneficial in gluten ataxia patients, irrespective of intestinal mucosal villous morphology [31]. In other words, in some cases having signs of early developing celiac disease, a long follow-up without treatment might be even harmful, because permanent tissue damage might develop (fig. 2).

Conclusions

Celiac disease clearly exists beyond small-bowel villous atrophy, and the current diagnostic criteria based on mucosal damage, excluding early developing celiac disease and also dermatitis herpetiformis, are no longer valid. Detection of serum and intestinal celiac autoantibodies helps in identifying patients who suffer from genetic gluten intolerance and who might benefit from early treatment with a gluten-free diet. In celiac disease, gluten-induced symptoms may occur outside the intestine. When patients found to have early signs of celiac disease are left on a gluten-containing diet, the wide clinical spectrum of the disease should be kept in mind during the regular follow-up.

References

1 Sollid LM: Coeliac disease: dissecting a complex inflammatory disorder. Nat Rev Immunol 2002;2:647–655.

2 Walker-Smith JA, Guandalini S, Schmitz J, Shmerling DH, Visakorpi JK: Revised criteria for diagnosis of coeliac disease. Arch Dis Child 1990;65:909–911.

3 Marsh MN: Gluten, major histocompatibility complex, and the small intestine: a molecular and immunobiologic approach to the spectrum of gluten sensitivity ('celiac sprue'). Gastroenterology 1992;102:330–354.

4 Collin P, Helin H, Mäki M, Hällström O, Karvonen A-L: Follow-up of patients positive in reticulin and gliadin antibody tests with normal small bowel biopsy findings. Scand J Gastroenterol 1993;28: 595–598.

5 Corazza GR, Andreani ML, Biagi F, Bonvicini F, Bernardi M, Gasbarrini G: Clinical, pathological, and antibody pattern of latent celiac disease: report of three adult cases. Am J Gastroenterol 1996;91:2203–2207.

6 Troncone R: Latent coeliac disease in Italy. Acta Paediatr 1995;84:1252–1257.

7 Salmi TT, Collin P, Järvinen O, Haimila K, Partanen J, Laurila K, Korponay-Szabo I, Huhtala H, Reunala T, Mäki M, Kaukinen K: Immunoglobin A autoantibodies against transglutaminase 2 in the small intestinal mucosa predict forthcoming coeliac disease. Aliment Pharmacol Ther 2006;24:541–552.

8 Mohamed BM, Feighery C, Coates C, O'Shea U, Delaney D, O'Brian S, Kelly J, Abuzakouk M: The absence of a mucosal lesion on standard histological examination does not exclude diagnosis of celiac disease. Dig Dis Sci 2008;53:52–61.

9 Salazar de Sousa J, Ramos de Almeida JM, Monteiro MV, Magalhaes Ramalho P: Late onset coeliac disease in the monozygotic twin of a coeliac child. Acta Paediatr Scand 1987;76:172–174.

10 Hervonen K, Karell K, Holopainen P, Collin P, Partanen J, Reunala T: Concordance of dermatitis herpetiformis in monozygous twins. J Invest Dermatol 2000;115:990–993.

11 Kakar S, Nehra V, Murray JA, Dayharsh GA, Burgar LJ: Significance of intraepithelial lymphocytosis in small bowel biopsy samples with normal mucosal architecture. Am J Gastroenterol 2003; 98:2027–2033.

12 Lähdeaho ML, Kaukinen K, Collin P, Ruuska T, Partanen J, Haapala AM, Mäki M: Celiac disease – from inflammation to atrophy: a long-term follow-up study. J Pediatr Gastroenterol Nutr 2005;41:44–48.

13 Sulkanen S, Halttunen T, Laurila K, Kolho K-L, Korponay-Szabo I, Sarnesto A, Savilahti E, Collin P, Mäki M: Tissue transglutaminase autoantibody enzyme-linked immunosorbent assay in detecting celiac disease. Gastroenterology 1998;115:1322–1328.

14 Dickey W, Hughes DF, McMillan SA: Patients with serum IgA endomysial antibodies and intact duodenal villi: clinical characteristics and management options. Scand J Gastroenterol 2005;40: 1240–1243.

15 Paparo F, Petrone E, Tosco A, Maglio M, Borrelli M, Salvati VM, Miele E, Greco L, Auricchio S, Troncone R: Clinical, HLA, and small bowel immunohistochemical features of children with positive serum antiendomysium antibodies and architecturally normal small intestinal mucosa. Am J Gastroenterol 2005;100:2294–2298.

16 Westerlund A, Ankelo M, Simell S, Ilonen J, Knip M, Simell O, Hinkkanen AE: Affinity maturation of immunoglobulin A anti-tissue transglutaminase autoantibodies during development of coeliac disease. Clin Exp Immunol 2007;148:230–240.

17 Marzari R, Sblattero D, Florian F, Tongiorgi E, Not T, Tommasini A, Ventura A, Brandbury A: Molecular dissection of tissue transglutaminase autoantibody response in celiac disease. J Immunol 2001;166:4170–4176.

18 Picarelli A, Maiuri L, Frate A, Greco M, Auricchio S, Londei M: Production of antiendomysial antibodies after in-vitro gliadin challenge of small intestine biopsy samples from patients with coeliac disease. Lancet 1996;348:1065–1067.

19 Korponay-Szabo IR, Halttunen T, Szalai Z, Laurila K, Kiraly R, Kovacs JB, Fesus L, Mäki M: In vivo targeting of intestinal and extraintestinal transglutaminase 2 by coeliac autoantibodies. Gut 2004;53:641–648.

20 Salmi TT, Collin P, Korponay-Szabo I, Laurila K, Partanen J, Huhtala H, Kiraly R, Lorand L, Reunala T, Mäki M, Kaukinen K: Endomysial antibody-negative coeliac disease: clinical characteristics and intestinal autoantibody deposits. Gut 2006;55:1746–1753.

21 Kaukinen K, Peräaho M, Collin P, Partanen J, Woolley N, Kaartinen T, Nuutinen T, Halttunen T, Mäki M, Korponay-Szabo I: Small bowel mucosal transglutaminase 2-specific IgA deposits in coeliac disease without villous atrophy: a prospective and randomized study. Scand J Gastroenterol 2005;40:564–572.

22 Hogberg L, Stenhammar L, Falth-Magnusson K, Grodzinsky E: Anti-endomysium and anti-gliadin antibodies as serological markers for a very late mucosal relapse in a coeliac girl. Acta Paediatr 1997;86:335–336.

23 Mäki M, Lahdeaho ML, Hällström O, Viander M, Visakorpi JK: Postpubertal gluten challenge in coeliac disease. Arch Dis Child 1989;64:1604–1607.

24 Matysiak-Budnik T, Malamut G, Patey-Mariaud de Serre N, Grosdidier E, Seguier S, Brousse N, Caillat-Zucman S, Cerf-Bensussan N, Schmitz J, Cellier C: Long-term follow-up of 61 patients diagnosed in childhood: evolution towards latency is possible on a normal diet. Gut 2007;56:1379–1386.
25 Fry L, Seah PP, McMinn RMH, Hoffbrand AV: Lymphocytic infiltration of epithelium in diagnosis of gluten-sensitive enteropathy. BMJ 1972; 3:371–374.
26 Savilahti E, Reunala T, Mäki M: Increase of lymphocytes bearing the gamma/delta T cell receptor in the jejunum of patients with dermatitis herpetiformis. Gut 1992;33:206–211.
27 Aine L, Mäki M, Reunala T: Coeliac-type dental enamel defects in patients with dermatitis herpetiformis. Acta Derm Venereol 1992;72:25–27.
28 Kaukinen K, Mäki M, Partanen J, Sievänen H, Collin P: Celiac disease without villous atrophy: revision of criteria called for. Dig Dis Sci 2001;46: 879–887.
29 Freeman HJ, Chiu BK: Multifocal small bowel lymphoma and latent celiac sprue. Gastroenterology 1986;90:1992–1997.
30 Hadjivassiliou M, Gibson A, Davies-Jones GAB, Lobo AJ, Stephenson TJ, Milford-Wars A: Does cryptic gluten sensitivity play a part in neurological illness? Lancet 1996;347:369–371.
31 Hadjivassiliou M, Davies-Jones GAB, Sanders D, Grunewald RA: Dietary treatment of gluten ataxia. J Neurol Neurosurg Psychiatry 2003;74: 1221–1224.
32 Hadjivassiliou M, Mäki M, Sanders D, Williamsson CA, Grunewald RA, Woodroofe NM, Korponay-Szabo I: Autoantibody targetting of brain and intestinal transglutaminase in gluten ataxia. Neurology 2006;66:373–377.

Prof. Markku Mäki
Pediatric Research Center, Medical School
University of Tampere, Building Finn-Medi 3
FI–33014 University of Tampere (Finland)
Tel. +358 3 3551 8400, Fax +358 3 3551 8402, E-Mail markku.maki@uta.fi

Fasano A, Troncone R, Branski D (eds): Frontiers in Celiac Disease.
Pediatr Adolesc Med. Basel, Karger, 2008, vol 12, pp 18–22

The Changing Clinical Presentation of Celiac Disease

E. Lebenthal · E. Shteyer · D. Branski

Pediatric Gastroenterology, Division of Pediatrics, Hadassah University Hospitals, Jerusalem, Israel

Abstract

The incidence, the age at presentation and the features of celiac disease (CD) in children have changed considerably over the past 20 years. CD is now believed to be the most common genetically predetermined condition in humans with a prevalence of 1%. Only approximately one third of the patients presents with diarrhea while one third is diagnosed upon screening, and one fifth presents with nonspecific recurrent abdominal pain. Furthermore, it is apparent that most children with CD remain undiagnosed. Another trend is the presentation later in life with atypical symptoms such as anemia, bone disorder and growth failure. The increasing number of CD-associated autoimmune disorders, like insulin-dependent diabetes mellitus, dermatitis herpetiformis, alopecia, Sjögren's syndrome, autoimmune thyroiditis, autoimmune hepatitis, and atrophic gastritis, is apparent. Currently most patients present with subtle or non-gastrointestinal manifestations at a later age. Median age at presentation of children has shifted from 4 to 8 years.

The incidence, age at presentation and the features of celiac disease (CD) in children have changed considerably over the past 20 years. In the past, CD presented most commonly either very early in life, between 9 and 24 months, or in the third or fourth decade of life [1–6]. In contrast to the equal sex ratio in children, twice to thrice as many females were diagnosed in adulthood [6].

Clinical Presentation – Past and Present

In the past infants and toddlers presented primarily with gastrointestinal manifestations and malabsorption characterized by diarrhea, steatorrhea, abdominal distention, wasted buttocks, hypotonia, growth failure, weight loss, anemia, anorexia, irritability, malnutrition and associated nutritional deficiencies (fat-soluble vitamins, electrolytes, etc.). Some, however, manifested with recurrent vomiting or constipation even with rectal prolapse and intussusception.

In contrast, in recent studies the gastrointestinal manifestations are less prominent at diagnosis. Only 36–42% presented with diarrhea while 26% were diagnosed upon targeted screening and 16% presented with nonspecific recurrent abdominal pain [7, 8]. Furthermore, it is apparent that most children with CD remain undiagnosed.

Another trend is the presentation later in life with atypical symptoms such as anemia, bone disorders or autoimmune diseases [6].

Diagnosis of Celiac Disease

CD is characterized by small-intestinal mucosal injury and nutrient malabsorption. It is activated in genetically susceptible individuals by the dietary ingestion of proline- and glutamine-rich proteins that are found in wheat, rye, and barley, and are widely termed 'gluten'. Although approximately 1% of the population of the United States is affected by CD, most affected individuals remain undiagnosed [9]. This probably reflects the fact that patients with CD can manifest a spectrum of intestinal and/or extra-intestinal symptoms and, in some cases, they can be relatively asymptomatic, with their disease first being detected by antibody screening because they were identified as being at high risk of developing CD (for example, by being a family member of an affected patient). Presumed disease is best detected by serologic screening for the presence of IgA antibodies specific for tissue transglutaminase, and endomysium, this should be followed by biopsy of the mucosa of the small intestine to establish the ultimate diagnosis [9]. Immunoglobulin A deficiency is 10–15 times more common in patients with CD than in healthy subjects [10]. In such cases, immunoglobulin G (IgG) antibodies should be determined [10]. Life-threatening complications, although relatively rare, can include the development of refractory CD and enteropathy-associated T-cell lymphomas [9].

Prevalence and Incidence

In 1998 Jenkins et al. [11] presented an incidence of CD of 1:2,500 whereas in a recent study the prevalence among screened healthcare professionals was 1:166 [12].

CD is now believed to be the most common genetically predetermined condition in humans with a childhood prevalence of 1% [13]. In the past CD was considered primarily a disorder of European and Western populations. Currently there are more and more reports that CD is emerging as a global problem [14].

The incidence of CD in various autoimmune disorders has increased 10- to 30-fold when compared to the general population, and autoimmune disease is associated with clinically asymptomatic CD in many patients [15].

Associated Autoimmune Diseases

The increasing number of CD-associated autoimmune diseases, like insulin-dependent diabetes mellitus, dermatitis herpetiformis, alopecia, Sjögren's syndrome, autoimmune thyroiditis, autoimmune hepatitis, atrophic gastritis and more, raises the question whether or not the changes in clinical presentation and increase in prevalence of autoimmune disorders are related to changing practices in breastfeeding, infant feeding, including time of gluten introduction into the diet, quantity of gluten consumption, and late diagnosis of CD [16]. In a recent publication, Norris et al. [17] reported a lower incidence of developing CD autoimmunity when gluten is introduced between 4 and 6 months of age while the infant is still being breastfed.

A significant protection affect on the incidence of CD was suggested by the duration of breastfeeding (exclusive breastfeeding as well as partial breastfeeding). The data do not support the influence of age at first dietary gluten exposure. On the other hand it appears to affect the age at onset of symptoms and, is associated with the appearance and increase of CD-associated autoimmune diseases [18].

On the other hand diabetes type 1 and other associated autoimmune diseases have an increased intestinal permeability [19]. In addition, diabetes type 1 patients have upregulation of zonulin, a protein that modulates intestinal permeability [20]. Zonulin upregulation seems to precede the onset of disease. There might be a possible link between increased intestinal permeability, gluten antigens and the development of autoimmunity [20].

Another plausible cause for the increase in associated autoimmune diseases and the change in clinical manifestations can be due to a change in the incidence and prevalence of episodes of acute gastroenteritis early in life and a change in the response of the gut immune system and T cells [21]. A prospective study in children who carried CD human leukocyte antigens DQ2 and DQ8 [22] revealed that a high frequency of rotavirus infections may increase the risk of CD autoimmunity in childhood in genetically predisposed individuals [22].

Furthermore, a decrease in severe and prolonged diarrhea requiring hospitalization early in life might be a cause for the current modified symptoms, appearance and late diagnosis of CD [22].

The Modified Clinical Presentation

In recent studies in children, only 36–42% had gastrointestinal manifestations (diarrhea and protuberant abdomen) at presentation [7, 8], whereas in adults the gastrointestinal manifestations were 43%. On the other hand, larger numbers present with relatively nonspecific and subtle symptoms, such as recurrent abdominal pain, anemia and even constipation [7, 8]. Target screening of high risk groups (insulin-dependent diabetes mellitus, Down's syndrome or autoimmune thyroiditis, autoimmune liver disease, etc.) reveal an increasing number of asymptomatic patients with CD.

Currently, most patients present with subtle or non-gastrointestinal manifestations at a later age [7, 8]. The median age at presentation of children shifted from 4 to 8 years [7]. Data from studies on adults with CD are similar to children [23] reporting only 43% with gastrointestinal manifestations in 1993, compared to 73% prior to 1993, and delay in the diagnosis of CD. The Canadian Celiac Health survey [24] reported 2,681 adult patients in whom there was a mean delay in diagnosis of 11.7 years. In 40% of these patients the diagnoses prior to the ultimate diagnosis of CD were anemia (40%), stress (31%), and irritable bowel syndrome (29%), while osteoporosis and low bone density were found in a high percentage (35%) [24].

Disorders Associated with Celiac Disease

Over the years there have been descriptions of many conditions associated with CD (table 1). The increasing number of associated autoimmune diseases in long-standing CD patients raises concerns about the association to the delayed and late diagnosis of CD, as well as the implementation, use and compliance with a gluten-free diet. The relationship between the increased frequency of autoimmune diseases and CD is attributed to a common genetic and immunological mechanism, as well as the presence of CD itself [25]. Gluten withdrawal does not prevent the development of autoimmune diseases [26]; however, insulin-dependent diabetes and thyroid-specific autoantibodies may disappear in patients after they start a gluten-free diet [26], suggesting a relationship between the autoimmune process and gluten exposure [27]. Improvement may occur in cardiomyopathy, thyroiditis and peripheral neuropathy on a gluten-free diet [24]. However, associated autoimmune disorders generally do not improve with a gluten-free diet [25].

Genetic diseases associated with an increased prevalence of CD, such as Down's syndrome or Turner's syndrome, are raising questions related to the genetic defects in CD that have not been explored.

Conclusion

Only a small number of patients present with the 'classical' symptoms of marked weight loss, malnutrition, and steatorrhea. In contrast, many individuals with CD manifest predominantly extra-intestinal symptoms and nonspecific findings of growth failure, unexplained iron deficiency anemia, recurrent abdominal pain, and osteoporosis, or are relatively asymptomatic like individuals identified only because they have affected family members or associated diseases.

Table 1. Disorders associated with celiac disease (CD) with approximate percentage of positive CD in screening

Autoimmune disorders	
Insulin-dependent diabetes	8–10%
Sjögren's syndrome	10%
Dermatitis herpetiformis	6–7%
Addison's disease	8%
Autoimmune hepatitis	6%
Autoimmune cholangitis	3.5%
Alopecia areata	3–4%
Connective tissue disease	2–3%
Atrophic gastritis	
Syndromes	
Down's syndrome	5–10%
Turner's syndrome	6%
Beckwitt-Wiedemann syndrome	
Neurological disorders	
Neuropathy	5%
Celiac ataxia	
Intractable epilepsy and parieto-occipital calcifications	
Migraine	
Liver diseases	
Primary biliary cirrhosis	5–10%
Elevated transaminase levels	9%
Cardiac diseases	
Autoimmune myocarditis	4%
Idiopathic dilated cardiomyopathy	2–4%
Pericarditis	
Endocrinological diseases	
Secondary hypopituitarism	
Amenorrhea	
Hypogonadism	
Bone diseases	
Osteoporosis	2–7%
Bone fractures	
Enamel hypoplasia	
Skin diseases	
Atopic dermatitis	
Chronic urticaria	
Cutaneous vasculitis	
Psoriasis	
Hematological and immunologic disorders	
Iron deficiency anemia	
IgA deficiency	
Hyposplenism	
Nephrological manifestations	
IgA nephropathy/Henoch-Schönlein purpura	
Immune complex glomerulonephritis	
Nephrotic syndrome	
Pulmonary manifestations	
Autoimmune fibrosing alveolitis	
Lymphocytic interstitial pneumonia	
Desquamative interstitial pneumonitis	
Gastrointestinal diseases	
Crohn's disease	
Ulcerative colitis	
Microscopic colitis	
Enteropathy-associated T-cell lymphoma	
Others	
Aphthous stomatitis	

References

1 American Gastroenterological Association medical position statement: celiac sprue. Gastroenterology 2001;120: 1522–1525.
2 Fasano A, Catassi C: Current approaches to diagnosis and treatment of celiac disease: an evolving spectrum. Gastroenterology 2001;120:636–651.
3 Feighery C: Fortnightly review: celiac disease BMJ 1999;319:236–239.
4 Citritira PJ, King AL, Fraser JS: AGA technical review on celiac sprue. American Gastroenterological Association. Gastroenterology 2001;120: 1526–1540.
5 Maki M, Colin P: Coeliac disease. Lancet 1997;349:1755–1759.
6 Van Heel DA, West J: Recent advances in coeliac disease. Gut 2006;55:1037–1046.
7 Ravikumara M, Tuthill DP, Jenkins HR: The changing clinical presentation of coeliac disease. Arch Dis Child 2006;91:969–971.

8 Beattie RM: The changing face of coeliac disease. Arch Dis Child 2006;91: 955–956.
9 Kagnoff MF: Celiac disease: pathogenesis of a model immunogenetic disease. J Clin Invest 2007;117:41–49.
10 Kumar V, Jarzabek-Chorzelska M, Sulej J, et al: Celiac disease and immunoglobulin A deficiency: how effective are the serological methods of diagnosis? Clin Diagn Lab Immunol 2002;9: 1295–1300.
11 Jenkins HR, Hawkes N, Swift GL: Incidence of coeliac disease. Arch Dis Child 1998;79:198–199.
12 El-hadi S, Tuthill D, Lewis E, et al: Unrecognized coeliac disease is common in healthcare students. Arch Dis Child 2004;89:842.
13 Fasano A: Clinical presentation of coeliac disease in the paediatric population. Gastroenterology 2005;128: S68–S73.
14 Lebenthal E, Branski D: Celiac disease: an emerging global problem. J Pediatr Gastroenterol Nutr 2002;35:474–474.
15 Kumar V, Rajadhyaksha M, Wortsman J: Celiac disease-associated autoimmune endocrinopathies. Clin Diagn Lab Immunol 2001;8:678–685.
16 Ventura A, Magazzu G, Greco L: Duration of exposure to gluten and risk for autoimmune disorders in patients with celiac disease. Gastroenterology 1999;117:297–303.
17 Norris JM, Barriga K, Hoffenberg EJ, et al: Risk of celiac disease autoimmunity and timing of gluten introduction in the diet of infants at increased risk of disease. JAMA 2005;293:2343–2351.
18 Peters U, Schneeweiss S, Trautwein EA, Erbersdobler HF: A case control study of the effect of infant feeding on celiac disease. Ann Nutr Metab 2001;45: 135–142.
19 Kuitunen M, Saukkonen T, Ilonen J, et al: Intestinal permeability to mannitol and lactulose in children with type I diabetes with thte HLA-DQB1*02 allele. Autoimmunity 2002;35:365–368.
20 Sapone A, de Magistris L, Pietzak M: Zonulin upregulation is associated with increased gut permeability in subjects with type I diabetes and their relatives. Diabetes 2006;55:1443–1449.
21 Wildin RS, Ramsdell F, Peake J, et al: X-linked neonatal diabetes mellitus, enteropathy and endocrinopathy syndrome is the human equivalent of mouse scurfy. Nat Genet 2001;27:18–20.
22 Stene LC, Honeyman MC, Hoffenberg EJ, et al: Rotavirus infection frequency and risk of celiac disease autoimmunity in early childhood: a longitudinal study. Am J Gastroenterol 2006;101: 2333–2340.
23 Fasano A, Berti I, Gerarduzzi T, et al: Prevalence of celiac disease in at-risk and not-at-risk groups in the United States: a large multicenter study. Arch Intern Med 2003;163:286–292.
24 Cranney A, Zazkadas M, Graham ID, et al: The Canadian celiac health survey. Dig Dis Sci 2007;52:1087–1015.
25 Green PHR, Jabri B: Celiac disease. Annu Rev Med 2006;57:207–221.
26 Sategna Guietti C, Solerio E, Scaglione N, et al: Duration of gluten exposure in adult celiac disease does not correlate with the risk of autoimmune disorders. Gut 2001;49:502–505.
27 Ventura A, Neri E, Ughi C, et al: Gluten-dependent diabetes-related and thyroid-related autoantibodies in patients with celiac disease. J Pediatr 2000;137:263–265.

David Branski, MD
Division of Pediatrics, Hadassah University Hospitals
POB 12000
Jerusalem 91120 (Israel)
Tel. +972 2 6777 543, Fax +972 2 6434 579, E-Mail branski@hadassah.org.il

Fasano A, Troncone R, Branski D (eds): Frontiers in Celiac Disease.
Pediatr Adolesc Med. Basel, Karger, 2008, vol 12, pp 23–31

The Global Village of Celiac Disease

Carlo Catassi[a,b] · Surender Kumar Yachha[c]

[a]Department of Pediatrics, Università Politecnica delle Marche, Ancona, Italy; [b]Center for Celiac Research, University of Maryland School of Medicine, Baltimore, Md., USA; [c]Department of Pediatric Gastroenterology, Sanjay Gandhi Postgraduate Institute of Medical Sciences, Lucknow, India

Abstract

Celiac disease (CD) is one of the commonest lifelong disorders in countries populated by individuals of European origin, affecting approximately 1% of the general population. This is a common disease also in North Africa, the Middle East and India. The huge prevalence of CD in the Saharawi people (5.6%) is an outlier finding probably related to strong genetic predisposition and abrupt dietary changes during the last few centuries. CD in the Saharawi children, as well as in those of other developing countries, is sometimes a severe disease, characterized by chronic diarrhea, stunting, anemia and increased mortality. Further studies are needed to quantify the incidence of the celiac condition in apparently 'celiac-free' areas as sub-Saharan Africa and the Far East. In many developing countries the frequency of CD is likely to increase in the near future, given the diffuse tendency to adopt Western, gluten-rich dietary patterns. As most cases currently escape diagnosis all over the world, an effort should be done to increase the awareness of CD polymorphism. A cost-effective case-finding policy could significantly reduce the morbidity and mortality associated with untreated disease.

In the past, celiac disease (CD) was considered a rare disorder, mostly affecting individuals of European origin, usually characterized by onset during the first years of life. At that time diagnosis was entirely based on the detection of typical gastrointestinal symptoms and confirmation by small-intestinal biopsy. The emergence of highly sensitive and specific serological tools, first the antigliadin and later the antiendomysium (EMA) and the antitransglutaminase (tTG) antibodies, showed an unsuspected frequency of clinically atypical or even silent forms of CD. Using these sensitive serological tools, a huge number of studies have recently shown that CD is one of the commonest, lifelong disorders affecting mankind all over the world. This widespread diffusion is not surprising at all, given that causal factors, i.e. HLA predisposing genotypes (DQ2 and DQ8) and consumption of gluten-containing cereals, show a worldwide distribution (table 1). CD is not only frequent in developed countries, but is increasingly reported in areas of the developing world, especially North Africa, the Middle East and India. CD can contribute substantially to childhood morbidity and mortality in many developing countries [1].

The knowledge of CD geographical distribution can help to clarify the complex interaction between genetic and environmental factors underlying this complex disorder. The aim of this paper is to present an updated picture of CD epidemiology, in both the general population and at-risk groups, with a special focus on the emerging problem of CD in developing countries.

Table 1. Frequency (%) of selected haplotypes predisposing to CD in different populations

Population	DQ2 (cis)	DQ8	Population	DQ2 (cis)	DQ8
Saharawi	23.0	2.7	South African blacks	6.2	2.8
Sardinia	22.4	5.0	Inuit	6.1	0
Iran	20.0	12.0	Gipsy	6.0	0
Turkey	18.0	22.0	Mongolia	5.2	4.4
USA	13.1	4.2	North American Indians	4.5	25.3
Algeria	11.2	2.2	Japan	0.6	7.6
Scandinavia	11.0	15.0	Mexico	0	28.3
North India	9.0	15.6	Cayapa	0	41
Italy	9.0	2.0	Bushman	0	30.2
Cameroon	9.0	0.6	Highlanders (Papua New Guinea)	0	0

Celiac Disease Prevalence in the General Population

In Countries Mostly Populated by Individuals of European Origin

Italy was the homeland of the new 'era' of CD epidemiology during the early nineties. On a sample of 17,201 healthy Italian students, we firstly showed that CD is much more common than previously thought and that most atypical cases remain undiagnosed unless actively searched by serological screening [2]. The prevalence of active CD in screened subjects was 4.77 per 1,000 (95% CI 3.79–5.91), 1 in 210 subjects. The overall prevalence of CD (including known CD cases) was 5.44 per 1,000 (95% CI 4.57–6.44), 1 in 184 subjects. The ratio of known (previously diagnosed) to undiagnosed CD cases was as high as 1:7. These results pointed to the existence of a 'celiac iceberg', with a minority of cases being diagnosed on clinical grounds (visible part) and a larger portion remaining undiagnosed unless actively searched by serological screening (submerged iceberg). A wide spectrum of clinical presentation and poor awareness of CD among doctors were (and remain nowadays) the main reasons for underdiagnosis.

Serological screenings performed on general population samples confirmed that the prevalence of CD in Europe is high [3–9], mostly ranging between 0.75 and 0.4% of the general population, with a trend toward higher figures (1% or more) among groups that have been genetically isolated, e.g. in Northern Ireland [10], Finland [11] and Sardinia [12].

A large international, multicenter study investigated a wide population sample in 4 different European countries: Finland (n = 6,403 adults), Northern Ireland (n = 1,975 children + 4,656 adults), Germany (n = 8,806 adults) and Italy (n = 4,779 adults + 2.649 children). The prevalence of EMA positivity (roughly equivalent to CD prevalence) was 2.0% in Finland (95% CI 1.7–2.3), 1.2% in Italy (95% CI 0.8–1.6), 0.9% in Northern Ireland (95% CI 0.5–1.3) and 0.3% (0.1–0.5%) in Germany. This study confirmed that many CD cases would remain undetected without active serological screening. While confirming that CD is a very common disorder in the European Union, wide and unexplained variations between countries (7-fold difference in CD prevalence between Finland and Germany) were also disclosed [13].

Until recently CD has generally been perceived to be less common in North America than in Europe. This misconception has been clarified by a large US prevalence study including 4,126 subjects sampled from the general population [14].

The overall prevalence of CD in this US population sample was 1:133, actually overlapping the European figures. Similar disease frequencies have been reported from developed countries mostly populated by individuals of European origin, e.g. Canada, Australia and New Zealand.

The presence of CD has long been established in many South American countries that are mostly populated by individuals of European origin. Among Brazilian blood donors, the prevalence of CD ranged between 1:681 [15] and 1:214 [16]. It is worth noting that studies on blood donors tend to underestimate the prevalence of CD, as these individuals represent the 'healthiest' segment of the population and are mostly males (while CD is more common among women). In Argentina, Gomez et al. [17] found an overall prevalence of 1 in 167 of 2,000 adults involved in a prenuptial examination.

In Countries Mostly Populated by Individuals of Non-European Origin

The highest CD prevalence in the world has been described in an African population originally living in Western Sahara, the Saharawi, of Arab-Berber origin. In a sample of 990 Saharawi children screened by EMA testing and intestinal biopsy, we found a CD prevalence of 5.6%, which is almost 10-fold higher than in most European countries [18]. The reasons for this spiking CD frequency are unclear but could be primarily related to genetic factors, given the high level of consanguinity of this population. The main susceptibility genotypes, HLA-DQ2 and -DQ8, exhibit one of the highest frequencies in the world in the general background Saharawi population [19]. Gluten consumption is very high as well, since wheat flour is the staple food of the Saharawi refugees. CD in the Saharawi children can be a severe disease, characterized by chronic diarrhea, stunting, anemia and increased mortality.

We have recently completed a screening project on school children in Cairo City, Egypt [20]. Blood samples were obtained from 1,500 children attending school in Cairo City between October 2001 and June 2004. Small-bowel biopsies were collected if the serological screening demonstrated either (a) positive results for both IgA class anti-tTG and EMA antibodies or (b) positive results for IgG anti-tTG in children with IgA deficiency. The prevalence of CD in this sample of Egyptian students was 53% (95% CI 0.17–0.89). This estimate may be low, as more CD cases could be diagnosed at the follow-up, e.g. in the group currently showing a positive tTG IgA and a negative EMA.

Besides Western Sahara and Egypt, there are no data on the frequency of CD in the general African population. However, indirect evidence suggests that this is not a rare disorder in Northern African countries. Large series of clinically diagnosed patients have been reported from Algeria, Tunisia, and Libya. Furthermore, CD is one of the commonest disorders diagnosed in children born from North-African immigrants in both France and Italy.

The Middle East holds a special place in the history of CD. Domestication of ancient grains began in Neolithic settlements from wild progenitors *Triticum monococcum bocoticcum* and *T. monococcum uratru* in the north-eastern region (Turkey, Iran and Iraq) and *Triticum turgidum dicoccoides* in the south-western region (Israel/Palestine, Syria and Lebanon) of the so-called Fertile Crescent area. This extends from the Mediterranean Coast on its western extreme to the great Tigris-Euphrates plain eastward. Cultivation of wheat and barley was first exploited and intensively developed in the Levant and western Zagros (Iran) some 10,000–12,000 years ago. From the Fertile Crescent, farming spread and reached the Western European edge some 6,000 years ago. During the eighties, Simoons [21] theorized that this pattern of agriculture spreading could explain the higher CD incidence in some Western countries, particularly Ireland. Mapping the prevalence of HLA-B8 antigen (the first HLA antigen known to be associated with CD) across Europe, he noted an east-west gradient, with a consistent increase in antigen frequency with decreasing length of time since farming was adopted. Simoons then hypothesized that the HLA-B8 antigen may once have been prevalent throughout pre-agricultural Europe. According to this theory, spreading of wheat consumption exerted a negative selective pressure on CD-associated genes, such as the HLA-B8. Higher B8 frequency in North Eastern Europe, and consequently higher CD frequency, may therefore be attributable to a lack of exposure to cereals until relatively recently [21]. This theory did not survive the recent developments of both CD genetics and epidemiology. On one side, it is now well established that the main genetic predisposition to CD is not linked to HLA-B8 but to some DQ genotypes (DQ2 and DQ8) which are in linkage disequilibrium with B8. Both DQ2 and DQ8 do not show any clear-cut east-west prevalence gradient. On the other hand, the overall CD prevalence is not lower in Middle East countries than in Europe, as should be the case if the longer history of agriculture tended to eliminate the genetic backbone predisposing to CD.

Rather CD is a frequent disorder in the Middle East and along the 'silk road' countries. One of the higher prevalences of CD in blood donors has indeed been reported in Iran (1 on 167). In the same country, 12% of cases with a diagnosis of irritable bowel syndrome for many years have actually CD [22]. In studies from Iran, Iraq, Saudi Arabia and Kuwait, CD accounted for 20 and 18.5% of cases with chronic diarrhea in adults and children, respectively. In a study from Jordan, the high incidence of CD was related to the large wheat consumption of the population (135 kg/head/year).

With the availability of improved and more accessible diagnostic tools for CD, this disorder is being more and more frequently recognized in India, both in children and in adults. The overall prevalence of CD in India is not known but is likely to be high in the so-called celiac belt, a part of North India where wheat is a staple food [23]. CD cases reported from India were 130 between the years 1966 and 2000 versus 517 between the years 2001 and 2005. The major factors that resulted in increased reports of CD from India were use of serological testing to overcome diagnostic overlap with tropical sprue, tuberculosis and small-bowel bacterial overgrowth.

CD constitutes 26% (35/137) of all malabsorption syndrome cases in Indian children (91% cases >2 years of age) [24]. CD was responsible for 16.6% of the 246 cases of chronic diarrhea [25]. Among malabsorption syndrome in Indian adults, 9% is constituted by CD [26]. By using a case-finding approach (serological testing on symptomatic subjects), Sood et al. [27] reported a prevalence of newly diagnosed CD of 1 in 310 children out of a sample of 4,347 school-age children from Punjab, India. An epidemiological study in Leicestershire (UK) revealed that CD among subjects of Punjabi and Gujarati communities of Indian origin had an incidence of 6.9 and 0.9 per 10^5/year, respectively, with a higher relative risk among the Punjabi community (2.9 to Europeans and 8.1 to Gujaratis) [28].

CD in Indian children is predominantly associated with the DQ2 allele, often in linkage disequilibrium with the A26-B8-DR3 alleles (the so-called Indian haplotype, a variant of the ancestral Caucasian haplotype A1-B8-DR3-DQ2) [29]. There is a regional difference of CD occurrence in India that is possibly linked to genetic differences coupled with variation in difference in staple diet (wheat in north India and rice in south India). The DR3 allele frequency of 14.9% from north India (Delhi) is comparable to that from south India (Tamil Nadu) of 14.3% among Yadhavas and 11.6% among Piramalai Kallars castes. However, a major difference in DQ2 allele frequency exists between the two regions: north India 31.9% and south India 12.8% (Piramalai Kallars) and 9% (Yadhavas) [23].

Clinical series from India usually describe typical or 'hypertypical' cases, with chronic diar-

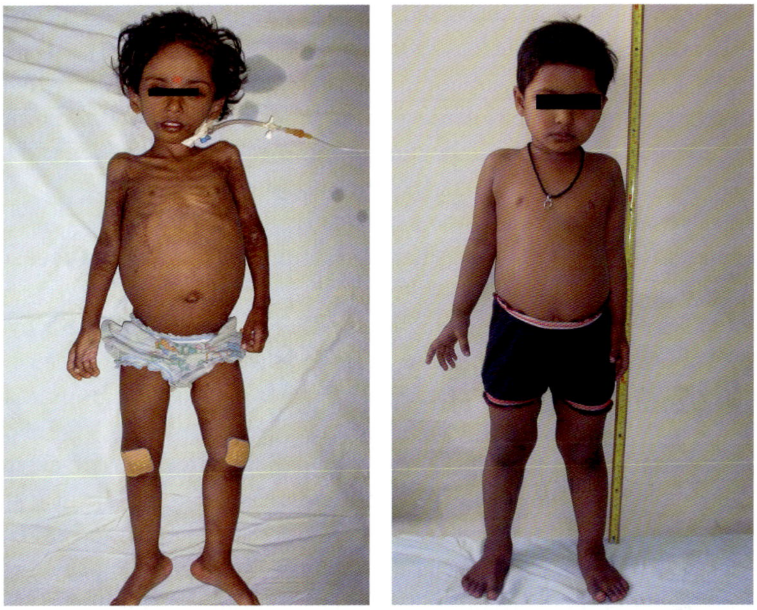

Fig. 1. a This is an Indian girl presenting at the age of 3.5 years with chronic diarrhea and severe malnutrition. Investigations showed the positivity of CD serological markers and flat mucosa at the small-intestinal biopsy. **b** After 6 months of gluten-free diet, an impressive improvement of the nutritional status of this child was evident.

rhea, anemia and stunting being the commonest symptoms in children (fig. 1). Recently atypical CD cases (18/42 celiacs) presenting with short stature, anemia, abdominal distention, rickets, constipation, diabetes mellitus and delayed puberty have been reported. Children with atypical CD are significantly older (median age 10.4 vs. 5.5 years) than classical cases [30].

Finally, there are only anecdotic reports of CD in Far East countries. Given the low prevalence of HLA predisposing genes DQ2/DQ8 and the low/absent gluten consumption, reduced disease prevalence should be expected in those populations.

Celiac Disease in Developing Countries

The burden of disease caused by CD in developing countries has been largely underestimated in the past. This situation depends on several reasons, particularly (1) common belief that CD does not exist in developing countries, (2) poor awareness of the clinical variability of CD, (3) scarcity of diagnostic facilities and (4) more emphasis on other causes of small-intestinal damage, such as intestinal tuberculosis and environmental enteropathy. It is also possible that the prevalence of CD is increasing in some developing countries because of the widespread diffusion of Western dietary habits, with increasing consumption of gluten-containing cereals. We suggested that the abrupt modification of dietary habits is one of the causes of the huge prevalence of CD among the Saharawis. Historically, the Bedouin diet was based on prolonged breastfeeding, camel milk and meat, dates, sugar, and small amounts of cereals and legumes. Over the last century, however, the Saharawi dietary habits have changed dramatically because of the European colonization, and products made with wheat flour, especially bread, have become the staple food.

Clinically the typical child with CD in a developing country resembles the picture of chronic protein-energy malnutrition known as 'kwashiorkor' (fig. 1). Chronic diarrhea, abdominal distention, stunting (height for age lower than 2 SD) and anemia are frequent findings. Severe stunting is associated with an increased risk of mortality, especially among children with protracted diarrhea. The risks of developing severe diarrhea and of dying from dehydration are greatest among the youngest children, especially during summer.

The reliability of serological CD autoantibodies in developing countries was a matter of debate. Different studies in South America, North Africa and India have recently shown that both the EMA and anti-tTG antibodies are highly specific indicators of celiac autoimmunity also in subjects with a high rate of infectious and/or parasitic diarrhea [31]. As a matter of fact, the 'weight' of these tests is even stronger than in developed countries, as a certain degree of nonspecific, celiac-like damage of the small intestinal mucosa (with increased intraepithelial lymphocyte count and reduced villous height/crypt depth ratio) is a frequent finding at the biopsy (so-called environmental enteropathy). The recent introduction of a reliable quick test for the point-of-care determination of IgA class anti-tTG antibodies on a drop of whole blood could overcome, at least in part, problems related to the scarcity of sophisticated diagnostic equipments [32].

Treatment of CD is based on lifelong exclusion from the diet of gluten-containing cereals, i.e. wheat, barley and rye. In most developed countries this is easily accomplished by using both cereals that do not contain gluten (e.g. rice and maize) and palatable gluten-free, commercially available products that are specifically designed for patients with CD. In contrast, treating the disease in the context of a developing country can be extremely difficult. To be effective, implementation of a gluten-free diet has to take local dietary habits into account, e.g. by using naturally gluten-free products that are locally available, such as millet, manioc and rice. However, in order to avoid cross-contamination with gluten, dedicated machinery needs to be used to mill these starchy foods. The treatment strategy should also include educational courses for doctors, nurses, dieticians, school personnel, affected families and the general population. Finally the implementation of patients' groups can help affected individuals to cope with the daily difficulties of treatment and to maintain contacts with other national societies and international agencies.

Celiac Disease Prevalence in At-Risk Groups

Studies all over the world have shown that the prevalence of CD is definitely increased in specific population subgroups. The risk of CD in first-degree relatives has been reported to be 6–7% on average, mostly ranging from 3 to 10 [1]. In a Finnish study on 380 patients with celiac disease and 281 patients with dermatitis herpetiformis, the mean disease prevalence was 5.5%, distributed as follows: 7% among siblings, 4.5% among parents and 3.5% among children [33]. The prevalence of CD is increased also in second-degree relatives, highlighting the importance of genetic predisposition as a risk factor.

CD prevalence is increased in autoimmune diseases, especially type 1 diabetes and thyroiditis, but also in less common disorders, e.g. Addison's disease or autoimmune myocarditis. The average prevalence of CD among children with type 1 diabetes is 4.5% (0.97–16.4%) [34]. Usually diabetes is diagnosed first, while CD is often subclinical and only detectable by serological screening. The increased frequency of CD in several thyroid diseases (Hashimoto's thyroiditis, Graves' disease and primary hypothyroidism) is well established. A 3- to 5-fold increase in CD prevalence has been reported in subjects with autoimmune thyroid disease. On the other hand, CD-associated hypothyroidism may sometimes lack features of an autoimmune process. Interestingly, treatment of CD by gluten withdrawal may lead to normalization of subclinical hypothyroidism [35].

An increased frequency of CD is found in some genetic diseases, especially Down's, Turner's and Williams' syndromes. In a multicenter Italian study on 1,202 subjects with Down's syndrome, 55 CD cases were found, with a prevalence of this disease association of 4.6% [36]. In Down's children CD is not detectable on the basis of clinical findings alone and is therefore underdetected. Even when there are symptoms, they may be considered clinically insignificant or possibly attributed to Down's syndrome itself. Nevertheless, the reported amelioration of gastrointestinal complaints on a gluten-free diet for all symptomatic patients suggests that identification and treatment can improve the quality of life for these children.

Selective IgA deficiency (total serum IgA lower than 5 mg%) predisposes to CD development, and this primary immunodeficiency is 10- to16-fold more common in patients with CD than the general population [37]. Patients with selective IgA deficiency and CD are missed by using the class A anti-tTG test (or any other IgA-based test, e.g. EMA) for screening purposes. For this reason it is appropriate to (1) check the total level of serum IgA in patients screened for CD and (2) perform an IgG-based test (e.g. IgG anti-tTG and/or IgG antigliadin) if total IgA is lower than normal.

The Celiac Iceberg

The epidemiology of CD is efficiently conceptualized by the iceberg model, which retains its validity across different populations in the world [1]. The prevalence of CD can be conceived as the overall size of the iceberg, which is not only influenced by the frequency of the predisposing genotypes in the population, but also by the pattern of gluten consumption. In many countries the prevalence of CD is roughly in the range of 0.5–1% of the general population. A sizable portion of these cases is properly diagnosed because of suggestive complaints (e.g. chronic diarrhea, unexplained iron deficiency) or other reasons (e.g. family history of CD). These cases make up the visible part of the celiac iceberg, in quantitative terms expressed by the incidence of the disease. In developed countries, for each diagnosed case of CD, an average of 5–10 cases remain undiagnosed (the submerged part of the iceberg), usually because of atypical, minimal or even absent complaints. These undiagnosed cases remain untreated and are therefore exposed to the risk of long-term complications. The 'water line', namely the ratio of diagnosed to undiagnosed cases, mostly depends on the physician's tendency to request serological CD markers in situations of low clinical suspicion, i.e. awareness of CD clinical polymorphism.

The best approach to the iceberg of undiagnosed CD seems to be a systemic process of case finding focused on at-risk groups, a procedure that minimizes costs and is ethically appropriate. Increased awareness of the clinical polymorphism of CD, coupled with a low threshold for serological testing, can efficiently uncover a large portion of the submerged CD iceberg, primary care being the natural setting of this selective screening. A primary care practice provides the best opportunity to first identify individuals who are at risk for CD and need referral for definitive diagnosis. We have recently completed a multicenter, prospective, case-finding study using serological testing (IgA class anti-tTG antibody determination) of adults who were seeking medical attention from their primary care physician in the USA and Canada [38]. By applying simple and well-established criteria for CD case-finding on a sample of adults, we achieved a 32- to 43-fold increase in the diagnostic rate of this condition. The most frequent risk factors for undiagnosed CD were: (a) thyroid disease, (b) positive family history for CD, (c) persistent gastrointestinal complaints and (d) iron deficiency with or without anemia. Many newly diagnosed cases of CD reported a long-standing history of symptoms (usually of years) that should have raised the suspicion of CD well before.

Conclusions

CD is one of the commonest lifelong disorders in countries populated by individuals of European origin, affecting approximately 1% of the general population. This is a common disease also in North Africa, the Middle East and India. The huge prevalence of CD in the Saharawi people (5.6%) is an outlier finding probably related to strong genetic predisposition and abrupt dietary changes (fig. 2). CD in the Saharawi children, as well as in other developing countries, is sometimes a severe disease, characterized by chronic diarrhea, stunting, anemia, and increased mortality. Further studies are needed to quantify the incidence of the celiac condition in apparently 'celiac-free' areas as sub-Saharan Africa and the Far East. In many developing countries the frequency of CD is likely to increase in the near future, given the diffuse tendency to adopt a Western, gluten-rich dietary pattern. As most cases currently escape diagnosis all over the world, an effort should be made to increase the awareness of CD polymorphism. A cost-effective case-finding policy could significantly reduce the morbidity and mortality associated with untreated disease.

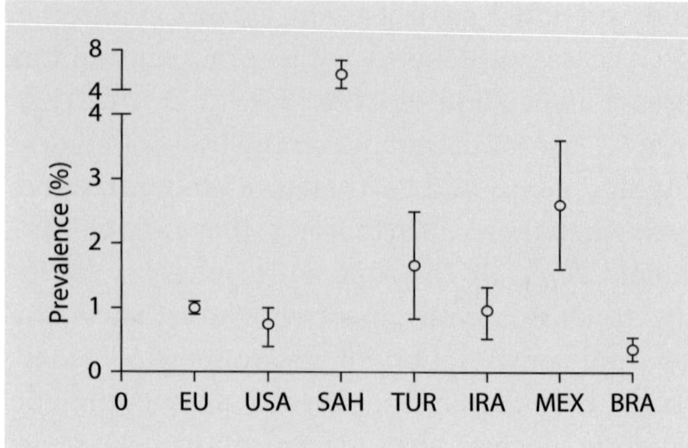

Fig. 2. Prevalence (and 95% CI) of CD in different countries. EU = European Union; USA = United States of America; SAH = Saharawi; TUR = Turkey; IRA = Iran; MEX = Mexico; BRA = Brazil.

References

1 Fasano A, Catassi C: Current approaches to diagnosis and treatment of celiac disease: an evolving spectrum. Gastroenterology 2001;120:636–651.

2 Catassi C, Fabiani E, Rätsch IM, Coppa GV, Giorgi PL, Pierdomenico R, et al: The coeliac iceberg in Italy: a multicentre antigliadin antibodies screening for coeliac disease in school-age subjects. Acta Paediatr Suppl 1996;412:29–35.

3 Volta U, Bellentani S, Bianco Bianchi F, Brandi G, De Franceschi L, Miglioli L, et al: High prevalence of celiac disease in Italian general population. Dig Dis Sci 2001;46:1500–1505.

4 Henker J, Losel A, Conrad K, Hirsch T, Leupold W: Prevalence of asymptomatic coeliac disease in children and adults in the Dresden region of Germany. Dtsch Med Wochenschr 2002;127:1511–1515.

5 Korponay-Szabo IR, Kovacs JB, Czinner A, Goracz G, Vamos A, Szabo T: High prevalence of silent celiac disease in preschool children screened with IgA/IgG antiendomysium antibodies. J Pediatr Gastroenterol Nutr 1999;28:26–30.

6 Csizmadia CGDS, Mearin ML, von Blomberg BME, Brand R, Verloove-Vanhorick SP: An iceberg of childhood coeliac disease in the Netherlands. Lancet 1999;353:813–814.

7 Riestra S, Fernandez E, Rodrigo L, Garcia S, Ocio G: Prevalence of coeliac disease in the general population of northern Spain: strategies of serologic screening. Scand J Gastroenterol 2000;35:398–402.

8 Ivarsson A, Persson LA, Juto P, Peltonen M, Suhr O, Hernell O: High prevalence of undiagnosed coeliac disease in adults: a Swedish population-based study. J Intern Med 1999;245:63–68.

9 West J, Logan RF, Hill PG, Lloyd A, Lewis S, Hubbard R, et al: Seroprevalence, correlates, and characteristics of undetected coeliac disease in England. Gut 2003;52:960–965.

10 Johnston SD, Watson RGP, McMillan SA, Sloan J, Love AHG: Coeliac disease detected by screening is not silent – simply unrecognized. Q J Med 1998;91:853–860.

11 Mäki M, Mustalahti K, Kokkonen J, Kulmala P, Haapalahti M, Karttunen T, et al: Prevalence of celiac disease among children in Finland. N Engl J Med 2003;348:2517–2524.

12 Meloni G, Dore A, Fanciulli G, Tanda F, Bottazzo GF: Subclinical coeliac disease in schoolchildren from northern Sardinia. Lancet 1999;353:37.

13 Mustalahti K: Oral presentation. Xth International Meeting on Coeliac Disease, Belfast, April 28–30, 2004.

14 Fasano A, Berti I, Gerarduzzi T, Not T, Colletti RB, Drago S, et al: Prevalence of celiac disease in at-risk and non at-risk groups: a large, multicentre study. Arch Intern Med 2003;163:286–292.
15 Gandolfi L, Pratesi R, Cordoba JC, Tauil PL, Gasparin M, Catassi C: Prevalence of celiac disease among blood donors in Brazil. Am J Gastroenterol 2000;95: 689–692.
16 Oliveira RP, Sdepanian VL, Barreto JA, Cortez AJ, Carvalho FO, Bordin JO, et al: High prevalence of celiac disease in Brazilian blood donor volunteers based on screening by IgA antitissue transglutaminase antibody. Eur J Gastroenterol Hepatol 2007;19:43–49.
17 Gomez JC, Selvaggio GS, Viola M, Pizarro B, la Motta G, de Barrio S: Prevalence of celiac disease in Argentina: screening of an adult population in the La Plata area. Am J Gastroenterol 2001;96:2700–2704.
18 Catassi C, Rätsch IM, Gandolfi L, Pratesi R, Fabiani E, El Asmar R, et al: Why is coeliac disease endemic in the people of Sahara? Lancet 1999;354: 647–648.
19 Catassi C, Doloretta Macis M, Rätsch IM, De Virgilis S, Cucca F: The distribution of DQ genes in the Saharawi population provides only a partial explanation for the high celiac disease prevalence. Tissue Antigens 2001;58: 402–406.
20 Abu-Zekry M, Kryszak D, Diab M, Catassi C, Fasano A: Prevalence of celiac disease among schoolage children in Egypt: preliminary results of a pilot study (abstract). J Pediatr Gastroenterol Nutr 2008, in press.
21 Simoons FJ: Celiac disease as a geographic problem; in Walcher DN, Kretchmer N (eds): Food, Nutrition and Evolution. New York, Masson, 1981, pp 179–199.
22 Shahbazkhani B, Forootan M, Merat S, Akbari MR, Nasserimoghadam S, Vahedi H, et al: Coeliac disease presenting with symptoms of irritable bowel syndrome. Aliment Pharmacol Ther 2003;18:231–235.
23 Yachha SK: Celiac disease: India on the global map. J Gastroenterol Hepatol 2006;21:1511–1513.
24 Yachha SK, Misra S, Malik A, Nagi B, Mehta S: Spectrum of malabsorption syndrome in North Indian children. Indian J Gastroenterol 1993;12:120–125.
25 Mohindra S, Yachha SK, Srivastava A, Krishnani N, Aggarwal R, Ghoshal UC, et al: Coeliac disease in Indian children: assessment of clinical, nutritional and pathologic characteristics. J Health Popul Nutr 2001;19:204–208.
26 Ranjan P, Ghoshal UC, Aggarwal R, Pandey R, Misra A, Naik S, et al: Etiological spectrum of sporadic malabsorption syndrome in northern Indian adults at a tertiary hospital. Indian J Gastroenterol 2004;23:94–98.
27 Sood A, Midha V, Sood N, Avasthi G, Sehgal A: Prevalence of celiac disease among school children in Punjab, North India. J Gastroenterol Hepatol 2006;21:1622–1625.
28 Sher KS, Fraser RC, Wicks AC, Mayberry JF: High risk of celiac disease in Punjabis: epidemiological study in the South Asian and European populations of Leicestershire. Digestion 1993;54:178–182.
29 Kaur G, Sarkar N, Bhatnagar S, Kumar S, Rapthap CC, Bhan MK, et al: Pediatric celiac disease in India is associated with multiple DR3-DQ2 haplotypes. Hum Immunol 2002;63:677–682.
30 Sharma A, Poddar U, Yachha SK, Khanna V: Time to recognize atypical celiac disease in Indian children. Indian J Gastroenterol 2006;25(suppl 2):A5.
31 Yachha SK, Aggarwal R, Srinivas S, Srivastava A, Somani SK, Itha S: Antibody testing in Indian children with celiac disease. Indian J Gastroenterol 2006;25:132–135.
32 Raivio T, Kaukinen K, Nemes E, Laurila K, Collin P, Kovacs JB, et al: Self transglutaminase-based rapid coeliac disease antibody detection by a lateral flow method. Aliment Pharmacol Ther 2006;24:147–154.
33 Hervonen K, Hakanen M, Kaukinen K, Collin P, Reunala T: First-degree relatives are frequently affected in coeliac disease and dermatitis herpetiformis. Scand J Gastroenterol 2002;37:51–55.
34 Holmes GKT: Screening for coeliac disease in type 1 diabetes. Arch Dis Child 2002;87:495–499.
35 Sategna-Guidetti C, Volta U, Ciacci C, et al: Prevalence of thyroid disorders in untreated adult celiac disease patients and effect of gluten withdrawal: an Italian multicenter study. Am J Gastroenterol 2001;96:751–757.
36 Bonamico M, Mariani P, Danesi HM, Crisogianni M, Failla P, Gemme G, et al: Prevalence and clinical picture of celiac disease in Italian Down syndrome patients: a multicenter study. J Pediatr Gastroenterol Nutr 2001;33:139–143.
37 Cataldo F, Marino V, Ventura A, et al: Prevalence and clinical features of selective immunoglobulin A deficiency in coeliac disease: an Italian multicentre study. Italian Society of Paediatric Gastroenterology and Hepatology (SIGEP) and 'Club del Tenue' Working Groups on Coeliac Disease. Gut 1998;42: 362–365.
38 Catassi C, Kryszak D, Jacques OL, Duerksen D, Hill I, Crowe SE, et al: Detection of celiac disease in primary care: a multicenter case-finding study in North America. Am J Gastroenterol 2007;102:1–7.

Prof. Carlo Catassi
Department of Pediatrics, Università Politecnica delle Marche
Via F. Corridoni 11
IT–60123 Ancona (Italy)
Tel. +39 071 596 2364, Fax +39 071 36 281, E-Mail catassi@tin.it

Fasano A, Troncone R, Branski D (eds): Frontiers in Celiac Disease.
Pediatr Adolesc Med. Basel, Karger, 2008, vol 12, pp 32–45

HLA and Non-HLA Genes in Celiac Disease

A. Zhernakova[a] · C. Wijmenga[a,b]

[a]Complex Genetics Section, DBG-Department of Medical Genetics, University Medical Center Utrecht, Utrecht, and [b]Department of Genetics, University Medical Center Groningen, Groningen, The Netherlands

Abstract

Celiac disease (CD) is a multifactorial disorder in which the combination of several genetic factors together with an environmental trigger is necessary for development of the disease. Genetic predisposition to CD is complex and includes the HLA-*DQA1*05/ DQB1*02* and HLA-*DQA*0301/ DQB*0302* genes as major factors; these are estimated to explain some 40% of the heritability of the disease. The other 60% of the genetic susceptibility to CD is shared between an unknown number of non-HLA genes, each of which is estimated to contribute only a small risk effect. In the past 30 years, two strategies of genetic research – linkage studies and association studies – have led to the discovery of several susceptibility loci and genes, such as a region on 5q (CELIAC2 locus), *MYO9B* and *CTLA4*. A recently performed genome-wide association study and follow-up have identified eight new risk regions, seven of which harbor genes controlling the immune response. In this chapter we will review the progress that has been made in genetic research into celiac disease and discuss future strategies and research perspectives.

Celiac disease (CD) is a multifactorial disorder with a complex genetic predisposition. The strong genetic component in CD has been demonstrated by the much higher concordance rates for CD in monozygous twins (83–86%) than in dizygous twins (17–20%) [1, 2]. The recurrence risk for siblings of CD patients to develop the disease is about 10%. Assuming the prevalence of CD in the general population to be 0.5%, this leads to an estimation of *sibling relative risk* (λs) of 20. The inheritance patterns seen in families do not follow Mendelian inheritance rule, which suggests that multiple genes are involved in CD.

The genetic predisposition to CD has been studied since 1974 when the association with HLA molecules was detected [3]. HLA-DQ2 molecules are the major genetic risk factor for CD and can explain at least 40% of the heritability of this disease. The pathophysiological role of HLA molecules in CD has been well investigated [4, 5]. However, characterizing the remaining 60% of non-HLA heritability of CD has been a major challenge for the past 30 years and the subject of intensive genetic research. A number of candidate genes have been suggested although they only explain part of the heritability of CD.

There are four possible approaches to genetic research into CD and these can be presented as a pyramid (fig. 1). (i) The easiest and most straightforward method that has been widely used is the **functional candidate genes association study.** Molecules that are known to play an important functional role in CD can be investigated in such association studies. (ii) This approach becomes more powerful when several genes included in a

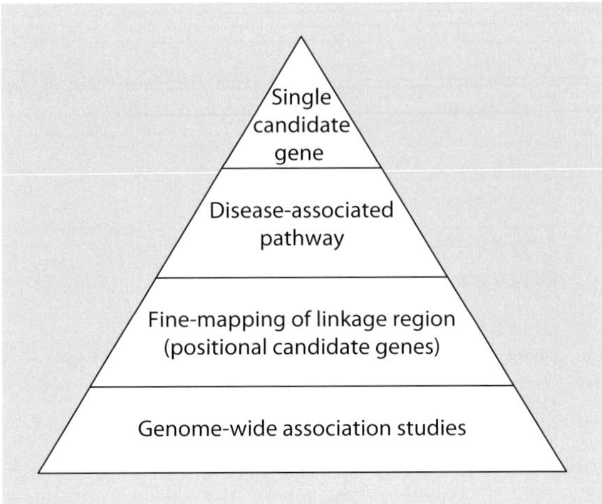

Fig. 1. The four strategies of genetic research applied to celiac disease.

pathway involved in the disease are investigated **(pathway association study)**. (iii) As an alternative to the first two hypothesis-driven methods, a **linkage study** investigates the distorted transmission of particular chromosomal loci through the whole genome and it is followed by fine-mapping of linkage regions containing tens to hundreds of positional candidate genes. (iv) Advanced technologies offer the possibility of performing hypothesis-free **genome-wide association studies**. We will discuss the results of all these approaches in detail in the following sections.

HLA Genes (CELIAC1 Locus on 6p21)

The *HLA* region is located on 6p21 and contains some 200 genes. The major HLA haplotype that is expressed in more than 90% of CD patients is DQ2 *(DQA*0501–DQB*0201*; corresponding to DQ2.5), a minority of CD cases are associated with DQ8 (*DQA*0301–DQB1*0302*) [6]. The primary function of the DQ heterodimer is to present the triggering environmental factor – the gluten molecules – to the T–cell helper cells. Gluten proteins are modified by the intestinal enzyme tissue transglutaminase so that they fit to the binding grooves of HLA-DQ2 and HLA-DQ8 molecules and can then be efficiently presented to the CD4+ T cells.

The HLA-DQ2 heterodimer could be encoded in cis where both *DQA1*0501* and *DQB1*0201* are located on the same DR3-DQ2 haplotype, and in trans where these two molecules are located on different haplotypes (in a combination of DR5-DQ7(*DQA1*0501-DQB1*0301*) and DR7-DQ2 (*DQA1*0201-DQB1*0202*) haplotypes) (table 1) [6]. Both cis and trans DQ2.5 differ in one residue in the leader peptide of DQA1 (*DQA1*0501* vs. *DQA1*0505*) and in one residue in the membrane-proximal domain of DQB1 (*DQB1*0201* vs. *DQB1*0202*), and they are considered to convey a similar disease risk.

Functional studies prove that disease susceptibility depends on the dosage effect of the DQ2.5 dimer [7]. Homozygosity for the DR3-DQ2 haplotype leads to the formation of two copies of DQ2.5 dimer in cis, whereas the combination of the DR2-DQ2 haplotype with DR7-DQ2 gives the DQ2.5 dimer in both the cis and trans forms. Both these genotypes confer the highest risk to CD (relative risk (RR) 10.1–13.1) [Monsuur et al., unpublished data]. The presence of one copy of DR3-DQ2 together with the other non-susceptible haplotype, or heterozygosity for DR5-DQ7/DR7-DQ2 leads to the formation of one functional DQ2.5 dimer in cis or trans respectively, corresponding to a medium risk for CD predisposition (RR 1.3–1.8) [7; Monsuur et al., unpublished data]. The dosage effect of the DQB1*0201 molecule has further been proved in genotype-phenotype clinical studies [8], while a dosage effect for DQ8 molecules have also been suggested [9].

Interestingly, the homozygosity for the DR3-DQ2 haplotype is highly increased in a small subgroup of CD patients who do not response to a gluten-free diet and who show aberrant intestinal

Table 1. HLA genotypes associated with disease (CD) and genetic risk

Haplotype (1/2)	DQA1-DQB1 alleles for the two homologous chromosomes	Possible DQ haplotype	Genetic risk (Monsuur et al., in preparation)
DR3-DQ2/ DR3-DQ2	DQA*0501-DQB*0201/ DQA*0501-DQB*0201/	DQ2.5 cis, DQ2.5 cis	13.1
DR3-DQ2/ DR7-DQ2	DQA*0501-DQB*0201/ DQA*0201-DQB*0202	DQ2.5 cis, trans DQ2.2 cis, trans	10.1
DR5-DQ7/ DR7-DQ2	DQA*0505-DQB*0301/ DQA*0201-DQB*0202	DQ2.5 trans, Other	1.8
DR3-DQ2/ Other	DQA*0501-DQB*0201/ Other	DQ2.5 cis, Other	1.3

T cells (these patients have so-called RCDII – refractory celiac disease) [10]. 44–62% of RCDII patients are homozygous for DR3-DQ2 compared to 20–24% of uncomplicated CD patients [10, 11]. This might reflect a correlation of the DQ2.5 dose with the severity of the disease.

The association of CD with DQ2 molecules is extremely strong in all populations. From a large group of 1,008 European patients with CD, only 4 did not have either a full or part of DQ2 or DQ8 heterodimer [9]. However, 25–30% of healthy individuals also express DQ2 or DQ8, which implies that the HLA variant is necessary, but not sufficient in itself, for CD.

Apart from the genes encoding the DQ molecules, the HLA region also contains a large number of immune-related genes that might be good candidates for susceptibility to CD. Dissecting the separate effects of other genes located in the HLA complex is a hard task because of the high *linkage disequilibrium* in the HLA region. Several studies have suggested the presence of other susceptibility genes for CD in the HLA region, including *MICA*, *MICB* and *TNF* genes [12–16], however, the majority of these studies were unable to perform a proper conditioning on the DQ2 haplotype. Nonetheless, extensive fine mapping is necessary to determine whether the HLA region harbors other susceptibility factors in addition to the well-established HLA-DQ2 [17–19].

Genome-Wide Linkage Studies

Linkage studies are carried out in families with multiple individuals and aim to identify chromosomal regions containing disease-predisposing genes. The principle of genetic linkage studies lies in the analysis of the co-segregation of the disease under study with a genetic marker within families. For complex diseases the non-parametric method of linkage analysis is widely used that allows testing for allele sharing between affected siblings. For each marker, the identity-by-descent allele sharing between affected siblings is determined (0, 1 or 2 alleles could be shared) and compared to the expected allele sharing under the null hypothesis of no linkage. If the inheritance pattern in affected siblings is different from that expected by chance, this is seen as evidence for linkage to a particular marker. Chromosomal regions exhibiting increased allele sharing are likely to contain susceptibility genes [20]. Linkage results are usually reported as a *logarithm of the odds (LOD) score*. According to the criteria proposed by Lander and Kruglyak [21], a LOD score of >2.2 corresponds to suggestive linkage, whereas a LOD score of >3.6 corresponds to significant linkage.

So far 12 independent genetic linkage studies in different populations have been performed in CD. The majority of these studies confirmed the linkage to the HLA gene region (6p21). In addition, a number of genomic regions outside the HLA region have shown suggestive linkage, but only a few of these have been independently confirmed in different populations. Three genomic regions – on15q12, 19p13.1 and 2q23–32 – have shown significant linkage (LOD >3.6). Other potential true-positive regions found in multiple populations are 4p14–15, 5q31, 9p and 11p11 (table 2).

A number of loci with significant linkage and those discovered in different populations have been examined more closely in fine-mapping studies; the results are described below.

The CELIAC2 Locus on 5q31–q33

The 5q31 region has been detected in independent genome scans in Scandinavian and Italian populations [22–26], and achieved a genome significance in a meta-analysis of European CD patients [27]. This locus partly overlaps with linkage regions of other autoimmune or inflammatory diseases – inflammatory bowel disease (IBD5) [28], type 1 diabetes (IDDM18) [29] and asthma [30] – and shows an overrepresentation of immune-related genes, many of which could serve as attractive functional candidates. However, studies performed on several candidate genes from this region, including the Crohn's disease-associated IBD5 locus (with *SLC22A4* and *SLC22A5* genes), the T1D-associated *IL12B* gene, and other immune-related genes (such as *IRF1*, *IL4*, *IL5*, *IL9*, *IL13*, *IL17B* and *NR3C1*) showed negative results [31–35]. One explanation might be that multiple genes from the 5q region, each with a minor effect, play a role in susceptibility to the disease. Fine mapping of the 5q region with a dense set of *single nucleotide polymorphisms (SNPs)* might help to find the causal gene and the exact functional variants.

The CELIAC3 Locus on 2q33

Significant linkage to the 2q33 region has been reported in a Scandinavian population [36] and evidence of linkage has been observed in several other studies [37–39]. According to the meta- and mega-analysis in European CD families, the overall evidence of linkage in chromosome 2q33 region is weak [27]. A cluster of attractive functional candidates *(CD28*, *CTLA4* and *ICOS)* is located under the CELIAC3 linkage peak and has been widely studied in different populations. *CD28* and *CTLA4* are both co-stimulatory molecules that bind to the B7 family receptors on the surface of antigen-presenting cells, and, together with the antigen-specific T-cell receptor, are necessary for T-cell activation. *CD28* functions as a positive regulator of T cells, whereas *CTLA4* provides the inhibiting negative signal. The association of *CTLA4* with other autoimmune diseases has been proved [40]. Based on the strong association with *CTLA4* that was originally found in French CD patients [41], this gene region was intensively investigated in a number of association studies in different populations [for review, see 42]. The results remain contradictory – whereas in British and Scandinavian populations a convincing association with the *CD28-CTLA4-ICOS* block has been observed [43–45], in other populations only borderline significance or no association could be detected [46–49].

Interestingly, in populations with linkage to this region, the maximum LOD score on chromosome 2 is observed for markers located 2–3 Mb centromeric to the *CTLA4* region [38, 50, 51]; therefore it is highly possible that linkage to the CELIAC3 region could be explained by a gene outside the *CD28-CTLA4-ICOS* block. The *STAT1* gene, a functional candidate gene located under the CELIAC3 linkage peak has recently been tested in the Dutch CD cohort, but was also shown not be associated [52]. Other clusters of immune-related genes, including apoptose-related *CASP8* and *CASP10* genes, are located

Table 2. Results of genome wide linkage studies performed in celiac disease (CD) excluding the HLA region

Population References	Number of families (1st/2nd/3rd)	Study design	Suggestive linkage (LOD > 2.2)	Significant linkage (LOD > 3.6)	Other loci with positive linkage
West Ireland Zhong et al. [65], 1996	15	Affected sibpairs	6p23, 11p11, 7qchr, 22centr	–	15q
Italy Greco et al. [22, 23], 1998, 2001 Percopo et al. [26], 2003	39/71/89	Affected sibpairs	5q	–	11qter
UK King et al. [66, 67], 2000, 2001	16/34	Extended families	11p11	–	6p12, 17q12, 18q23, 22q13.3
Sweden/Norway Naluai et al. [25], 2001	70/36	Affected sibpairs	–	–	5q, 9p, 11q
Finland Liu et al. [24], 2002	60/38	Affected sibpairs	–	–	1p36, 4p15, 5q31, 7q21, 9p21–23, 16q12
Finland Woolley et al. [69], 2002	9/1	Population isolate	–	15q12	–
North Europe Popat et al. [72], 2002	24	Extended families	–	–	4p14, 19p13.3, 5p15.1
North America Neuhausen et al. [87], 2002	62	Extended families	3p, 5p, 18q	–	10p, 12p, 12q, 13q
The Netherlands Van Belzen et al. [53], 2003	67/15	Affected sibpairs	6q21–22	19p13.1	–
Finland Rioux et al. [36], 2004	54	Affected sibpairs	10p	2q23–32	–
The Netherlands Van Belzen et al. [70], 2004	1	Large pedigree	9p21–p13	–	–
North America Garner et al. [71], 2006	160	Affected sibpairs	7q, 9q	–	–

under the CELIAC3 locus and might be attractive candidates for further genetic studies.

The CELIAC4 Locus on 19p13.1

Strong linkage to 19p13.1 was observed in the Dutch CD population (multiple maximum LOD score 4.43) [53] and was further suggested in a meta-analysis of European CD consortium data which did not include the Dutch cohort [27]. In a dense SNP fine mapping of the LOD-1.5 region (i.e. the 99% confidence interval) performed in Dutch CD patients, a single peak of association was observed in the 3′ end of the myosin IXb (*MYO9B)* gene [54]. Association to the MYO9B gene has also been reported in Spanish CD patients and Hungarian patients with dermatitis herpetiformis (DH) [55, 56]. The role of *MYO9B* in CD pathogenesis probably lies in impairing the intestinal barrier via the regulation of the Rho-dependent signaling pathway. The *MYO9B* gene is strongly associated in Dutch CD, and this has been confirmed in two independent case-control data sets included in the original study [54]. However these findings were not replicated in several other populations [57–60], which makes it difficult to interpret the role of *MYO9B* in susceptibility to CD. Interestingly, the 19p13.1 region has also been linked to another inflammatory intestinal disease: Crohn's disease (IBD6) in two independent genome scans [28, 61]. Similar to CD, the association of *MYO9B* to IBD has been confirmed in a multicentre study including Dutch, British and Canadian/Italian IBD cohorts [62], but it could not be confirmed in Scandinavian patients [63]. This implies heterogeneity between populations, which is also seen for other IBD genes (*DLG5* and *CARD15*) [64].

Searching for the Other Celiac Disease Genes

Other notable regions from the linkage scans that have been found in multiple populations include: 11p [65–67]; 11q [23, 25, 68]; 15q12 [69]; 9p21 [24, 70]; 7q [24, 65, 71], and 4p14 [24, 72]. Fine mapping of these regions has not yet been performed, and no candidate genes under these peaks have been established as risk factors predisposing to CD. A meta-analysis including all the linkage scans performed so far could help in prioritizing the most important susceptible CD loci.

From Linkage Results to Susceptibility Genes

The results of linkage studies usually include large chromosomal regions that span several megabases in size and may contain tens to hundreds of genes each. One possible strategy to define the causal variant might be to fine map each locus with a dense set of SNPs. This strategy has been successfully performed in the CELIAC4 region [54], however, it is expensive and requires substantial facilities. An alternative strategy would be to prioritize the genes under the linkage peak based on their biological function. Additional data, such as expression of the gene in a tissue of interest, differential expression in patient and control samples, and the presence of regulatory elements, should also be taken into account. Recent advances in bioinformatic tools now permit automatic prioritizing. The principle of these tools is to make a ranking of genes under the linkage loci based on their functional interaction with other genes located under different linkage peaks, or their functional or expression similarities [for review, see 73].

Candidate Gene Association Studies

The candidate gene *association studies* allow quick testing of the best candidate at low cost and have therefore been widely used. Decisions to test candidate genes are based on the known pathogenesis of the disease (functional candidates) and/or their location under the linkage peak (positional candidate). Most of the candidate genes so far studied for association with CD belong to the group of adaptive immunity genes, while a minority of the candidates are involved in gluten digestion and intestinal barrier function. Table 3 lists the genes that have been tested for association with CD so far, with positive results in at least one study.

Other genes that have been tested with only negative results include two genes involved in the digestion process of gluten, *PGPEP* [74] and *PREP* [75], and a number of immune-related genes: *MMP1* [76], *IL12B* [31], *IRF1* [35], *STAT1* [52], *RANTES* (*CCL5*) [77], a cluster of immune-related genes on chr5 (*IL4, IL5, IL9, IL13, IL17B* and *NR3C1*) [34], *IL1α*, *IL1β*, *IL1RN*, *IL18* and *MCP-1* [78] and *TGM2* [79].

Table 3. Candidate genes that show a positive association with celiac disease

Gene (risk factor)	Chromosomal position	Positive studies population [ref]	Negative studies population [ref]	Remarks
ICAM-1	19p13.2	French [88]	n/a	Association found only in subgroup of adult patients
MMP3	11q22.3	Italy [89]	Scandinavia [76]	Association found only in male patients
CD209	19p13	Spain [90]	n/a	Association found only with DQ2-negative subgroup
FOXP3	Xp11.23	Norway/ Sweden [91]	Spain [92]	Observed association is borderline significant and was not evident after multiple testing
CYP4F3, CYP4F2	19p13	The Netherlands [32]	n/a	
IFNG	12q14	Spain [93] Italy [94]	Finland [18] The Netherlands [95]	
KIR2DL5B	19q	Spain [96]	Finland [18]	
Leiden fV	1q23	Italy [97]	n/a	Observed in one family
MIF	22q11.23	Spain [98]	n/a	
PTPN22	1p13.1	The Netherlands [99] Scandinavia [100]	Spain [101] Europe [102]	Borderline association, in Dutch – only found in subgroup of patients with early age of manifestation
CTLA4	2q33	Many populations	Many populations	See section on linkage (p 35)
IL10	1q31	Sweden [103]	Finland [18] Italy [94] Caucasian [104]	
FAS	10q24.1	The Netherlands [105]	n/a	Associated with the severity of villous atrophy

However, it is too early to exclude all these genes as potential candidates, since the genetic analysis of many of them was not comprehensively designed. The majority of these analyses were performed before the completion of *HapMap*, a repository of all common SNP variations together with the known allelic associations between SNPs (i.e. *linkage disequilibrium*). So that often only one marker or potentially functional SNP was tested and these candidate gene studies therefore only investigated part of the underlying genetic variation. Moreover, most of the studied candidate genes are located outside the linkage peaks so that their risk effect is expected to be minor. Sufficiently large cohorts are needed to prove or exclude variants with only modest effects, and most of the negative studies mentioned above did not have enough power for this.

Pathway Analysis

Based on the linkage studies we could conclude that the HLA genotype is the only major factor in the genetics of CD, with the remaining 60% of the heritability shared between dozens of risk genes with small effect. This leads us to the polygenic model of CD, in which large numbers of susceptibility alleles are necessary for the disease to manifest in HLA-susceptible individuals. It would be logical to suggest that these minor susceptibility variants might be clustered in genes along only a few particular pathways, therefore leading to their impaired function. For example, the association with the negative co-stimulatory molecule CTLA4 has been observed in some populations. It is tempting to suggest that variants in other molecules of the co-stimulatory pathways, such as CTLA4 ligands B7H1 and B7H2 and positive co-stimulatory molecule CD28, might also influence susceptibility to CD via the same mechanism. In this example, the combination of susceptible variants, each with a weak effect in a number of genes on the co-stimulatory pathway, could together lead to the impairment of the negative co-stimulation of T cells and therefore to increased hyperactivation of T cells. If each of these hypothetical variants has only a weak effect, their separate detection by genetic association studies would require an impossibly large patient cohort. Another alternative could be a pathway analysis that would allow calculating the joint probability of observed variations in a number of genes from the same pathway. Pathway analysis remains a challenging task for bioinformatics, but recent publications have described a number of analytical tools [80, 81].

One successful example of pathway analysis in CD was the investigation of tight junction (TJ) genes. TJ molecules form the complex that determines the cell–cell junction and mediate intestinal permeability. An association study performed in 41 TJ genes discovered two genes (*PARD3* and *MAGI2*) that showed association with CD in multiple populations [82].

Genome-Wide Association Studies

Advanced technologies now allow performing association studies with hundreds of thousands of SNPs simultaneously. The HAPMAP project already provides access to over 6 million SNPs in the whole genome and allows counting on the LD structure of the human genome [83]. This makes it possible to perform *genome-wide association studies (GWAS)* aimed at covering all the common variants in the genome. Recently, the first GWAS in CD was performed in 778 CD cases and 1,422 population controls from the United Kingdom. Above the strong and extended association to the HLA region, the 4q27 genomic locus, including two immune related genes *IL2* and *IL21*, was associated at the genome-wide significance level ($p = 2.0 \times 10^{-7}$). Association with the *IL2/IL21* gene locus was subsequently confirmed in three independent CD populations from UK, Ireland and the Netherlands [84]. Moreover, similar association of the *IL2/IL21* gene region was observed in other autoimmune diseases (type 1 diabetes, rheumatoid arthritis), suggesting it as a common autoimmune locus [85]. Both IL2 and IL21 molecules are widely expressed cytokines, important for T-cell maturation and proliferation, and are therefore attractive candidates for CD pathogenesis.

In a more extensive follow up of the 1,020 top GWAS associated SNPs in multiple independent cohorts from three populations, seven additional new risk regions were identified [Hunt et al., Nat. Genet, in press]. Six of the new CD loci contain genes controlling adaptive immune responses, including *RGS1* (1q31), *IL18RAP* (2q11-2q12), *CCR3* (3p21), *IL12A* (3q25-q26), *TAGAP* (6q25) and *SH2B3* (12q24). The last associated locus located on 3q28 harbors the LPP gene that might play role in maintaining cell adhesion and motility. Three novel CD loci (*IL2/IL21*, *CCR3* and *SH2B3*) are also associated to type 1 diabetes, whereas association to the *IL18RAP* locus is also observed for another intestinal inflammatory condition namely Crohn's disease. [Hunt et al., Nat. Genet, in press;

Zhernakova et al., unpublished data]. Novel findings of GWAS dramatically improved our knowledge and understanding of the genetics of CD.

GWAS studies undoubtedly have advantages, but they also have some limitations. As a result of such studies, many false-positive SNPs are observed by chance and filtering them out will require replication work in multiple large cohorts. At the same time, true associated variants with a moderate effect could be overlooked because of the highly significant false-positives and they might not be included in the replication studies. The GWAS strategy is successful only if the risk polymorphisms occur with a reasonable frequency (*the common disease – common variant hypothesis (CD/CV)*) [86]. There is substantial evidence that the CD/CV hypothesis is valid for common diseases – which was proved by the recent GWAS results in CD and multiple examples in other common disorders. However, it is still possible that there are rare gene variants not sufficiently covered by existing approaches to GWAS which influence susceptibility to common diseases. The next level of zooming-in technologies, such as deep-sequencing should be able to define a more exact picture of genetic susceptibility to common diseases.

Conclusions and Future Perspectives

CD is a complex disease with a strong genetic component. The functional effect of one of the genetic factors, HLA, is well understood and this molecule can explain some 40% of the genetic susceptibility to CD. Genome-wide linkage studies have identified several disease susceptibility loci, but many of these have not been replicated in other populations. Hence, except for the *MYO9B* gene on 19p13.1, other underlying susceptibility genes in these regions have not yet been identified. The contribution of all the non-HLA genes to CD susceptibility is expected to be modest. Finding susceptibility genes with moderate effects by testing single candidate genes is a daunting task, so that pathway analyses are expected to be a more powerful tool, especially as our knowledge of the disease process increases. However, pathways can contain tens to hundreds of genes and selecting true susceptibility genes from such pathways remains difficult. Much of this type of genetic research is still hypothesis-based but with the advance of genome-wide studies it is now possible to take a completely unbiased and hypothesis-free approach. A recently performed GWAS followed by extensive replication in multiple populations, led to the identification of eight novel CD susceptibility genes. Future fine mapping and functional studies are required to identify the causative genes and the CD predisposing mutations. This could lead to the development of new non-invasive diagnostic tools and such genes may eventually provide new targets for therapeutic intervention.

Glossary

Association study: a study that aims to identify the joint occurrence of two genetically encoded characteristics in a population. Often, an association between a genetic marker and a phenotype (disease) is assessed.

Common disease/common variant (CD/CV): hypothesis that states that many genetic variants that underlie complex diseases are common, and therefore susceptible to detection by population-association study designs. An alternative possibility is that genetic contributions to complex diseases arise from many variants, all of which are rare.

HapMap: a catalogue of common genetic variants in the human genome, compiled by the International HapMap Project.

Human leukocyte antigen (HLA): 4-Mb region of chromosome 6 containing many genes of immunological function.

Linkage analysis: analysis of the co-segregation of the disease under study with a genetic marker within families. Linkage is based on the assumption that affected individuals within families share the predisposing genetic variants. Linkage analysis determines whether the affected individuals share the genetic information in a given region more often than would be expected by chance.

Linkage disequilibrium: the non-random association of alleles of genetic markers. Two markers are in linkage disequilibrium when some combinations of alleles in a population occur more or less frequently than would be expected at random.

LOD score: A statistical estimate that measures the probability of two loci being close together and consequently being inherited together.

Sibling relative risk (λs): risk of a patient's sibling to develop the disease. It is used as a measure of genetic component in complex disorders.

Single nucleotide polymorphism (SNP): single nucleotide variation on the DNA sequence.

GWAS: genome-wide association study, a large-scale genotyping analysis of markers in cases and controls. The first GWAS study in CD is performed on a 300k Illumina chip, and it includes typing of 300,000 SNPs across the whole genome.

Acknowledgements

The authors received funding from the Netherlands Organization of Scientific Research, the Dutch Digestive Diseases Foundation, and the Celiac Disease Consortium, an Innovative Cluster approved by the Netherlands Genomics Initiative, and were partially funded by the Dutch Government (BSIK03009). We thank Jackie Senior for critically reading the manuscript.

References

1 Greco L, Romino R, Coto I, Di Cosmo N, Percopo S, Maglio M, Paparo F, Gasperi V, Limongelli MG, Cotichini R, D'Agate C, Tinto N, Sacchetti L, Tosi R, Stazi MA: The first large population based twin study of coeliac disease. Gut 2002;50:624–628.

2 Nistico L, Fagnani C, Coto I, Percopo S, Cotichini R, Limongelli MG, Paparo F, D'Alfonso S, Giordano M, Sferlazzas C, Magazzu G, Momigliano-Richiardi P, Greco L, Stazi MA: Concordance, disease progression, and heritability of coeliac disease in Italian twins. Gut 2006;55:803–808.

3 Mulder DJ: Letter: HL-A antigens and coeliac disease. Lancet 1974;2:727.

4 Louka AS, Sollid LM: HLA in coeliac disease: unravelling the complex genetics of a complex disorder. Tissue Antigens 2003;61:105–117.

5 Jabri B, Sollid LM: Mechanisms of disease: immunopathogenesis of celiac disease. Nat Clin Pract Gastroenterol Hepatol 2006;3:516–525.

6 Sollid LM: Coeliac disease: dissecting a complex inflammatory disorder. Nat Rev Immunol 2002;2:647–655.

7 Vader W, Stepniak D, Kooy Y, Mearin L, Thompson A, van Rood JJ, Spaenij L, Koning F: The HLA-DQ2 gene dose effect in celiac disease is directly related to the magnitude and breadth of gluten-specific T cell responses. Proc Natl Acad Sci USA 2003;100:12390–12395.

8 Karinen H, Karkkainen P, Pihlajamaki J, Janatuinen E, Heikkinen M, Julkunen R, Kosma VM, Naukkarinen A, Laakso M: Gene dose effect of the DQB1*0201 allele contributes to severity of coeliac disease. Scand J Gastroenterol 2006;41: 191–199.

9 Karell K, Louka AS, Moodie SJ, Ascher H, Clot F, Greco L, Ciclitira PJ, Sollid LM, Partanen J: HLA types in celiac disease patients not carrying the DQA1*05-DQB1*02 (DQ2) heterodimer: results from the European Genetics Cluster on Celiac Disease. Hum Immunol 2003;64:469–477.

10 Al-Toma A, Goerres MS, Meijer JW, Pena AS, Crusius JB, Mulder CJ: Human leukocyte antigen-DQ2 homozygosity and the development of refractory celiac disease and enteropathy-associated T-cell lymphoma. Clin Gastroenterol Hepatol 2006;4:315–319.

11 Wolters VM, Verbeek WH, Zhernakova A, Onland-Moret C, Schreurs MW, Monsuur AJ, Verduijn W, Wijmenga C, Mulder CJ: The MYO9B gene is a strong risk factor for developing refractory celiac disease. Clin Gastroenterol Hepatol 2007;5:1399–1405, 1405. e1–e2.

12 de la Concha EG, Fernandez-Arquero M, Vigil P, Rubio A, Maluenda C, Polanco I, Fernandez C, Figueredo MA: Celiac disease and TNF promoter polymorphisms. Hum Immunol 2000;61:513–517.

13 Lopez-Vazquez A, Rodrigo L, Fuentes D, Riestra S, Bousono C, Garcia-Fernandez S, Martinez-Borra J, Gonzalez S, Lopez-Larrea C: MICA-A5.1 allele is associated with atypical forms of celiac disease in HLA-DQ2-negative patients. Immunogenetics 2002;53:989–991.

14 Rueda B, Pascual M, Lopez-Nevot MA, Koeleman BP, Ortega E, Maldonado J, Lopez M, Martin J: Association of MICA-A5.1 allele with susceptibility to celiac disease in a family study. Am J Gastroenterol 2003;98:359–362.

15 Gonzalez S, Rodrigo L, Lopez-Vazquez A, Fuentes D, Agudo-Ibanez L, Rodriguez-Rodero S, Fdez-Morera JL, Martinez-Borra J, Lopez-Larrea C: Association of MHC class I related gene B (MICB) to celiac disease. Am J Gastroenterol 2004;99:676–680.
16 Rodriguez-Rodero S, Rodrigo L, Fdez-Morera JL, Martinez-Borra J, Lopez-Vazquez A, Fuentes D, Lopez-Arbesu R, Lopez-Soto A, Gonzalez S, Lopez-Larrea C: MHC class I chain-related gene B promoter polymorphisms and celiac disease. Hum Immunol 2006;67:208–214.
17 Bolognesi E, Karell K, Percopo S, Coto I, Greco L, Mantovani V, Suoraniemi E, Partanen J, Mustalahti K, Maki M, Momigliano-Richiardi P: Additional factor in some HLA DR3/DQ2 haplotypes confers a fourfold increased genetic risk of celiac disease. Tissue Antigens 2003;61:308–316.
18 Woolley N, Mustalahti K, Maki M, Partanen J: Cytokine gene polymorphisms and genetic association with coeliac disease in the Finnish population. Scand J Immunol 2005;61:51–56.
19 Louka AS, Lie BA, Talseth B, Ascher H, Ek J, Gudjonsdottir AH, Sollid LM: Coeliac disease patients carry conserved HLA-DR3-DQ2 haplotypes revealed by association of TNF alleles. Immunogenetics 2003;55:339–343.
20 Dawn Teare M, Barrett JH: Genetic linkage studies. Lancet 2005;366: 1036–1044.
21 Lander E, Kruglyak L: Genetic dissection of complex traits: guidelines for interpreting and reporting linkage results. Nat Genet 1995;11:241–247.
22 Greco L, Babron MC, Corazza GR, Percopo S, Sica R, Clot F, Fulchignoni-Lataud MC, Zavattari P, Momigliano-Richiardi P, Casari G, Gasparini P, Tosi R, Mantovani V, De Virgiliis S, Iacono G, D'Alfonso A, Selinger-Leneman H, Lemainque A, Serre JL, Clerget-Darpoux F: Existence of a genetic risk factor on chromosome 5q in Italian coeliac disease families. Ann Hum Genet 2001;65:35–41.
23 Greco L, Corazza G, Babron MC, Clot F, Fulchignoni-Lataud MC, Percopo S, Zavattari P, Bouguerra F, Dib C, Tosi R, Troncone R, Ventura A, Mantavoni W, Magazzu G, Gatti R, Lazzari R, Giunta A, Perri F, Iacono G, Cardi E, de Virgiliis S, Cataldo F, De Angelis G, Musumeci S, Clerget-Darpoux F, et al: Genome search in celiac disease. Am J Hum Genet 1998;62:669–675.
24 Liu J, Juo SH, Holopainen P, Terwilliger J, Tong X, Grunn A, Brito M, Green P, Mustalahti K, Maki M, Gilliam TC, Partanen J: Genomewide linkage analysis of celiac disease in Finnish families. Am J Hum Genet 2002;70:51–59.
25 Naluai AT, Nilsson S, Gudjonsdottir AH, Louka AS, Ascher H, Ek J, Hallberg B, Samuelsson L, Kristiansson B, Martinsson T, Nerman O, Sollid LM, Wahlstrom J: Genome-wide linkage analysis of Scandinavian affected sib-pairs supports presence of susceptibility loci for celiac disease on chromosomes 5 and 11. Eur J Hum Genet 2001;9: 938–944.
26 Percopo S, Babron MC, Whalen M, De Virgiliis S, Coto I, Clerget-Darpoux F, Landolfo F, Greco L: Saturation of the 5q31-q33 candidate region for coeliac disease. Ann Hum Genet 2003;67: 265–268.
27 Babron MC, Nilsson S, Adamovic S, Naluai AT, Wahlstrom J, Ascher H, Ciclitira PJ, Sollid LM, Partanen J, Greco L, Clerget-Darpoux F: Meta and pooled analysis of European coeliac disease data. Eur J Hum Genet 2003;11:828–834.
28 Rioux JD, Silverberg MS, Daly MJ, Steinhart AH, McLeod RS, Griffiths AM, Green T, Brettin TS, Stone V, Bull SB, Bitton A, Williams CN, Greenberg GR, Cohen Z, Lander ES, Hudson TJ, Siminovitch KA: Genomewide search in Canadian families with inflammatory bowel disease reveals two novel susceptibility loci. Am J Hum Genet 2000;66:1863–1870.
29 Morahan G, Huang D, Ymer SI, Cancilla MR, Stephen K, Dabadghao P, Werther G, Tait BD, Harrison LC, Colman PG: Linkage disequilibrium of a type 1 diabetes susceptibility locus with a regulatory IL12B allele. Nat Genet 2001;27:218–221.
30 Moffatt MF, Cookson WO: The genetics of asthma. Maternal effects in atopic disease. Clin Exp Allergy 1998;28(suppl 1):56–61; discussion 65–56.
31 Louka AS, Torinsson Naluai A, D'Alfonso S, Ascher H, Coto I, Ek J, Giordano M, Gudjonsdottir AH, Mellai M, Momigliano-Richiardi P, Percopo S, Samuelsson L, Wahlstrom J, Greco L, Sollid LM: The IL12B gene does not confer susceptibility to coeliac disease. Tissue Antigens 2002;59:70–72.
32 Curley CR, Monsuur AJ, Wapenaar MC, Rioux JD, Wijmenga C: A functional candidate screen for coeliac disease genes. Eur J Hum Genet 2006;14: 1215–1222.
33 Ryan AW, Thornton JM, Brophy K, Daly JS, O'Morain C, McLoughlin RM, Kennedy NP, Abuzakouk M, Stevens FM, Feighery C, Kelleher D, McManus R: Haplotype variation at the IBD5/SLC22A4 locus (5q31) in coeliac disease in the Irish population. Tissue Antigens 2004;64:195–198.
34 Ryan AW, Thornton JM, Brophy K, Daly JS, McLoughlin RM, O'Morain C, Abuzakouk M, Kennedy NP, Stevens FM, Feighery C, Kelleher D, McManus R: Chromosome 5q candidate genes in coeliac disease: genetic variation at IL4, IL5, IL9, IL13, IL17B and NR3C1. Tissue Antigens 2005;65:150–155.
35 Seegers D, Borm ME, van Belzen MJ, Mulder CJ, Bailing J, Crusius JB, Meijer JW, Wijmenga C, Pena AS, Bouma G: IL12B and IRF1 gene polymorphisms and susceptibility to celiac disease. Eur J Immunogenet 2003;30:421–425.
36 Rioux JD, Karinen H, Kocher K, McMahon SG, Karkkainen P, Janatuinen E, Heikkinen M, Julkunen R, Pihlajamaki J, Naukkarinen A, Kosma VM, Daly MJ, Lander ES, Laakso M: Genomewide search and association studies in a Finnish celiac disease population: Identification of a novel locus and replication of the HLA and CTLA4 loci. Am J Med Genet A 2004;130:345–350.
37 Holopainen P, Naluai AT, Moodie S, Percopo S, Coto I, Clot F, Ascher H, Sollid L, Ciclitira P, Greco L, Clerget-Darpoux F, Partanen J: Candidate gene region 2q33 in European families with coeliac disease. Tissue Antigens 2004; 63:212–222.
38 Naluai AT, Nilsson S, Samuelsson L, Gudjonsdottir AH, Ascher H, Ek J, Hallberg B, Kristiansson B, Martinsson T, Nerman O, Sollid LM, Wahlstrom J: The CTLA4/CD28 gene region on chromosome 2q33 confers susceptibility to celiac disease in a way possibly distinct from that of type 1 diabetes and other chronic inflammatory disorders. Tissue Antigens 2000;56:350–355.

39 Popat S, Hearle N, Hogberg L, Braegger CP, O'Donoghue D, Falth-Magnusson K, Holmes GK, Howdle PD, Jenkins H, Johnston S, Kennedy NP, Kumar PJ, Logan RF, Marsh MN, Mulder CJ, Torinsson Naluai A, Sjoberg K, Stenhammar L, Walters JR, Jewell DP, Houlston RS: Variation in the CTLA4/CD28 gene region confers an increased risk of coeliac disease. Ann Hum Genet 2002;66:125–137.
40 Ueda H, Howson JM, Esposito L, Heward J, Snook H, Chamberlain G, Rainbow DB, Hunter KM, Smith AN, Di Genova G, Herr MH, Dahlman I, Payne F, Smyth D, Lowe C, Twells RC, Howlett S, Healy B, Nutland S, Rance HE, Everett V, Smink LJ, Lam AC, Cordell HJ, Walker NM, Bordin C, Hulme J, Motzo C, Cucca F, Hess JF, Metzker ML, Rogers J, Gregory S, Allahabadia A, Nithiyananthan R, Tuomilehto-Wolf E, Tuomilehto J, Bingley P, Gillespie KM, Undlien DE, Ronningen KS, Guja C, Ionescu-Tirgoviste C, Savage DA, Maxwell AP, Carson DJ, Patterson CC, Franklyn JA, Clayton DG, Peterson LB, Wicker LS, Todd JA, Gough SC: Association of the T-cell regulatory gene CTLA4 with susceptibility to autoimmune disease. Nature 2003;423:506–511.
41 Djilali-Saiah I, Schmitz J, Harfouch-Hammoud E, Mougenot JF, Bach JF, Caillat-Zucman S: CTLA-4 gene polymorphism is associated with predisposition to coeliac disease. Gut 1998;43: 187–189.
42 van Heel DA, Hunt K, Greco L, Wijmenga C: Genetics in coeliac disease. Best Pract Res Clin Gastroenterol 2005;19:323–339.
43 Amundsen SS, Naluai AT, Ascher H, Ek J, Gudjonsdottir AH, Wahlstrom J, Lie BA, Sollid LM: Genetic analysis of the CD28/CTLA4/ICOS (CELIAC3) region in coeliac disease. Tissue Antigens 2004;64:593–599.
44 Hunt KA, McGovern DP, Kumar PJ, Ghosh S, Travis SP, Walters JR, Jewell DP, Playford RJ, van Heel DA: A common CTLA4 haplotype associated with coeliac disease. Eur J Hum Genet 2005;13: 440–444.
45 Haimila K, Smedberg T, Mustalahti K, Maki M, Partanen J, Holopainen P: Genetic association of coeliac disease susceptibility to polymorphisms in the ICOS gene on chromosome 2q33. Genes Immun 2004;5:85–92.
46 Rueda B, Zhernakova A, Lopez-Nevot MA, Gomez-Garcia M, Ortega E, Pinero A, Correro F, Brieva JA, Nieto A, Koeleman BP, Martin J: CTLA4/CT60 polymorphism is not relevant in susceptibility to autoimmune inflammatory intestinal disorders. Hum Immunol 2005;66:321–325.
47 Zhernakova A, Eerligh P, Barrera P, Wesoly JZ, Huizinga TW, Roep BO, Wijmenga C, Koeleman BP: CTLA4 is differentially associated with autoimmune diseases in the Dutch population. Hum Genet 2005;118:58–66.
48 Martin-Pagola A, Perez de Nanclares G, Vitoria JC, Bilbao JR, Ortiz L, Zubillaga P, Castano L: No association of CTLA4 gene with celiac disease in the Basque population. J Pediatr Gastroenterol Nutr 2003;37:142–145.
49 Mora B, Bonamico M, Indovina P, Megiorni F, Ferri M, Carbone MC, Cipolletta E, Mazzilli MC: CTLA-4 +49 A/G dimorphism in Italian patients with celiac disease. Hum Immunol 2003;64:297–301.
50 Holopainen P, Arvas M, Sistonen P, Mustalahti K, Collin P, Maki M, Partanen J: CD28/CTLA4 gene region on chromosome 2q33 confers genetic susceptibility to celiac disease. A linkage and family-based association study. Tissue Antigens 1999;53: 470–475.
51 King AL, Moodie SJ, Fraser JS, Curtis D, Reid E, Dearlove AM, Ellis HJ, Ciclitira PJ: CTLA-4/CD28 gene region is associated with genetic susceptibility to coeliac disease in UK families. J Med Genet 2002;39:51–54.
52 Diosdado B, Monsuur AJ, Mearin ML, Mulder C, Wijmenga C: The downstream modulator of interferon-gamma, STAT1 is not genetically associated to the Dutch coeliac disease population. Eur J Hum Genet 2006;14: 1120–1124.
53 Van Belzen MJ, Meijer JW, Sandkuijl LA, Bardoel AF, Mulder CJ, Pearson PL, Houwen RH, Wijmenga C: A major non-HLA locus in celiac disease maps to chromosome 19. Gastroenterology 2003;125:1032–1041.
54 Monsuur AJ, de Bakker PI, Alizadeh BZ, Zhernakova A, Bevova MR, Strengman E, Franke L, van't Slot R, van Belzen MJ, Lavrijsen IC, Diosdado B, Daly MJ, Mulder CJ, Mearin ML, Meijer JW, Meijer GA, van Oort E, Wapenaar MC, Koeleman BP, Wijmenga C: Myosin IXB variant increases the risk of celiac disease and points toward a primary intestinal barrier defect. Nat Genet 2005; 37:1341–1344.
55 Koskinen LL, Korponay-Szabo IR, Viiri K, Juuti-Uusitalo K, Kaukinen K, Lindfors K, Mustalahti K, Kurppa K, Adany R, Pocsai Z, Szeles G, Einarsdottir E, Wijmenga C, Maki M, Partanen J, Kere J, Saavalainen P: Myosin ixb gene region and gluten intolerance: linkage to coeliac disease and a putative dermatitis herpetiformis association. J Med Genet 2007; [Epub ahead of print].
56 Sanchez E, Alizadeh BZ, Valdigem G, Ortego-Centeno N, Jimenez-Alonso J, de Ramon E, Garcia A, Lopez-Nevot MA, Wijmenga C, Martin J, Koeleman BP: MYO9B gene polymorphisms are associated with autoimmune diseases in Spanish population. Hum Immunol 2007;68:610–615.
57 Giordano M, Marano C, Mellai M, Limongelli MG, Bolognesi E, Clerget-Darpoux F, Momigliano-Richiardi P, Greco L: A family-based study does not confirm the association of MYO9B with celiac disease in the Italian population. Genes Immun 2006;7:606–608.
58 Amundsen SS, Monsuur AJ, Wapenaar MC, Lie BA, Ek J, Gudjonsdottir AH, Ascher H, Wijmenga C, Sollid LM: Association analysis of MYO9B gene polymorphisms with celiac disease in a Swedish/Norwegian cohort. Hum Immunol 2006;67:341–345.
59 Hunt KA, Monsuur AJ, McArdle WL, Kumar PJ, Travis SP, Walters JR, Jewell DP, Strachan DP, Playford RJ, Wijmenga C, van Heel DA: Lack of association of MYO9B genetic variants with coeliac disease in a British cohort. Gut 2006;55:969–972.
60 Nunez C, Marquez A, Varade J, Martinez A, Polanco I, Maluenda C, Fernandez-Arquero M, de la Concha EG, Urcelay E: No evidence of association of the MYO9B polymorphisms with celiac disease in the Spanish population. Tissue Antigens 2006;68: 489–492.

61 van Heel DA, Dechairo BM, Dawson G, McGovern DP, Negoro K, Carey AH, Cardon LR, Mackay I, Jewell DP, Lench NJ: The IBD6 Crohn's disease locus demonstrates complex interactions with CARD15 and IBD5 disease-associated variants. Hum Mol Genet 2003;12:2569–2575.
62 van Bodegraven AA, Curley CR, Hunt KA, Monsuur AJ, Linskens RK, Onnie CM, Crusius JB, Annese V, Latiano A, Silverberg MS, Bitton A, Fisher SA, Steinhart AH, Forbes A, Sanderson J, Prescott NJ, Strachan DP, Playford RJ, Mathew CG, Wijmenga C, Daly MJ, Rioux JD, van Heel DA: Genetic variation in myosin IXB is associated with ulcerative colitis. Gastroenterology 2006;131:1768–1774.
63 Amundsen SS, Vatn M, Wijmenga C, Sollid LM, Lie BA: Association analysis of MYO9B gene polymorphisms and inflammatory bowel disease in a Norwegian cohort. Tissue Antigens 2006;68:249–252.
64 Cavanaugh J: NOD2:ethnic and geographic differences. World J Gastroenterol 2006;12:3673–3677.
65 Zhong F, McCombs CC, Olson JM, Elston RC, Stevens FM, McCarthy CF, Michalski JP: An autosomal screen for genes that predispose to celiac disease in the western counties of Ireland. Nat Genet 1996;14:329–333.
66 King AL, Yiannakou JY, Brett PM, Curtis D, Morris MA, Dearlove AM, Rhodes M, Rosen-Bronson S, Mathew C, Ellis HJ, Ciclitira PJ: A genome-wide family-based linkage study of coeliac disease. Ann Hum Genet 2000;64:479–490.
67 King AL, Fraser JS, Moodie SJ, Curtis D, Dearlove AM, Ellis HJ, Rosen-Bronson S, Ciclitira PJ: Coeliac disease: follow-up linkage study provides further support for existence of a susceptibility locus on chromosome 11p11. Ann Hum Genet 2001;65:377–386.
68 Holopainen P, Mustalahti K, Uimari P, Collin P, Maki M, Partanen J: Candidate gene regions and genetic heterogeneity in gluten sensitivity. Gut 2001;48:696–701.
69 Woolley N, Holopainen P, Ollikainen V, Mustalahti K, Maki M, Kere J, Partanen J: A new locus for coeliac disease mapped to chromosome 15 in a population isolate. Hum Genet 2002;111:40–45.
70 van Belzen MJ, Vrolijk MM, Meijer JW, Crusius JB, Pearson PL, Sandkuijl LA, Houwen RH, Wijmenga C: A genome-wide screen in a four-generation Dutch family with celiac disease: evidence for linkage to chromosomes 6 and 9. Am J Gastroenterol 2004;99:466–471.
71 Garner CP, Ding YC, Steele L, Book L, Leiferman K, Zone JJ, Neuhausen SL: Genome-wide linkage analysis of 160 North American families with celiac disease. Genes Immun 2007;8:108–114.
72 Popat S, Bevan S, Braegger CP, Busch A, O'Donoghue D, Falth-Magnusson K, Godkin A, Hogberg L, Holmes G, Hosie KB, Howdle PD, Jenkins H, Jewell D, Johnston S, Kennedy NP, Kumar P, Logan RF, Love AH, Marsh MN, Mulder CJ, Sjoberg K, Stenhammar L, Walker-Smith J, Houlston RS: Genome screening of coeliac disease. J Med Genet 2002;39:328–331.
73 Elbers CC, Onland-Moret NC, Franke L, Niehoff AG, van der Schouw YT, Wijmenga C: A strategy to search for common obesity and type 2 diabetes genes. Trends Endocrinol Metab 2007;18:19–26.
74 Monsuur AJ, Stepniak D, Diosdado B, Wapenaar MC, Mearin ML, Koning F, Wijmenga C: Genetic and functional analysis of pyroglutamyl-peptidase I in coeliac disease. Eur J Gastroenterol Hepatol 2006;18:637–644.
75 Diosdado B, Stepniak DT, Monsuur AJ, Franke L, Wapenaar MC, Mearin ML, Koning F, Wijmenga C: No genetic association of the human prolyl endopeptidase gene in the Dutch celiac disease population. Am J Physiol Gastrointest Liver Physiol 2005;289:G495–G500.
76 Louka AS, Stensby EK, Ek J, Gudjonsdottir AH, Ascher H, Sollid LM: Coeliac disease candidate genes: no association with functional polymorphisms in matrix metalloproteinase 1 and 3 gene promoters. Scand J Gastroenterol 2002;37:931–935.
77 Zhernakova A, Alizadeh BZ, Eerligh P, Hanifi-Moghaddam P, Schloot NC, Diosdado B, Wijmenga C, Roep BO, Koeleman BP: Genetic variants of RANTES are associated with serum RANTES level and protection for type 1 diabetes. Genes Immun 2006;7:544–549.
78 Rueda B, Zhernakova A, Lopez-Nevot MA, Martin J, Koeleman BP: Association study of functional genetic variants of innate immunity related genes in celiac disease. BMC Med Genet 2005;6:29.
79 Popat S, Hogberg L, McGuire S, Green H, Bevan S, Stenhammar L, Houlston RS: Germline mutations in TGM2 do not contribute to coeliac disease susceptibility in the Swedish population. Eur J Gastroenterol Hepatol 2001;13:1477–1479.
80 Heidema AG, Boer JM, Nagelkerke N, Mariman EC, van der AD, Feskens EJ: The challenge for genetic epidemiologists: how to analyze large numbers of SNPs in relation to complex diseases. BMC Genet 2006;7:23.
81 Kristensen VN, Tsalenko A, Geisler J, Faldaas A, Grenaker G, Lingjaerde OC, Fjeldstad S, Yakhini Z, Lonning PE, Borresen-Dale AL: Multilocus analysis of SNP and metabolic data within a given pathway. BMC Genomics 2006;7:5.
82 Wapenaar MC, Monsuur A, van Bodegraven A, Weersma RK, Bevova M, Linskens R, Howdle P, Holmes G, Mulder CJ, Dijkstra G, van Heel DA, Wijmenga C: Associations with tight junction genes Pard3 and Magi2 in Dutch patients point to a common barrier defect for celiac disease and ulcerative colitis. Gut 2007; [Epub ahead of print].
83 International HapMap Consortium: A haplotype map of the human genome. Nature 2005;437:1299–1320.
84 van Heel DA, Franke L, Hunt KA, Gwilliam R, Zhernakova A, Inouye M, Wapenaar MC, Barnardo MC, Bethel G, Holmes GK, Feighery C, Jewell D, Kelleher D, Kumar P, Travis S, Walters JR, Sanders DS, Howdle P, Swift J, Playford RJ, McLaren WM, Mearin ML, Mulder CJ, McManus R, McGinnis R, Cardon LR, Deloukas P, Wijmenga C: A genome-wide association study for celiac disease identifies risk variants in the region harboring IL2 and IL21. Nat Genet 2007;39:827–829.
85 Zhernakova A, Alizadeh BZ, Bevova M, van Leeuwen MA, Coenen MJ, Franke B, Franke L, Posthumus MD, van Heel DA, van der Steege G, Radstake TR, Barrera P, Roep BO, Koeleman BP, Wijmenga C: Novel association in chromosome 4q27 region with rheumatoid arthritis and confirmation of type 1 diabetes point to a general risk locus for autoimmune diseases. Am J Hum Genet 2007;81:1284–1288.
86 Becker KG: The common variants/multiple disease hypothesis of common complex genetic disorders. Med Hypotheses 2004;62:309–317.

87 Neuhausen SL, Feolo M, Camp NJ, Farnham J, Book L, Zone JJ: Genome-wide linkage analysis for celiac disease in North American families. Am J Med Genet 2002;111:1–9.
88 Abel M, Cellier C, Kumar N, Cerf-Bensussan N, Schmitz J, Caillat-Zucman S: Adulthood-onset celiac disease is associated with intercellular adhesion molecule-1 (ICAM-1) gene polymorphism. Hum Immunol 2006;67: 612–617.
89 Mora B, Bonamico M, Ferri M, Megiorni F, Osborn J, Pizzuti A, Mazzilli MC: Association of the matrix metalloproteinase-3 (MMP-3) promoter polymorphism with celiac disease in male subjects. Hum Immunol 2005;66:716–720.
90 Nunez C, Rueda B, Martinez A, Maluenda C, Polanco I, Lopez-Nevot MA, Ortega E, Sierra E, Gomez de la Concha E, Urcelay E, Martin J: A functional variant in the CD209 promoter is associated with DQ2-negative celiac disease in the Spanish population. World J Gastroenterol 2006;12:4397–4400.
91 Bjornvold M, Amundsen SS, Stene LC, Joner G, Dahl-Jorgensen K, Njolstad PR, Ek J, Ascher H, Gudjonsdottir AH, Lie BA, Skinningsrud B, Akselsen HE, Ronningen KS, Sollid LM, Undlien DE: FOXP3 polymorphisms in type 1 diabetes and coeliac disease. J Autoimmun 2006;27:140–144.
91 Sanchez E, Rueda B, Orozco G, Oliver J, Vilchez JR, Paco L, Lopez-Nevot MA, Callejas JL, Sabio JM, Gomez-Garcia M, Nieto A, Delgado M, Martin J: Analysis of a GT microsatellite in the promoter of the foxp3/scurfin gene in autoimmune diseases. Hum Immunol 2005;66:869–873.
93 Rueda B, Martinez A, Lopez-Nevot MA, Mas-Fontao A, Paco L, Ortega E, Fernandez-Arquero M, Urcelay E, Gomez de la Concha E, Martin J: A functional variant of IFNgamma gene is associated with coeliac disease. Genes Immun 2004;5:517–519.
94 Lio D, Scola L, Forte GI, Accomando S, Giacalone A, Crivello A, Cataldo F: TNFalpha, IFNgamma and IL-10 gene polymorphisms in a sample of Sicilian patients with coeliac disease. Dig Liver Dis 2005;37:756–760.
95 Wapenaar MC, van Belzen MJ, Fransen JH, Sarasqueta AF, Houwen RH, Meijer JW, Mulder CJ, Wijmenga C: The interferon gamma gene in celiac disease: augmented expression correlates with tissue damage but no evidence for genetic susceptibility. J Autoimmun 2004;23:183–190.
96 Santin I, Castellanos-Rubio A, Perez de Nanclares G, Vitoria JC, Castano L, Bilbao JR: Association of KIR2DL5B gene with celiac disease supports the susceptibility locus on 19q13.4. Genes Immun 2007;8:171–176.
97 Mari T, Zullo A, Hassan C, Di Giulio L, Morini S: Genetic association between factor V Leiden and coeliac disease. Gut 2006;55:1677–1678.
98 Nunez C, Rueda B, Martinez A, Lopez-Nevot MA, Fernandez-Arquero M, de la Concha EG, Martin J, Urcelay E: Involvement of macrophage migration inhibitory factor gene in celiac disease susceptibility. Genes Immun 2007;8:168–170.
99 Zhernakova A, Eerligh P, Wijmenga C, Barrera P, Roep BO, Koeleman BP: Differential association of the PTPN22 coding variant with autoimmune diseases in a Dutch population. Genes Immun 2005;6:459–461.
100 Viken MK, Amundsen SS, Kvien TK, Boberg KM, Gilboe IM, Lilleby V, Sollid LM, Forre OT, Thorsby E, Smerdel A, Lie BA: Association analysis of the 1858C>T polymorphism in the PTPN22 gene in juvenile idiopathic arthritis and other autoimmune diseases. Genes Immun 2005;6:271–273.
101 Rueda B, Nunez C, Orozco G, Lopez-Nevot MA, de la Concha EG, Martin J, Urcelay E: C1858T functional variant of PTPN22 gene is not associated with celiac disease genetic predisposition. Hum Immunol 2005;66:848–852.
102 Lee YH, Rho YH, Choi SJ, Ji JD, Song GG, Nath SK, Harley JB: The PTPN22 C1858T functional polymorphism and autoimmune diseases – a meta-analysis. Rheumatology (Oxford) 2007;46: 49–56.
103 Hahn-Zoric M, Hytonen AM, Hanson LA, Nilsson LA, Padyukov L: Association of –1087 IL10 and –308 TNFA gene polymorphisms with serological markers of coeliac disease. J Clin Immunol 2003;23:291–296.
104 Barisani D, Ceroni S, Meneveri R, Cesana BM, Bardella MT: IL-10 polymorphisms are associated with early-onset celiac disease and severe mucosal damage in patients of Caucasian origin. Genet Med 2006;8: 169–174.
105 Wu J, Alizadeh BZ, Veen TV, Meijer JW, Mulder CJ, Pena AS: Association of FAS (TNFRSF6)-670 gene polymorphism with villous atrophy in coeliac disease. World J Gastroenterol 2004;10: 717–720.

Prof. Cisca Wijmenga
Department of Genetics, Room E2.030, University Medical Center Groningen
PO Box 30.001
NL–9700 RB Groningen (The Netherlands)
Tel. +31 50 361 7100, Fax +31 50 361 7230, E-Mail c.wijmenga@medgen.umcg.nl

Fasano A, Troncone R, Branski D (eds): Frontiers in Celiac Disease.
Pediatr Adolesc Med. Basel, Karger, 2008, vol 12, pp 46–56

Twins and Family Contribution to Genetics of Celiac Disease

L. Greco[a] · M.A. Stazi[b] · F. Clerget-Darpoux[c]

[a]Department of Pediatrics and European Laboratory for the Investigation of Food-Induced Diseases, University of Naples Federico II, Naples; [b]Istituto Superiore di Sanità, National Center for Epidemiology, Surveillance and Health Promotion, Rome, Italy, and [c]INSERM, U535, and Université de Paris-Sud, IFR69, UMR-S535, Villejuif, France

Abstract

Celiac disease has a multifactorial background, but there is no doubt that the genetic component contributes most to the disease. The incidence within families is ten times the incidence among unrelated individuals. Concordance between monozygotic twins is more than 80%, as compared to the relatively low concordance (<20%) among dizygotic twins. Dizygotic twins have a concordance rate similar to siblings reared at different times. These data suggest that the genetic component is so strong that unshared environmental factors play a minor role in the pathogenesis of the disease. Monozygotic and dizygotic twins share the same environment in infancy, but their concordance rate is very different: the common environment likely explains a minor part of the variance in the incidence of the disease. First-degree relatives of celiac patients have a disease incidence of 10%, but this familial risk is not shared equally among all families. The risk is strongly related to the profile of HLA class II genes transmitted within the family. A double dose of the *DQB1*02* gene is associated with a higher risk than a single dose of the same gene. The HLA profile of the proband allows a gross estimation of the risk of a new sibling, but the typing of parents gives a more accurate estimate of the risk of a newborn to develop celiac disease. Among families with a case, 40% will have a negligible risk of having an affected newborn, 30% will have a risk ranging from 1 to 10%, and 30% will have a risk of >20%.

Celiac disease (CD) is one of the most frequent food-induced diseases in humans as more than 1% of gluten-consuming individuals is affected [1]. CD is not due to a rare modification of genes essential to good function, but has a large genetic component. We are indeed dealing with a multigenic condition in which several common genetic polymorphisms synergically produce a peculiar immunologic answer to a very common food antigen.

From the epidemiologic viewpoint, it is quite impressive to note that this strong genetic component does eventually produce a very stable incidence of the disease across different populations: CD is equally present and manifest in Punjab as in Sweden, in Cuba as in Hungary, in North Africa as in Australia. Human species share most of the genome, but populations appear to be different because of the multiple patterns of variation in very common genes. This is not so for CD: different genes finally produce the same response to gluten, production of autoantibodies and damage to the small intestinal mucosa. The example of HLA is illuminating: northern European populations more frequently adopt the DR3-associated HLA pattern, while in southern Europe the association with DR5/DR7 is more frequent, but eventually the disease is not different in any aspect between the two regions [2].

How Many Genes – How Much Environment: Twin Studies

We are aware that CD is a multifactorial disease involving both genetic and environmental factors. Besides the HLA region, already known to bear one or more risk loci for CD, at least three additional susceptibility loci have been suggested to map on chromosomes 5q31–33, 2q33 and 19p13 [3–5].

The twin method constitutes a powerful tool to estimate the genetic and environmental causes of family resemblance for a given trait [6]. The genetic contribution to celiac disease was inferred from case series and anecdotal case reports of concordant twin pairs since the early 1980s, but the potential of twin studies was enormously increased by the establishment of population-based registries of data on twins that represent some of the best resources for genetic epidemiologic research [7]. Matching a twin register with disease records makes it feasible to collect twin pairs in which at least one member is affected; this results in samples that are largely representative of the general twin population, and also ensures a gain in terms of statistical power because of independence by selection bias.

By cross-linking the membership lists of the Italian CD patients support group with the Italian Twin Registry [8], we were able to examine 47 pairs with at least one affected twin and this led to the first large population-based twin study of CD. We evaluated the concordance rates and the relative risk of CD for the co-twins of probands, by zygosity and HLA status [9]. The study was then updated and, 4 years later using a sample of 73 pairs, we were also able to estimate the progression rate to disease in co-twins of probands and the heritability of CD [10].

Concordance

CD concordance was estimated by zygosity and sex, using proband-wise (P_C) and pair-wise (P_P) concordance rates under incomplete ascertainment [11]. In such a scenario, concordant affected pairs are distinguished between 'doubly' (D) ascertained, for which both twins were in the disease records, and 'singly' (S) ascertained, where only one twin was in the records and the second twin was found to be affected on further examination. P_C is defined as the probability that one twin in a pair is affected, given that his/her co-twin is affected. P_P is the probability that both twins in a pair are affected, given that at least one is affected.

In the 2006 study [10], 73 twin pairs were enrolled. Twenty-three pairs were monozygotic (MZ; 6 males, 17 females) and 50 were dizygotic (DZ; 12 males, 15 females and 23 opposite sex pairs). The MZ/DZ same sex/DZ opposite sex ratio was 0.9:1.1:0.9 and was not significantly different from that expected (1:1:1). Age at enrolment was similar in MZ and DZ twins (t test: $p = 0.3$).

Seventeen pairs were known to be concordant before entering the study. Five clinically silent co-twins (4 MZ and 1 DZ) were diagnosed during the study because they were positive to autoantibody screening and to intestinal biopsy. Age at diagnosis varied greatly (range 0–57 years), although 50% of all affected twins developed the disease within 3 years of age.

When patients or their parents were asked about symptoms that led to diagnosis, the most frequent answers were: diarrhea (51%), vomiting (39%), weight loss (29%), anemia (22%), and abdominal distension (19%). Thirteen affected twins (2 index and 11 co-twins) claimed to be seemingly symptomless and to have been screened for CD because of affected relatives.

Overall, 17 of 23 MZ and 5 of 50 DZ twin pairs were concordant for CD: proband-wise (P_C) and

Table 1. Concordance by zygosity and gender in twin pairs

	Concordance	Discordance	Total	Concordances, %			
				proband-wise	95% CI	pair-wise	95% CI
MZ male	5	1	6	90	71–100	81.8	49.7–100
MZ female	12	5	17	80	63.1–96.9	66.7	43.2–90.1
All MZ	17	6	23	82.9*	69.5–96.2	70.7**	52.3–90.2
DZ male	0	12	12	0		0	
DZ female	1	14	15	12.5	0–34.7	6.7	0–19.3
DZ opp. sex	4	19	23	26.9	5.2–48.7	15.6	1–30.1
All DZ	5	45	50	16.7*	3.6–29.8	9.1**	1.3–16.9
Total	22	51	73				

Test for difference between monozygotic (MZ) and dizygotic (DZ) twins: $*\chi^2 = 48.09$, $p = 4.1 \times 10^{-12}$; $**\chi^2 = 38.61$, $p = 5.2 \times 10^{-10}$.

pair-wise (P_P) concordances were significantly different between MZ and DZ twins, with point estimates of 83 and 71% in MZ twins, and 17 and 9% in DZ twins, respectively (table 1). Concordances by gender did not significantly differ in MZ twins. In DZ, 1 of 5 concordant pairs was female-female and 4 of 5 were opposite sex pairs. None of the 12 DZ male-male pairs was concordant (table 1). In 15 of 19 discordant opposite sex pairs the affected twins were females.

Risk and HLA Status

It was recently shown that HLA-CD association is better described by a risk hierarchy of DR-DQ genotypes rather than by DQ2-DQ8 molecules [12]. Accordingly, twin pairs were stratified into four genotype groups with decreasing risk for CD: the highest risk genotypes are DQ2-DQ2 (equivalent to DR3/DR3 and DR3/DR7) genotypes (group 1, G1); DQ2 in trans (DR5/DR7) confers one third less risk (G2); the relative risks of DQ2-DQX (DR3/X) heterozygous (G3) and of half DQ2 (DR7/DR7), DQ8 (DR4/DR4-DQB1*0302 DR4/DR7) genotypes (G4) are estimated to be approximately one fourth of the G1; finally, the fifth group (G5) includes all the other genotypes with very low risk of CD (1/50 of the G1).

All MZ twin pairs, but one, belonged to G1–G4 risk categories. Discordant MZ co-twins were DR3/7 (n = 2), DR5/7 (n = 3) and DR3/5 (n = 1). Unexpectedly, the low risk genotype groups (G3 and G4) had the highest proportion of concordant pairs, giving an odds ratio point estimate of 3.2 relative to the G1 genotype group. This is possibly attributable to random fluctuation and more twin pairs should be available to investigate whether concordance estimates do follow the risk hierarchy of the genotype groups previously described [12].

In DZ pairs, 48 of 50 index twins carried high to low risk HLA genotypes and 2 of 50 were DR1/7 and DR4/13 (G5). One concordant pair belongs to the group of six pairs with both twins having high risk DR-DQ genotypes (G1). All these G1 pairs inherited the same parental HLA chromosomes (identical by descent). The same proportion of concordant pairs (2 of 12) was observed in the group with both twins carrying low risk genotypes (G3–G4). In this category, 1 concordant and 5 discordant pairs were HLA identical by descent. Finally, in the two remaining concordant pairs one of the two twins was DR3/7 (G1) and the other DR3/5 (G3).

Among 45 unaffected DZ co-twins, approximately one third carried high or medium risk genotypes (G1–G2), one third was at low risk (G3–G4) and one third had very low risk genotypes (G5).

A logistic regression model, corrected for age, sex, number of shared HLA haplotypes, and zygosity, performed in the first twin study [9], showed that genotypes DQA1*0501/DQB1*0201 (DQ2) and DQA1*0301/DQB1*0302 (DQ8) conferred to the non-index twin a relative risk of contracting the disease of 3.3 and 1.4, respectively. The relative risk of being concordant for celiac disease for the non-index twin of an MZ twin pair was 17 (95% CI 2.1–134), independent of the DQ at-risk genotype, providing evidence for a very strong genetic component to celiac disease, only partially due to the HLA genotype.

Heritability

Heritability is defined as the proportion of the total phenotypic variance that is attributable to the genetic variance. We estimated genetic and environmental components of variance in CD using structural equation modeling. We considered a model incorporating parameters for additive genetic (A), common (shared) environmental (C), and individual-specific (unshared) environmental (E) components of variance [6]. Additive genetic factors are shared completely by MZ twins, who are genetically identical, and correlate 0.5 in DZ twins, who share on average 50% of their segregating genes. Common environmental factors are shared completely by the co-twins regardless of zygosity, while unshared environmental influences act separately on each twin and therefore are responsible for less than perfect resemblance between MZ twins. Under these assumptions, the expectations for the total variance (V) and the covariance within twin pairs are given by: $V = A + C + E$; $Cov(MZ) = A + C$ and $Cov(DZ) = 0.5*A + C$.

Heritability (h^2) is A/V.

The study relied on incomplete ascertainment of twins [11]. For the variance components to be estimated, the ascertainment probability ($0<\pi<1$; i.e. the probability that an affected twin is in the disease records) has to be taken into account. It can be approximated as $\pi = 2D/(2D+S)$ where D and S are numbers of concordant pairs doubly and singly ascertained as described above in the Concordance section; moreover, the threshold of liability has to be fixed at the value corresponding to the population prevalence of the disease.

In the study by Nisticò et al. [10] there were 13 and 4 doubly ascertained pairs among MZ and DZ twins, respectively, and 4 and 1 singly ascertained pairs among MZ and DZ twins, respectively. This resulted in an ascertainment probability of $\pi = (2*17)/(2*17 + 5) = 34/39 = 0.87$.

Given the so-called 'iceberg' structure of CD, which underlines the importance of the subclinical component, we fitted the same ACE model assuming for the population prevalence the values 1/1,000 (threshold 3.09) from clinical diagnosis data, and 1/91 (threshold 2.29) from screening data [1].

Under the ACE model with a population prevalence for CD of 1/1,000, 57% of the variation in liability to CD was explained by additive genetic factors, while 42 and 1% were the contributions of common and unique environmental factors, respectively. When we fitted the same ACE model with a population prevalence of 1/91, the heritability estimate became 87%, and the relative weight of common environmental factors decreased to 12%; the contribution of the unshared environmental component of variance remained at the 1% level.

Message from Twin Studies

Polanco et al. [13] failed to increase concordance in twins by supplementing 18 g of gluten/day in the diet. High concordance has been observed in dermatitis herpetiformis-affected twins [14] but differences in clinical expression in MZ twins have also been observed: genetically identical individuals may develop distinguished phenotypes of gluten sensitivity, either dermatitis herpetiformis or CD [15].

Holtmeier et al. [16] found a distinct δT cell repertoires in MZ twins concordant for CD, pointing to the importance of post-transcriptional factors in the modulation of gene expression.

As expected, concordances in MZ twins are significantly higher compared to DZ pairs and are very close to those previously reported on a smaller sample size [9]. In DZ, the proportion of affected co-twins (5 of 50 = 10%) is in line with the prevalences of 4–12% in first-degree relatives reported in several studies [17].

Concordance rates by gender are not significantly different within MZ and DZ groups. In DZ pairs, the highest point estimates in opposite sex twins is not due to mean follow-up time as it is similar to that of female pairs and even shorter than that of male pairs.

Six of 23 MZ pairs were disease discordant after a period of 4.5–27 years of follow-up. Discordance in MZ twins is usually attributed to differential exposure to environmental risk factors. An alternative explanation may be that differences between genetically identical individuals are due to epigenetic modifications, occurring after twin separation, that control expression and silencing of disease genes [18].

Disease concordance in MZ pairs with high risk G1 genotypes (DR3/7, DR3/3) is higher than that observed in six DZ pairs of the same group and with the same parental HLA (2 haplotypes identical by descent). This difference could be explained by the polygenic liability to the disease: apart from the HLA class II region, other loci on chromosomes 2 and 5 are associated with or linked to CD in the Italian population [3, 4].

In our concordant pairs, most of the co-twins developed CD shortly after their siblings, with a median discordance time of 1 month for both MZ and DZ twins; since median follow-up times in discordant pairs were 10.5 and 8.2 years for MZ and DZ, respectively, we do not expect any dramatic variation in the concordance rates as a consequence of an even longer follow-up.

It is well known that CD is frequently asymptomatic or silent. In our study, approximately half of MZ and DZ affected co-twins were positive to antibody screening and had flat gut mucosa despite the absence of symptoms. Thus, if CD diagnoses due to symptom appearance only were considered, disease incidence would be largely – and to a similar extent – underestimated in MZ and DZ non-index twins. On the other hand, the exclusion or inclusion of silent co-twins would not strongly affect the cumulative incidence ratio of MZ relative to DZ co-twins (5-year relative risks 0.5/0.04 = 12.5 versus 0.68/0.08 = 8.5).

The twin study shows a substantial heritability for CD, with point estimates indicating that approximately 60–90% of the variance in liability to the disease has a genetic origin. However, because of the limited power of these studies, which reflects on large confidence intervals, we have to be cautious in interpreting the point estimates. They simply suggest a major genetic role in determining individual phenotypic differences, but they tell us nothing about which genes are directly implicated in the emergence of the disease. Environmental factors might play a role on the expression of the genotype: the elimination of gluten from the diet is a typical example of environmental intervention that, in the case of CD, can result in a total recovery of gut function and a correction of most other consequences, despite a considerable heritability: it does act on the expression of the phenotype, and is likely to have no relation with the incidence of the disease.

Common environment cannot be completely ruled out as a contributing factor. Common environment refers to any shared environmental factor that contributes to the resemblance of members of a twin pair regardless of zygosity. It may include biological events like exposure to infectious agents, dietary characteristics, and other intrauterine factors that may influence the similarity of CD patterns within pairs. Moreover, it is clear that the common environment of members of twin pairs is most alike in utero and during the first postnatal period, while tends to diverge over time. Therefore, possible effects of common environment on liability to CD could be seen both in the short discordance time and in the young age at diagnosis observed in our sample for the majority of concordant pairs.

Family studies have been extensively used to unravel the genetic predisposition to CD [19, 20]. In principle they consist of comparing the risk for relatives of affected individuals with that in the general population and, unlike the twin method, they suffer the disadvantage of not providing information on the extent to which the observed familial resemblance has a genetic basis or is attributable to shared environmental exposures.

The heritability point estimate under a high prevalence scenario is quite in line with the figures found in twin studies on other HLA-mediated diseases, such as type 1 diabetes 88% [21], Graves' disease 79% [22] and psoriasis 80% [23]: this plausibly reflects shared pathogenetic mechanisms that may partially explain the co-morbidity of these conditions [24–26]. A new twin study looking at co-morbidity for HLA-mediated diseases will possibly show that the causes of phenotypic correlation among the different autoimmune conditions can be attributed to common genetic pathways.

Risk of Developing Celiac Disease

Familial Risk

Several studies have shown a higher prevalence of CD in siblings of celiac patients compared to the general population, with risk estimates falling between 8 and 12% [19, 27–29]. However, the meaning of these estimates is not completely clear since the CD phenotype was frequently not precisely defined and might or might not have include latent, silent or only symptomatic forms of the disease according to the ESPGHAN criteria [30–32].

In an Italian population, we are performing an extensive family study in order to evaluate the risk to a sibling of a symptomatic patient of developing CD, and to provide the parents of a CD child the risk for a future baby with the best possible precision. We estimate this risk according to familial and genetic information.

A cohort of 188 nuclear families was ascertained through a symptomatic CD patient (the proband) having at least one sibling. For the vast majority (184 of 188) of the probands, we had families with both parents available for typing. A total of 798 individuals were sampled: 614 first-degree relatives of 184 celiac probands. Among the 246 siblings of probands, 24 siblings were diagnosed as affected including latent, silent and symptomatic forms. The recurrence risks (R), which correspond to the risk of developing CD for a sibling of a proband was thus estimated by: R = 24/246 = 9.8% (6.1; 13.4). This estimate is consistent with the value of about 10% provided by the literature [27–29].

We also estimated the risk of a sibling in families in which two children are already known to be affected. One consequence of the last 10 years of genome scans by linkage analysis using the sib-pair method has been the recruiting of large samples of families with at least two celiac cases. In these family data, Gudjonsdottir et al. [30] estimated a risk of 26.3% for siblings and 13% for parents of sib-pair family members. Similarly, from US family data Book et al. [20] also reported a prevalence of 21.3% of CD in siblings of affected sib-pairs and an overall prevalence of 17.8% of disease in all relatives of sib-pairs. Indeed selecting families with two confirmed cases leads to select parents carrying more genetic risk factors.

Risk of CD According to HLA-DQ Information

Though our European network, a total of 470 European trio families, one affected child and

Table 2. Observed number and frequencies of the genotypic groups for the 311 Italian probands

DQ genotypes	Genotypic group	DQ	Corresponding DR genotypes	311 CD patients	Corresponding Italian population, %
H1/H1 H1/H2	G1	DQ2/DQ2 DQ2/½ DQ2	DR3/DR3 DR3/DR7	74 (24%)	4
H2/H3	G2	DQ2 trans	DR5/DR7	117 (38%)	7
H1/H3 H1/H4 H1/H5	G3	DQ2/DQX	DR3/DR5 DR3/DR4 DR3/DRX	79 (25%)	17
H2/H2 H2/H4 H4/H4	G4	½ DQ2/½ DQ2 ½ DQ2/DQ8 DQ8	DR7/DR7 DR7/DR4 DR4/DR4	13 (4%)	3
Others	G5		Others	28 (9%)	69

two parents, were collected from Italy (128 families), France (117 families), and Norway/Sweden (225 families). Each family member was DQ genotyped (1,410 individuals). The analysis of these data showed that the genetic risk of an individual to develop a symptomatic form can be stratified into five classes according his/her HLA-DQ genotype [12].

Let us consider five DQA1-DQB1 haplotypes:

H1: DQ2 = DQA1*05-DQB1*02
H2: ½ DQ2 = DQA1*05⁻-DQB1*02
H3: ½ DQ2 = DQA1*05-QB1*02⁻
H4: DQ8 = DQA1*301-DQB1*302
H5: other haplotypes

Three genotypic groups correspond to the DQ2 heterodimer carriers: group 1 (G1): H1/H1 and H1/H2 (*DQ2* heterodimer and double dose of DQB1*02); group 2 (G2): H2/H3 (*DQ2* heterodimer encoded in *trans*), and group 3 (G3): H1/H5 (one copy of *DQ2* heterodimer).

Two genotypic groups correspond to non-DQ2 heterodimer carriers: group 4 (G4): H2/H2, H2/H4 and H4/H4 (*DQ8* and double dose of the at risk *DQB1* alleles: i.e. DQB1*02 or DQB1*302), and group 5 (G5): other genotypes.

In all populations, G1 is the highest risk group whereas the relative risks for the other genotypes vary from one population to another.

Estimation of the Risk of CD According to HLA-DQ in the Italian Population

Table 2 gives the observed number and frequencies of the genotypic groups for the 311 Italian probands and for the representative Italian population.

Given that the recurrence risk in siblings of an Italian CD patient has been estimated as 0.098, we can compute the familial correlation not due to HLA-DQ to be $\lambda = 1.4$.

Estimation of the Risk to a Sibling of a Patient According to HLA-DQ Information in the Italian Population

Risk to a Sibling of a Proband According the DQ Genotype of the Proband

For each possible DQ genotype of a proband, table 3 gives the risk of being affected for a sibling of this proband. Results are classed by genotypic group.

Table 3. Risks of a sibling of a proband according to the DQ genotype of the proband

	DQ2/DQ2			DQ2/DQX			DQ8/½ DQ2			DQ2–/DQ8–					
Proband group	G1	G1	G2	G3	G3	G3	G4	G4	G4	G5	G5	G5	G5	G5	G5
Proband genotype	H_1H_1	H_1H_2	H_2H_3	H_1H_3	H_1H_4	H_1H_5	H_2H_2	H_2H_4	H_4H_4	H_2H_5	H_3H_3	H_3H_4	H_3H_5	H_4H_5	H_5H_5
Risk[1]	**0.14**	**0.14**	**0.11**	*0.07*	*0.07*	*0.06*	*0.09*	*0.06*	0.04	0.04	0.03	0.03	0.03	0.02	0.02

[1]Values in bold print indicate a risk of >10%; values in italic print indicate a risk of between 5 and 10%, and values in normal print indicate a risk of <5%.

Risk to a Sibling of a Proband According to the DQ Genotype of Parents

As shown in table 3, the risk for a future baby is quite different according to the HLA DQ of the proband. HLA typing may also be proposed to the parents if they want to be better informed. Figure 1 gives what may be concluded with the parental typing. In the colored boxes, the risk for the baby may be negligible (blue), moderate (green), or high (red). In 30% of cases the estimate of risk is quite robust and accurate. In contrast, there are situations (boxes with numbers) in which parental typing may lead to quite variable risk for the baby (a range from negligible to high). In such a case, typing the baby will be encouraged soon after birth to improve the safety of the estimation.

For example, a mother H2H2 (½DQ2/½DQ2), who already has a child with CD, has a 29% risk of having another one if the father is H1H1 (DQ2/DQ2), but only a 7% risk if the father is H2H2 (½DQ2/½DQ2).

Similarly a father H2H5 (½DQ2/DQX), who already has a child with CD, has a very small (2%) risk of having another CD child if the mother is H2H5 (½DQ2/DQX) but a higher (12%) risk if the mother is H3H3 (½DQ2/½DQ2).

Figure 1 also shows that the decision of genotyping a newborn baby depends more on the possible variability of the risk for the child than on the mean expectation obtained from the parent genotypes. For example, if parents are H1H1/H1H1 (DQ2/DQ2), H2H4/H2H4 (DQ2/DQ8) or H3H5/H4H5 (½DQ2/DQ8) there is no doubt about the risk to the child and genotyping the child is unnecessary. If parents are H2H4/ H1H3 a new child has a mean risk of 15% but his/her risk may vary from 1 to 29%. In this situation genotyping the child is necessary if we want to refine the risk.

Risk to a Sibling of a Proband According to His/Her Own DQ Genotype

Figure 2 gives the probability (in italics) for a sibling of a proband to belong to G1 and the corresponding risk (inside the bar), showing that it is expected that approximately 40% of siblings will belong to G5 and consequently will have a negligible risk (<1%). However about 30% will belong to G1 or G2 and will be predicted to have a risk >20%.

Genetic Counseling?

Genetic counseling in families with a proband affected by a multifactorial disease is generally inappropriate, due to the large uncertainty around the empirical risk of recurrence. In CD, prenatal genetic counseling is neither required nor suggested, but those who work with celiac families are often asked about the recurrence risk for a possible future child. We answer that the risk of recurrence is approximately 10%, but do not give any more accurate information. For many parents

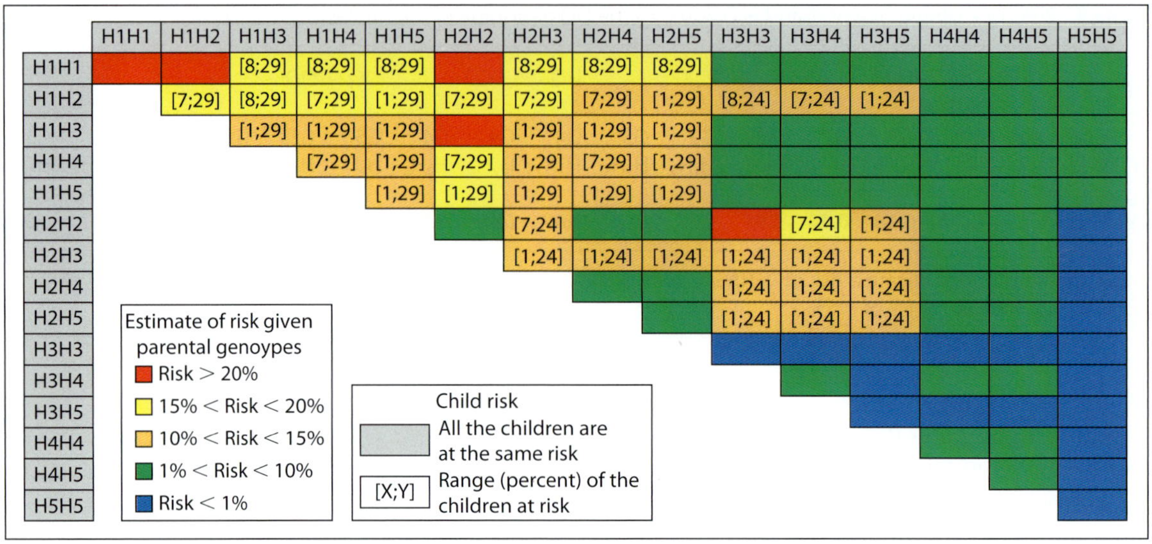

Fig. 1. Risk of a sibling of a proband according to the DQ genotype of the parents.

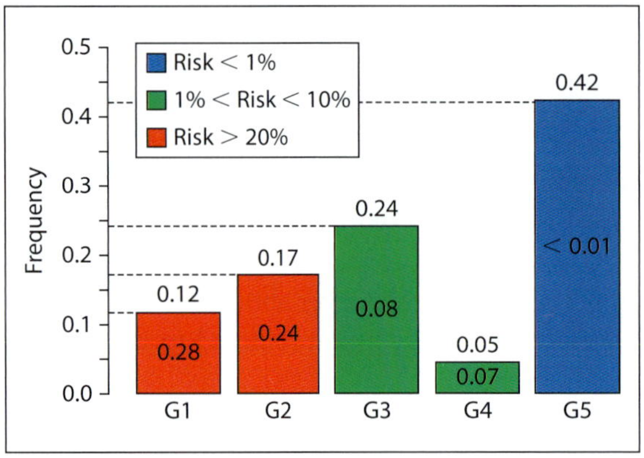

Fig. 2. Probability of a sibling of a proband to belong to a specific risk group.

a 10% risk of recurrence is intolerably high, and they feel discouraged to plan further pregnancies.

We have shown that a sibling of a celiac proband has an average recurrence risk of 10%, but this average has to be broken down according to the HLA DQ information on the proband. According to the HLA DQ of the proband the risk estimate for the sibling ranges from 2 to 14%. It is possible to provide better information to parents by performing their own HLA typing. In 30% of cases, the HLA parental typing will be sufficient to give an accurate estimate of their baby's risk. In other cases, for example when parents are H2H4 and H1H3, it may be advisable to genotype the baby after birth in order to precisely define his/her risk. Broadly, it is expected that approximately 40% of siblings of a celiac proband will have a negligible risk (<1%) of developing one form of the disease. Consequently about 40% of the families of a celiac proband will receive a very reassuring message by this procedure. Moreover, 30% of siblings are expected to have a risk of <10% and >1%, so it is possible for them to have a positive attitude about their recurrence risk.

Therefore, in one third of the families the risk of recurrence is high or very high (>20%). In these cases it is best is to share the information with the family in order to set up a plan to deal with this risk.

(1) Breastfeeding should be strongly supported [31], although it is well know that it does not prevent the diseases, but it affects only the phenotype by delaying the onset of symptoms [32].

(2) Gluten-containing foods should be introduced at weaning according to the usual practices adopted for infants from unaffected families, since there is no evidence that the time of gluten introduction may have any affect on the incidence of the disease. It is also desirable to unmask the disease as soon as possible and not delay to later ages when risk of complications increases [33]. It has been suggested that there is a 'window' of time for gluten introduction (4–6 months) when the child is 'protected' from developing the disease, but again this is likely to affect only the course of the disease [34]. Twin studies have indeed recently suggested that a non-familial environment has little or no effect on the onset of CD (see above) [10]. Gluten avoidance, which is environmental, may completely stop the pathogenesis of the disease, but this is not real life. Who, in our communities, will indeed accept spending a life on a gluten-free diet because of the genetic risk of developing the disease at the present estimates (never higher than 30%)?

(3) The easy availability of an anti-transglutaminase antibody test gives the possibility of anticipating the onset of the disease by measuring the antibody titer much in advance of clinical symptoms [35]. A secondary prevention may be put in place for subjects with a significant risk estimate: the vast majority of infants who will eventually develop the disease might be diagnosed before the disease becomes clinically manifest.

In conclusion for these infants at high risk of recurrence in celiac families, the doctors should encourage breastfeeding, ordinary weaning with gluten and an accurate follow-up after gluten introduction. A great amount of suffering, anxiety and the use of healthcare resources would really be prevented.

Given this solid base of risk estimation provided by HLA genotyping, it will be possible to improve the risk estimate by adding other genetic information. Currently, other susceptibility genes for CD have been suggested either by linkage or by association studies [3–5], but this information cannot be used in the risk estimation until susceptibility variants have been clearly identified. Our hope is that some of the predisposing variants will soon be identified: a multivariate combination of this information will then really improve the risk estimate, although it is possible that the information will not immediately provide better estimates because of the complexity of the genetic contribution of each locus.

References

1 Tommasini A, Not T, Kiren V, Baldas V, Santon D, Trevisiol C, Berti I, Neri E, Gerarduzzi T, Bruno I, Lenhardt A, Zamuner E, Spano A, Crovella S, Martellossi S, Torre G, Sblattero D, Marzari R, Bradbury A, Tamburlini G, Ventura A: Mass screening for coeliac disease using antihuman transglutaminase antibody assay. Arch Dis Child 2004;89:512–515.

2 Karell K, Louka AS, Moodie SJ, Ascher H, Clot F, Greco L, Ciclitira PJ, Sollid LM, Partanen J: HLA types in celiac disease patients not carrying the DQA1*05-DQB1*02 (DQ2) heterodimer: results from the european genetics cluster on celiac disease. Hum Immunol 2003;64:469–477.

3 Greco L, Babron MC, Corazza GR, Percopo S, Sica R, Clot F, Fulchignoni-Lataud MC, Zavattari P, Momigliano-Richiardi P, Casari G, Gasparini P, Tosi R, Mantovani V, De Virgiliis S, Iacono G, D'Alfonso A, Selinger-Leneman H, Lemainque A, Serre JL, Clerget-Darpoux F: Existence of a genetic risk factor on chromosome 5q in Italian coeliac disease families. Ann Hum Genet 2001;65:35–41.

4 Holopainen P, Naluai AT, Moodie S, Percopo S, Coto I, Clot F, Ascher H, Sollid L, Ciclitira P, Greco L, Clerget-Darpoux F, Partanen J; Members of the European Genetics Cluster on Coeliac Disease: Candidate gene region 2q33 in European families with coeliac disease. Tissue Antigens 2004;63:212–222.

5 Van Belzen MJ, Meijer JW, Sandkuijl LA, et al: A major non-HLA locus in celiac disease maps to chromosome 19. Gastroenterology 2003;125:1032–1041.

6 Neale MC, Cardon LR: Methodology for Genetic Studies of Twins and Families. Dordrecht, Kluwer Academic, 1992.

7 Boomsma D, Busjahn A, Peltonen L: Classical twin studies and beyond. Nat Rev Genet 2002;3:872–882.

8 Stazi MA, Cotichini R, Patriarca V, Brescianini S, Fagnani C, D'Ippolito C, Cannoni S, Ristori G, Salvetti M: The Italian Twin Project: from the personal identification number to a national twin registry. Twin Res 2002;5:382–386.

9 Greco L, Romino R, Coto I, Di Cosmo N, Percopo S, Maglio M, Paparo F, Gasperi V, Limongelli MG, Cotichini R, D'Agate C, Tinto N, Sacchetti L, Tosi R, Stazi MA: The first large population based twin study of coeliac disease. Gut 2002;50:624–628.
10 Nisticò L, Fagnani C, Coto I, et al: Concordance, disease progression, and heritability of coeliac disease in Italian twins. Gut 2006;55:803–808.
11 Witte JS, Carlin JB, Hopper JL: Likelihood-based approach to estimating twin concordance for dichotomous traits. Genet Epidemiol 1999;16:290–304.
12 Margaritte-Jeannin P, Babron MC, Bourgey M, et al: HLA-DQ relative risks for coeliac disease in European population: a study of the European Genetic Cluster on Coeliac Disease. Tissue Antigens 2004;63:562–567.
13 Polanco I, Mearin ML, Larrauri J, Biemond I, Wipkink-Bakker A, Pena AS: Effect of gluten supplementation in healthy siblings of children with celiac disease. Gastroenterology 1987;92: 678–681.
14 Anstey A, Wilkinson JD, Walshe MM: Dermatitis herpetiformis in monozygous twins – concordance for dermatitis herpetiformis and gluten-sensitive enteropathy. Clin Exp Dermatol 1991;16: 51–52.
15 Hervonen K, Karell K, Holopainen P, Collin P, Partanen J, Reunala T: Concordance of dermatitis herpetiformis and celiac disease in monozygous twins. J Invest Dermatol 2000;115: 990–993.
16 Holtmeier W, Rowell DL, Nyberg A, Kagnoff MF. Distinct delta T cell receptor repertoires in monozygotic twins concordant for coeliac disease. Clin Exp Immunol 1997;107:148–157.
17 Dubé C, Rostom A, Sy R, Cranney A, Saloojee N, Garritty C, Sampson M, Zhang L, Yazdi F, Mamaladze V, Pan I, Macneil J, Mack D, Patel D, Moher D: The prevalence of celiac disease in average-risk and at-risk Western European populations: a systematic review. Gastroenterology 2005;128:S57–S67.
18 Fraga MF, Ballestar E, Paz MF, Ropero S, Setien F, Ballestar ML, Heine-Suner D, Cigudosa JC, Urioste M, Benitez J, Boix-Chornet M, Sanchez-Aguilera A, Ling C, Carlsson E, Poulsen P, Vaag A, Stephan Z, Spector TD, Wu YZ, Plass C Carlsson E, Poulsen P, Vaag A, Stephan Z, Spector TD, Wu YZ, Plass C, Esteller M., Esteller M: Epigenetic differences arise during the lifetime of monozygotic twins. Proc Natl Acad Sci USA 2005;102: 10604–10609.
19 Högberg L, Fälth-Magnusson K, Grodzinsky E, Stenhammar L: Familial prevalence of coeliac disease: a twenty-year follow-up study. Scand J Gastroenterol 2003;38:61–65.
20 Book L, Zone JJ, Neuhausen SL: Prevalence of celiac disease among relatives of sib pairs with celiac disease in US families. Am J Gastroenterol 2003;98: 377–381.
21 Hyttinen V, Kaprio J, Kinnunen L, Koskenvuo M, Tuomilehto J: Genetic liability of type 1 diabetes and the onset age among 22,650 young Finnish twin pairs: a nationwide follow-up study. Diabetes 2003;52:1052–1055.
22 Brix TH, Kyvik KO, Christensen K, Hegedüs L: Evidence for a major role of heredity in Graves' disease: a population-based study of two Danish twin cohorts. J Clin Endocrinol Metab 2001; 86:930–934.
23 Duffy DL, Spelman LS, Martin NG: Psoriasis in Australian twins. J Am Acad Dermatol 1993;29:428–434.
24 Barera G, Bonfanti R, Viscardi M, Bazzigaluppi E, Calori G, Meschi F, Bianchi C, Chiumello G: Occurrence of celiac disease after onset of type 1 diabetes: a 6-year prospective longitudinal study. Pediatrics 2002;109:833–838.
25 Ch'ng CL, Biswas M, Benton A, Jones MK, Kingham JG: Prospective screening for coeliac disease in patients with Graves' hyperthyroidism using anti-gliadin and tissue transglutaminase antibodies. Clin Endocrinol (Oxf) 2005; 62:303–306.
26 Ojetti V, Aguilar Sanchez J, Guerriero C, Fossati B, Capizzi R, De Simone C, Migneco A, Amerio P, Gasbarrini G, Gasbarrini A: High prevalence of celiac disease in psoriasis. Am J Gastroenterol 2003;98:2574–2575.
27 Houlston RS, Ford D: Genetics of coeliac disease. Q J Med 1996;89:737–743.
28 Farrè C, Humbert P, Vilar P, et al: Serological markers and HLA-DQ2 haplotype among first-degree relatives of coeliac patient. Dig Dis Sci 1999;44: 2344–2349.
29 Korponay-Szabo I, Kovacs J, Lorincz M, et al: Families with multiple cases of gluten-sensitive enteropathy. Z Gastroenterol 1998;36:553–558.
30 Gudjonsdottir AH, Nilsson S, Ek J, Kristiansson B, Ascher H: The risk of celiac disease in 107 families with at least two affected siblings. J Pediatr Gastroenterol Nutr 2004;38:338–342.
31 Ivarsson A, Hernell O, Stenlund H, Persson A: Breast-feeding protects against coeliac disease. Am J Clin Nutr 2002;75:914–921.
32 Greco L, Auricchio S, Mayer M, Grimaldi M: Case control study on nutritional risk factors in coeliac disease. J Pediat Gastroenterol Nutr 1988;7: 395–399.
33 Ventura A, Magazu G, Gerarduzzi T, Greco L: Coeliac disease and the risk of autoimmune disorders. Gut 2002;51: 897; author reply 897–898.
34 Norris JM, Barriga K, Hoffenberg EJ, et al: Risk of coeliac disease autoimmunity and timing of gluten introduction in the diet of infants at increased risk of disease. JAMA 2005;293: 2310–2312.
35 Korponay-Szabo I R, Raivio T, Laurila K, et al: Coeliac disease case finding and diet monitoring by point-of-care testing. Aliment Pharmacol Ther 2005; 22:729–737.

Prof. Luigi Greco
Department of Pediatrics and European Laboratory for the Investigation of Food-Induced Diseases
University of Naples Federico II, Via Pansini 5
IT–80131 Naples (Italy)
Tel. +39 081 746 3275, Fax +39 081 546 9811, E-Mail ydongre@unina.it

Fasano A, Troncone R, Branski D (eds): Frontiers in Celiac Disease.
Pediatr Adolesc Med. Basel, Karger, 2008, vol 12, pp 57–65

Biochemistry and Biological Properties of Gliadin Peptides

M.V. Barone · S. Auricchio

Pediatric Department and European Laboratory for the Investigation of Food-Induced Diseases, University of Naples Federico II, Naples, Italy

Abstract

Gliadins, a family of wheat proteins, are central to the pathogenesis of celiac disease (CD). In addition to 'immunogenic' effects, gliadin directly affects cultured cells and intestine preparations, and produces damage in vivo via a separate 'toxic' peptide P31–43. We have shown that peptide P31–43, and the crude gliadin digest (PTG), fully reproduce the effects of epidermal growth factor (EGF) on actin cytoskeleton and cell cycle, through direct activation of the EGF pathway. Consistent effects may be observed in mucosa from CD patients. Based on these observations a new model can be proposed in which some of the gliadin 'toxic' effects may be explained by delayed receptor inactivation with consequent enhancement of the effects of trace amounts of EGF and, possibly, other growth factors, a novel prospective that may help to understand the pathogenesis of mucosal damage in CD.

Celiac disease (CD) is a permanent intolerance to cereal proteins characterized by chronic intestinal inflammation induced by the ingestion of dietary wheat gliadin and related prolamines from barley and rye. The disease occurs in genetically predisposed individuals: only HLA-DQ2- and/or DQ8-positive subjects are affected (or subjects carrying genes coding for at least one of the two DQ2 heterodimer molecules) [1]. Nonetheless, the inheritance is multifactorial; several other polymorphisms are likely to be involved, probably located in genomic areas identified by whole genome screening studies [2]. Altogether, these different polymorphisms are responsible for the genetic susceptibility to CD. Toxic prolamines have, among dietary proteins, a very peculiar structure. The proteins responsible for CD are characterized by a high percentage of proline (approximately 20%) and glutamine (approximately 38%) residues. Oat prolamines, which are likely to be tolerated by CD patients, have only 10% of proline residues. Several features of toxic prolamines are relevant to the pathogenesis of CD. In particular: (a) their low digestibility; (b) the presence of epitopes for intestinal T cells (α-gliadin 56–68 is a prototype), as well as their modification by tissue transglutaminase (TG2) and the resulting higher affinity to HLA molecules; (c) the presence of biologically active sequences not recognized by T cells (α-gliadin 31–43 is a prototype); (d) their ability to activate innate immunity, and (e) their ability to interfere with cellular growth, potentiating the activity of tyrosine kinase receptors.

Gliadin Biologically Active Sequences Not Recognized by T Cells

Although there is strong evidence in favor of a mucosal Th1 response to gliadin peptides in CD, it is also likely that other non-T-cell-mediated phenomena, related to physic/chemical properties of other gliadin peptides, play a role in the pathogenesis of the celiac lesion. During the last decades many biological activities have been associated with gliadin peptides in several cell types: agglutination of K562S cells [3]; interference with the differentiation of the in vitro developing fetal rat intestine [4]; increase in nitric oxide and γ-interferon-dependent cytokine production by mouse peritoneal macrophages [5]; maturation of bone marrow-derived dendritic cells [6], and reorganization of actin and increase in permeability in the intestinal epithelium [7–9]. Other effects have been specifically seen in celiac tissues. In untreated celiac patients P31–43 has been found to be able to prevent the restitution of enterocyte height which, in mucosal explants, normally occurs in 24–48 h of culture with medium alone [10]. The toxicity of P31–43 has been demonstrated both in vitro in organ culture of treated celiac biopsies [11] and in in vivo feeding studies [12]. Similar results have been obtained in vivo on small intestinal and oral mucosa with the α-gliadin peptide 31–49 [13, 14].

Until very recently, there was no molecular basis for understanding the biological effects of α-gliadin peptide 31–43. But two series of observations have renewed the interest for such biological effects: (1) an innate response to 31–43 (and other gliadin peptides) that seems to precede activation of pathogenic T cells, and (2) non-T-cell-mediated effect of gliadin peptide P31–43 that is able to interfere with the activity of epidermal growth factor (EGF) through modifications of the kinetics of its receptor (EGFR) trafficking.

Non-T-Cell-Mediated Properties of Gliadin Peptides

We have shown that gliadin peptides induce actin rearrangements and cell proliferation in a wide range of cell types, mimicking the effect of EGF [9]. The EGF pathway was in fact enhanced by gliadin; this phenomenon being due to delayed inactivation of EGF receptor. The effect was also present in a more complex system represented by the cultured small intestinal mucosa from patients with untreated CD. These observations add a new biological function to gliadin peptides in addition to their ability to activate the innate and adaptive immune response, which, in any case, is related to the role these proteins play in the remodeling of the celiac mucosa.

Gliadin Peptides Induce Rapid Actin Rearrangements

The ability of the peptic-tryptic digest of gliadin (PTG) and P31–43 to induce actin rearrangements in epithelial cell lines of intestinal origin [8] has been confirmed [9]. Moreover we have shown that also in other cell lines gliadin peptides can induce actin modifications. Both PTG and P31–43 can affect cells from a variety of different origins such as MCF7 cells, an epithelial cell line from a human mammary carcinoma and mouse skin fibroblasts NIH3T3(Cl7) (fig. 1). They act very rapidly (10–15 min) and produce similar morphological changes in the cell, leading to highly characteristic membrane ruffling. The effect was strongly reminiscent of that induced by growth factors. Of the several growth factors tested, only EGF was able to mimic the effects of gliadin peptides on the cell lines tested. The involvement of EGF was consistent with the high expression of EGFR and the EGF production in these cell lines [15]. Gliadin-induced actin modifications can be prevented by EGFR on all cell lines tested [9].

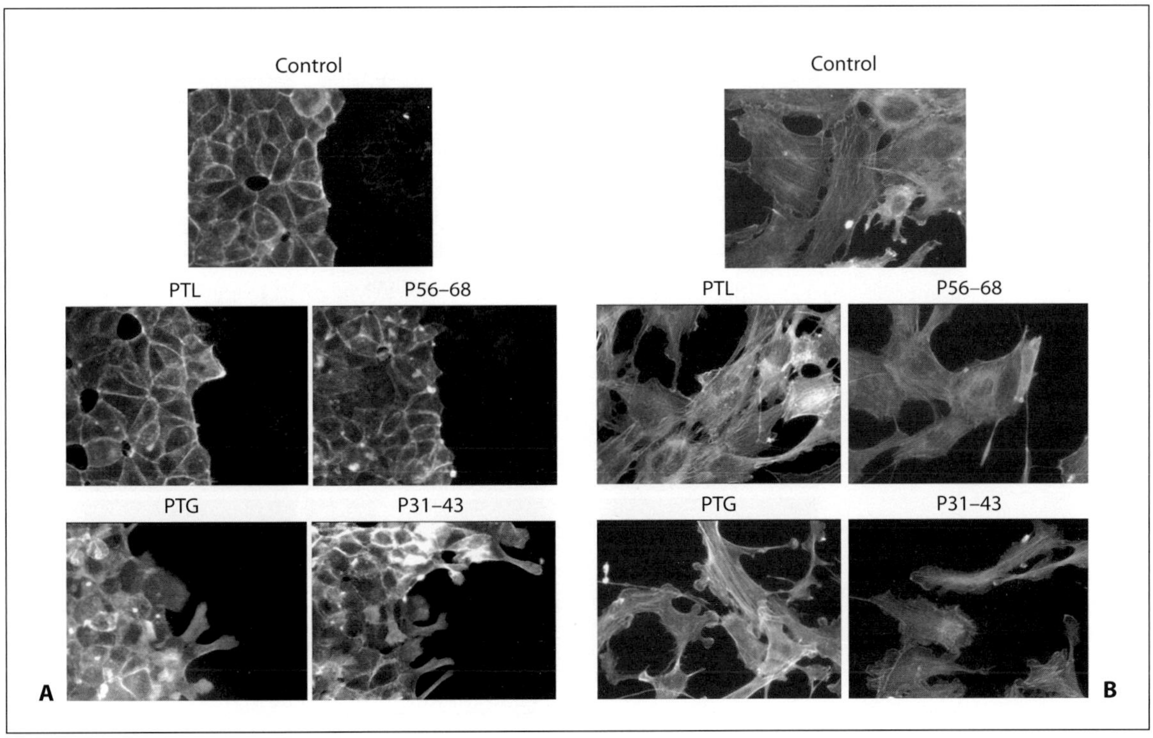

Fig. 1. PTG and P31–43 effects on actin rearrangement. Phalloidin staining of MCF7 (**A**) and NIH3T3 (**B**) cells 15 min after addition of PTG, PTL, P31–43, P56–68 as indicated.

Gliadin Peptides Exert EGF-Like Effects on G0→S Cell-Cycle Transition

Like EGF, PTG and P31–43 induced G0→S transition in resting NIH3T3 (Cl7) [16] cells measured as bromodeoxyuridine (BrdU) incorporation, confirming the hypothesis that gliadin peptides share other effects of EGF in addition to cytoskeletal modifications. The direct involvement of the EGFR pathway was proven by the ability of inhibitors such as PP2 (fig. 3), ZD1832 and anti-EGFR blocking antibody [9] to prevent the effects of gliadin peptides. In parallel, the peptides induced phosphorylation of the EGFR and the downstream effector signaling molecule Erk, indicating activation of the EGFR pathway [9].

Gliadin Peptides Interfere with EGFR Endocytosis

PTG and P31–43 are not known to bind EGFR, and similarity in the genomic data bank with the EGF sequence or any other growth factor was not found, suggesting that they do not act as direct ligands for the EGFR. Moreover, suboptimal concentrations of P31–43 and EGF showed a clear synergistic effect on S phase entry, rather than the additive effect that would be expected if they interacted with the same receptor [9]. Growth factor receptor activity can be regulated by ligand binding, and also by interference with degradation of activated receptors [17]. Endocytosis and receptor inactivation were indeed delayed in PTG- and P31–43-treated cells, with activated EGFR still

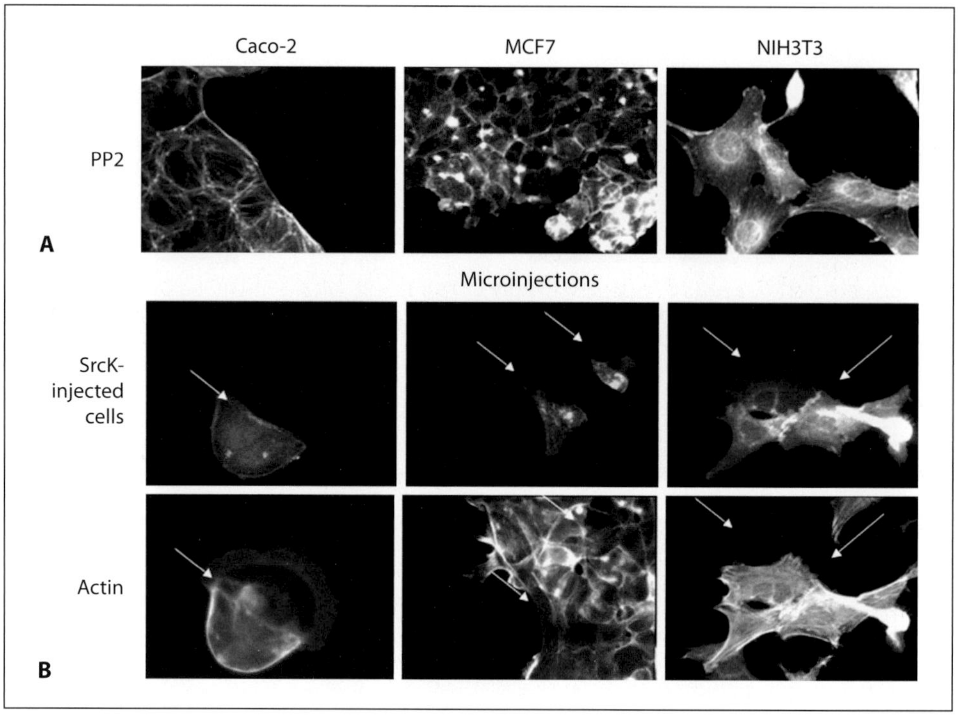

Fig. 2. Src activation is needed for PTG-induced actin rearrangement. **A** Phalloidin staining of Caco-2, MCF7 and NIH3T3 cells after 10 min pretreatment with PP2, followed by PTG addition for 15 min. Gliadin-induced actin modifications are completely prevented by PP2 treatment. **B** SrcK-microinjected Caco-2, MCF7 and NIH3T3 cells treated with gliadin peptides and stained with anti-Src antibody (aCST1) followed by secondary anti-rabbit-FITC (upper panel) and phalloidin/Texas-red (lower panel). Arrows indicate the injected cells which do not alter their actin staining after gliadin peptide treatment.

being present in Caco-2 cells 90 min after temperature shift, a time point when inactivation was complete in untreated cells [9]. Moreover, gliadin peptides interfere with the trafficking of vesicles carrying EGF-Alexa [9]. Although little is known about the viability of gliadin peptides, there are indications that they enter the enterocytes [18–20]. Mounted in Ussing chambers, biopsy specimens from untreated celiac patients allow transcellular transport of peptide 31–43 [18]. Furthermore data from our and other laboratories suggest that gliadin peptides enter the cells and interact with the vesicular compartment [19, 20] (manuscript in preparation).

Effects of Gliadin Peptides in Intestinal Biopsies from CD Patients

EGF Delay in Endocytic Vesicles

A delay of EGF in the early endocytic vesicles can be observed by labeling EGF with fluorochromes, such as Alexa-488. Pulse-chase experiments performed with Alexa-488-labelled EGF in mucosa from untreated patients in the active phase of the disease have shown a delayed trafficking of the EGF-carrying vesicles in epithelial cells after treatment with PTG and P31–43 [9], both in the epithelial cells of the crypts and the villi. Suggesting that gliadin peptide interference with

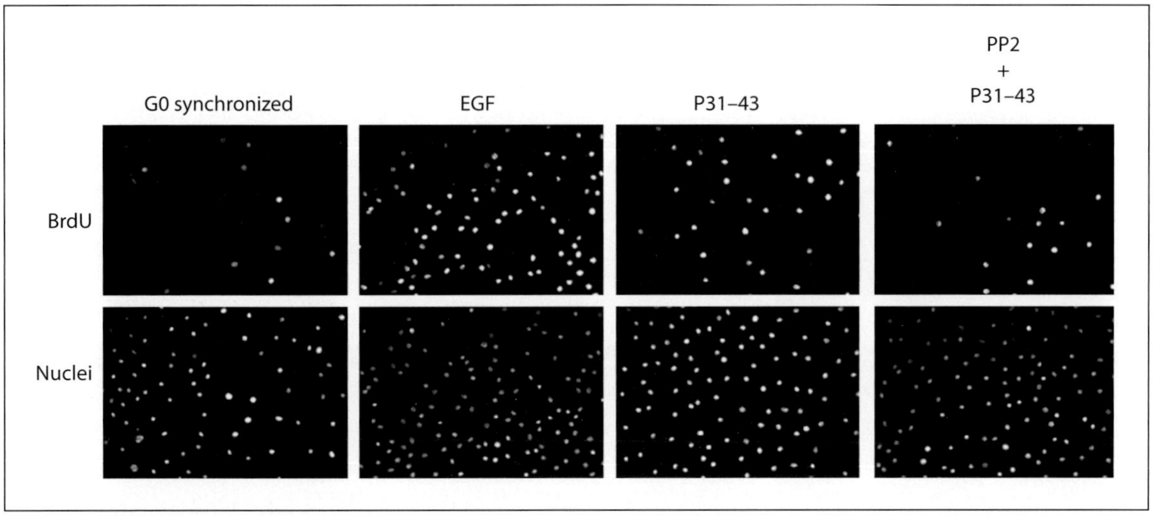

Fig. 3. Gliadin peptides can mimic full EGF-like effects on cell proliferation. Nuclei incorporating BrdU (upper panel) and total nuclei stained with Hoechst (lower panel). P31–43 can increase BrdU incorporation of G0 synchronized NIH3T3. Src inhibitor PP2 can prevent P31–43-induced proliferation. BrdU incorporation was calculated as the percentage of BrdU incorporating nuclei respective to total nuclei. BrdU incorporation of synchronized NIH3T3 was 5 ± 4% (mean ± standard deviation), with gliadin peptides 38 ± 6%, with gliadin peptides together with blocking anti-EGFR (528) 6 ± 5%.

EGF trafficking can be described, not only in isolated cells, but also in the intestines of CD patients.

Morphology and Cytoskeletal Changes in Epithelial Cells

Following gliadin challenge, the observation of EGF-Alexa-488 delay in biopsies from CD patients raises the possibility that some typical alterations in CD atrophic mucosa, such as villous atrophy and an increase in cryptic proliferation, can be ascribed to increased EGFR activity. Gliadin peptides, such as PTG and P31–43, induce changes in the length and shape of enterocytes, with shorter and disorganized cells; in contrast biopsies kept in medium without the addition of gliadin peptides show longer, more organized, enterocytes (fig. 4A) [11]. Similarly cytoskeletal rearrangements in enterocytes treated with gliadin peptides PTG and P31–43 produce a deeply disorganized picture with the appearance of several circular formations at the lateral side of the enterocytes, unlike in biopsies kept in medium alone in which these alterations are clearly reduced or absent (fig. 4B) [21]. Both morphological and cytoskeletal modifications can be prevented by adding EGFR inhibitors as shown in figure 4B.

Induction of Proliferation in Crypt Epithelial Cells

Proliferation of the cryptic compartment in mucosa from untreated CD patients is a diagnostic landmark. In biopsies from these patients, cultured in the absence of gliadin, BrdU incorporation is detectable in about 15% of epithelial cells; addition of gliadin peptides PTG or P31–43 raises this to 43%, a rate typical of an actively growing population. Treatment with EGFR inhibitors prevents the BrdU increase induced by gliadin peptides: BrdU incorporation is kept to 12% [9]. Peptides PTL and P56–68, used as a control, have no effect on any of the previously described assays [9] (fig. 4C).

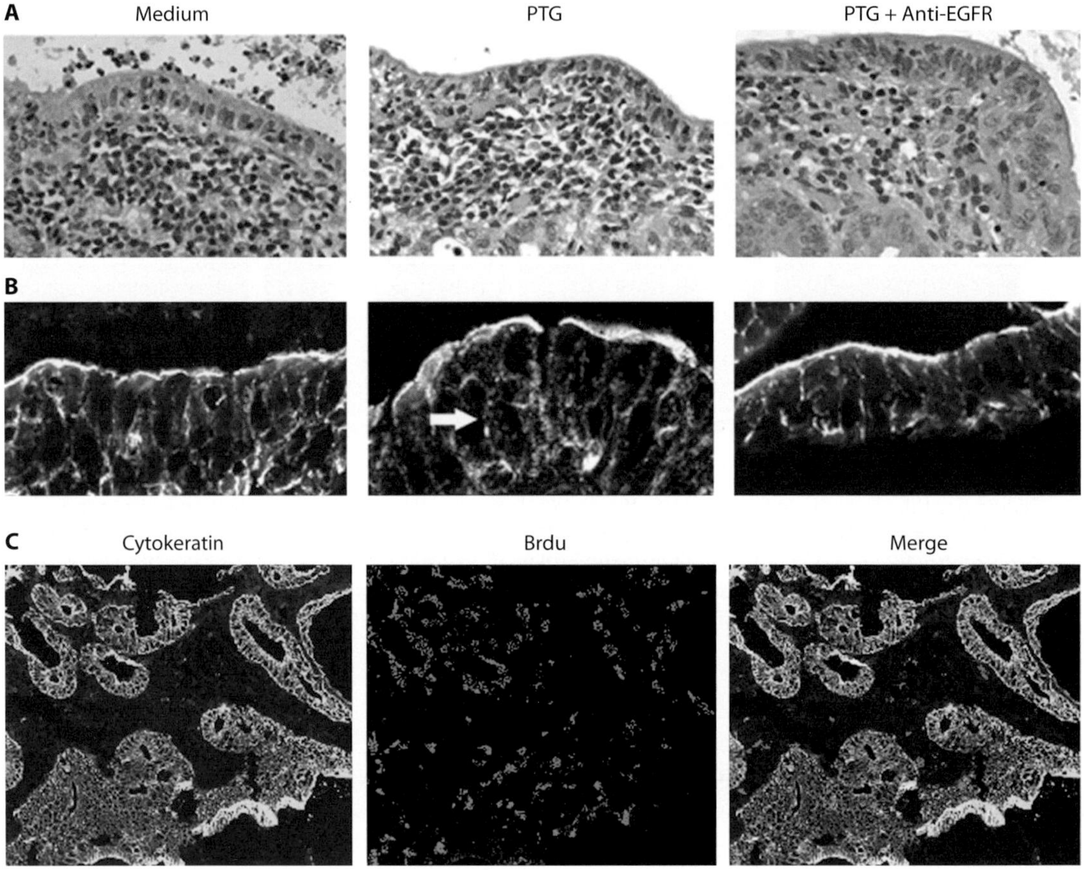

Fig. 4. EGFR inhibitor anti-EGFR528 prevents gliadin-induced morphology alteration and induction of S-phase entry in cultured biopsies from CD patients. **A** Ematossilin eosin staining of cultured biopsies from CD patients before a gluten-free diet. Lengths of 20 enterocytes were measured from at least 5 biopsies. Mean ± standard deviation was calculated: medium alone 23 ± 2 μm; gliadin peptides 18 ± 2.6 μm, and gliadin peptides together with blocking anti-EGFR (528) 22 ± 2.7 μm. **B** Confocal images of phalloidin staining of enterocytes from biopsies in culture. White arrow indicates circular actin formation at the periphery of the enterocyte in the presence of gliadin peptides. **C** Representative field of a biopsy from a CD patient before a gluten-free diet cultivated in the presence of P31–43. Cytokeratin staining to highlight epithelial cells and BrdU staining; merge is the overlay of these two panels. The percentage of BrdU-incorporating cells was calculated from at least 10 biopsies from CD patients. BrdU incorporation of enterocytes (cytokeratin positive) from biopsies cultivated with medium alone was 8 ± 6%, with gliadin peptides 43 ± 5%, with gliadin peptides together with blocking anti-EGFR (528) 12 ± 5%.

Conclusion

The evidence provided here is the first attempt to explain the molecular mechanism of these early direct effects of gliadin on actin cytoskeleton and cell cycle, and to link the activity of P31–43 to the activation of the EGF pathway. Delayed degradation of activated EGFR, caused by inhibition of the endocytotic trafficking of the EGF and possibly other growth factors, can explain the results.

P31–43, causing delayed maturation of early endosomes into late endosomes, might be responsible of multiple metabolic effects very likely depending on the kind of receptors present in the cells. In cells carrying EGFR the persistence of its activated state may have different consequences in different cell types, as it influences several pathways and different functions (cell reproduction and survival, permeability, motility, endocytosis, etc.) [22, 23]. It is likely that it also has consequences on the innate immune response and cytokine metabolism. In the human skin sterile wounding initiates an innate immune response that increases defensins and resistance to infection with a mechanism that needs activation of the EGFR [24]. Moreover growth signals induced by EGF are shared by IL-15 and other cytokine signal transduction pathways [25], and cooperation between tyrosine kinases and cytokines has already been described [26].

EGF pathway activation provides an opportunity to explain aspects of the pathogenesis of CD, related to the development of early mucosal damage, to the maintenance of an altered mucosal state, and to some complications.

Activation of the EGF pathway can induce a broad range of downstream effects from changes in cell morphology and cytoskeleton to activation of early responsive genes such as c-myc and c-fos and finally cell proliferation. Compatible with the EGF pathway activation, some known early effects of gliadin treatment can be observed in intestinal mucosa from CD patients: alteration of the villous architecture, disorganization of the inter-microvillus pit region [27], cytoskeletal modification [28] and an increase in the early responsive gene c-myc [29]. Electron microscopy observation of intestinal mucosa from CD patients in remission shows an increase in lysosome-like bodies in the apical cytoplasm of the luminal enterocytes 2.5 h after gliadin treatment [27], confirming a role for gliadin in the delay of endocytosis.

The same mechanism could explain the remodeling of gut mucosa in CD patients during the florid stage of the disease. Mucosal atrophy in CD is not due to reduced epithelial cell production, but is rather associated with increased cell proliferation in the crypts mediated by the presence of growth factors [30] generally ascribed to an immune response [8]. Our results introduce an alternative interpretation: EGFR, and possibly other receptors, is physiologically present in the crypts [31] showing a basal level of activation required for normal turnover and wound healing of the intestinal mucosa; in this scenario, delayed EGFR endocytosis, induced by the presence of gliadin, would be directly responsible for cell proliferation. A T-cell-mediated immune response would play a major role later in the stabilization and development of CD lesions.

Gliadin-induced activation of the EGF pathway could also be expected to result in other effects. One of the most dangerous complications of CD in adults is an increased risk of tumor insurgence such as lymphomas, oropharyngeal, esophageal and small intestine carcinomas; the risk is reduced by a strict gluten-free diet [32, 33], thus indicating that the gliadin-induced proliferative behavior could be related to tumor development, especially in a strongly responsive background such as in CD patients. Should such risk also apply to normal individuals? Gliadin, although incapable of producing CD in non-genetically predisposed individuals, is nonetheless able to show effects in healthy individuals: adult mice [34] fed a gluten-rich diet show proliferating crypts as do newborn mice. In addition, higher levels of EGFR have been demonstrated [35] in human volunteers with intestinal atrophic lesions produced in vivo after high dietary gluten uptake [36, 37]. However high levels of gluten were used in these cases and the newborn mice were fed gluten at a life stage in which only milk is physiologically given. Much lower levels are required in predisposed individuals to produce CD; genetic factors are probably responsible for the higher sensitivity to gliadin and its effects shown by CD patients.

Clearly gliadin is largely tolerated as demonstrated by the low incidence of these tumors in the general population. On the other hand, it is not inconceivable that, given the right circumstances such as a genetic predisposition or other environmental factors, gliadin could play a role in tumor development also in subjects not suffering from CD. Of course detailed study of the relationship between genetic background, gliadin intake, gliadin sensitivity and mucosal damage will be required to further clarify these points and gain a full understanding of the subject.

References

1 Karel K, Louka AS, Moodie SJ, Hascher H, Clot F, Greco L, Ciclitira PJ, Sollid LM, Partanen J: European Genetics Cluster on Celiac Disease: HLA types in celiac disease patients not carrying the DQA1*05-DQB1*02 (DQ2) heterodimer: results from the European Genetics Cluster on Celiac Disease. Hum Immunol 2003;64:469–477.

2 Babron MC, Nilsson S, Adamovic S, Naluai AT, Wahlstrom J, Ascher H, Ciclitira PJ, Sollid LM, Partanen J, Greco L, Clerget-Darpoux F: European Genetics Cluster on Coeliac Disease: Meta and pooled analysis of European coeliac disease data. Eur J Hum Genet 2003;11:828–834.

3 Auricchio S, De Ritis G, De Vincenti M, Mancini E, Minetti M, Sapora O, Silano V: Agglutinating activity of gliadin-derived peptides from bread wheat: implications for coeliac disease pathogenesis. Biochem Biophys Res Commun 1984;121:428–433.

4 Auricchio S, De Ritis G, De Vincenti M, Occorsio P, Silano V: Effect of gliadin-derived peptides from bread and durum wheats on small intestine cultures from rat fetus and coeliac children. Pediatr Res 1982;16:1004–1010.

5 Tuckova L, Novotna J, Novak P, Flegelova Z Kveton T, Jelinkova L, et al: Activation of macrophages by gliadin fragments isolation and characterization of active peptide. J Leukoc Biol 2002; 71:625–631.

6 Nikulina M, Habich C, Flohè B, Scott F, Kolb H: Wheat gluten causes dendritic cell maturation and chemokine secretion J Immunol 2004;173:1925–1933.

7 Thomas KE, Sapone A, Fasano A, Vogel SN: Gliadin stimulation of murine macrophage inflammatory gene expression and intestinal permeability are MyD88-dependent: role of the innate immune response in celiac disease. J Immunol 2006;176: 2512–2521.

8 Clemente MG, De Virgiliis S, Kang JS, Macatagney R, Musu MP, Di Pierro MR, Drago S, Congia M, Fasano A: Early effects of gliadin on enterocyte intracellular signalling involved in intestinal barrier function. Gut 2003;52: 218–223.

9 Barone MV, Gimigliano A, Castoria G, Paolella G, Maurano F, Paparo F, Maria M, Nanayakkara M, Mineo A, Miele E, Troncone R, Auricchio S: Growth factor-like activity of gliadin, an alimentary protein: implications for coeliac disease. Gut 2007;56:480–488.

10 De Ritis G, Auricchio S, Jones HV, Lew EJ, Bemardin IE, Kasarda DD: In vitro (organ culture) studies of the toxicity of specific A-gliadin peptides in celiac disease. Gastroenterology 1988;94: 41–49.

11 Maturi L, Troncone R, Mayer M, Coletta S, Picarelli A, De Vincenti M, Pavone V, Auricchio S: In vitro activities of A-gliadin related synthetic peptides: damaging effect on the atrophic coeliac mucosa and activation of mucosal immune response in the treated coeliac mucosa. Scand J Gastroenterol 1996;31:247–253.

12 Marsh M, Morgan S, Ensary A, Wardle T, Lobley R, Milla C, et al: In vivo activation of peptide 31–43, 56–68 of alpha-gliadin in gluten sensitive enteropathy (GSE) (abstract 8). Gastroenterology 1995;108:71.

13 Ciclitira PJ, Ellis Hl: In vivo gluten ingestion in celiac disease. Dig Dis 1998;16:337–340.

14 Lahteenoja H, Maki M, Viander M, Raiha I, Villja P, Rantala I, et al: Local challenge on oral mucosa with an alpha-gliadin related synthetic peptide in patient with celiac disease. Am J Gastroenterol 2000;95:2880–2887.

15 Auricchio A, Di Domenico M, Castoria G, Bilancio A, Migliaccio A: Epidermal growth factor induces protein tyrosine phosphorylation and association of p190 with ras-GTP-ase activating protein in Caco-2 cells. FEBS Lett 1994; 353:16–20.

16 Barone MV, Courtneidge SA: Src is required for myc, but not fos induction in response to PDGF. Nature 1995;387: 509–512.

17 Burke P, Schooler K, Wiley HS: Regulation of epidermal growth factor receptor by endocytosis and intracellular trafficking. Mol Biol Cell 2001;12: 1897–1910.

18 Matysiak-Budnik T, Candalh C, Duvage C, et al: Alterations of the intestinal transport and processing of gliadin peptides in celiac disease. Gastroenterology 2003;125:696–707.

19 Zimmer KP, Naim H, Weber P, et al: Targeting of gliadin peptides, CD8, alpha/beta-TCR, and gamma/delta-TCR to Golgi complexes and vacuoles within celiac disease enterocytes. FASEB J 1998;12:1349–1357.

20 Friis S, Dabelsteen E, Sjostrom H, et al: Gliadin uptake in human enterocytes. Differences between coeliac patients in remission and control individuals. Gut 1992;33:1487–1492.

21 Wilson S, Volkov Y, Feighery C: Investigation of enterocyte microfilaments in celiac disease, P100. 11th Int Symp Coeliac Disease, Belfast, 2004.
22 Hackel PO, Zwick E, Prenzel N, Ullrich A: Epidermal growth factor receptors: critical mediators of multiple receptor pathways. Curr Opin Cell Biol 1999;11: 184–189.
23 Citri A, Yarden Y: EGF-ERBB signalling: towards the systems level. Nat Rev Mol Cell Biol 2006;7:505–516.
24 Sorensen OE, Thapa DR, Roupe KM, Valore EV, Sjobring U, Roberts AA, Schmidtchen A, Ganz T: Injury-induced innate immune response in human skin mediated by transactivation of the epidermal growth factor receptor. J Clin Invest 2006;116: 1878–1885.
25 Yano S, Komine M, Fujimoto M, et al: Interleukin 15 induces the signals of epidermal proliferation through ERK and PI 3-kinase in a human epidermal keratinocyte cell line, HaCaT. Biochem Biophys Res Commun 2003;301: 841–847.
26 Budagian V, Bulanova E, Orinska Z, Thon L, Mamat U, Bellosta P, Basilico C, Adam D, Paus R, Bulfone-Paus S: A promiscuous liaison between IL-15 receptor and Axl receptor tyrosine kinase in cell death control. EMBO J 2005;24:4260–4270.
27 Bailey DS, Freedman AR, Price SC, Chescoe D, Ciclitira PJ: Early biochemical responses of the small intestine of celiac patients to wheat gluten. Gut 1989;1:78–85.
28 Holmgren Peterson K, Magnusson K-E, Stenhammar L, Falth-Magnusson K: Confocal laser scanning microscopy of small-intestinal mucosa in celiac disease. Scand J Gastoenterol 1995;30: 228–234.
29 Ciclitira PJ, Stewart J, Evan G, Wight DG, Sikora K: Expression of c-myc oncogene in celiac disease. J Clin Pathol 1987;3:307–311.
30 Salvati VM, Bajaj-Elliott M, Poulsom R, Mazzarella G, Lundin KE, Nilsen EM, Troncone R, MacDonald TT: Keratinocyte growth factor and celiac disease. Gut 2001;49:176–181.
31 Playford RJ, Hanby AM, Gschmeissner S, Peiffer LP, Wright NA, McGarrity T: The epidermal growth factor receptor (EGF-R) is present on the basolateral, but not the apical, surface of enterocytes in the human gastrointestinal tract. Gut 1996;39:262–266.
32 Holmes GK, Prior P, Lane MR, Pope D, Allan RN: Malignancy in celiac disease-effect of a gluten free diet. Gut 1989;30:333–338.
33 Collin P, Reunala T, Pukkala E, Laippala P, Keyrilainen O, Pasternack A: Celiac disease-associated disorders and survival. Gut 1994;35:1215–1218.
34 Troncone R, Caputo N, Zibella A, Molitierno G, Maiuri L, Auricchio S: Effects of gluten enriched diet on the small intestinal mucosa of normal mice and mice with graft versus host reaction. Gut 1994;35:779–782.
35 Stepankova R, Kofronova O, Tuckova L, Kozakova H, Cebra JJ, Tlaskalova-Hogenova H: Experimentally induced gluten enteropathy and protective effect of epidermal growth factor in artificially fed neonatal rats. J Pediatr Gastroentrol Nutr 2003;36:96–104.
36 Ferguson A, Blackwell J, Barneston R: Effects of additional dietary gluten on the small intestinal mucosa of volunteers and patients with dermatitis herpetiformis. Scand J Gastroenteol 1987;22:543–549.
37 Doherty M, Barry RE: Gluten-induced mucosal changes in subjects without overt small-bowel disease. Lancet 1981;1:517–520.

Prof. S. Auricchio
Pediatric Department and European Laboratory for the Investigation of Food-Induced Diseases, University of Naples Federico II
Via S. Pansini 5, IT–80131 Naples (Italy)
Tel. +39 081 746 3382, Fax +39 081 546 9811, E-Mail salauric@unina.it

Fasano A, Troncone R, Branski D (eds): Frontiers in Celiac Disease.
Pediatr Adolesc Med. Basel, Karger, 2008, vol 12, pp 66–81

Innate Immunity and Celiac Disease

Bertrand Meresse[a,b] · Georgia Malamut[a–c] · Shira Amar[a,b] · Nadine Cerf-Bensussan[a,b]

[a]INSERM, Unité 793; [b]Faculté de Médecine, Université Paris Descartes, et [c]Service de Gastroentérologie, AP-HP, Hôpital Européen Georges Pompidou, Paris, France

Abstract

Celiac disease (CD) is an inflammatory enteropathy induced by cereal-derived prolamines (gluten) in genetically predisposed individuals. Prolamines, due to their high proline content, are incompletely digested by enzymes in the intestinal lumen and brush border, resulting in the release of large peptides that can enter the mucosa and be toxic for the patients. There is now definitive evidence that the toxicity of gluten-derived peptides is largely due to their capacity to bind the peptide groove of HLA-DQ2 and DQ8, two related HLA molecules that confer the major genetic risk. Gluten peptides can thereby drive the activation of intestinal CD4+ T cells that induce intestinal damage. A second set of more recent data suggests the complementary contribution of innate immunity orchestrated by the proinflammatory cytokine IL-15. This cytokine drives the expansion of intraepithelial lymphocytes, arm the latter lymphocytes to direct an autoimmune attack against the epithelium, and promotes the onset of T lymphomas. Moreover, IL-15 can block the regulatory pathway of TGF-β and thereby unleash and perpetuate the activation of CD4+ T cells and intraepithelial lymphocytes. The role of gluten peptides and of other endogenous or exogenous factors in the abnormal upregulation of IL-15 is discussed.

A Role for Innate Immunity in Celiac Disease?

The immune system, built up progressively during evolution to fight pathogens, involves both innate and adaptive mechanisms. The innate system appeared very early, in primitive multicellular organisms, and has progressively gained in complexity to assume a dual function in mammals: a role of immediate barrier albeit with low specificity and no memory, and a second role of antigen-presentation to the adaptive immune system via major histocompatibility complex (MHC) molecules. The adaptive immune system emerged much later in vertebrates and relies on B and T lymphocytes to permit a delayed but highly specific response endowed with long-term memory. While the immune system has evolved to allow efficacious protection against pathogens of increasing sophistication, the counterpart has been the appearance of detrimental immune responses against self antigens or harmless antigens derived from the environment. Celiac disease (CD) is one example in which an environmental product, cereal derived-gluten, can induce an inappropriate immune reaction in genetically predisposed individuals and simultaneously promote immune reactivity against self antigens.

Since the discovery in the 1990s that MHC class II HLA-DQ2/8 molecules are the main genetic risk factor for CD [1], it has been convincingly established that adaptive immunity, orchestrated by CD4+ lamina propria T cells recognizing gluten-derived peptides specifically bound to HLA-DQ2/8 molecules, plays a central role in the intestinal inflammation characteristic of CD. Adaptive immunity provides an undisputable link between the two main genetic and environmental factors. The discovery that tissue transglutaminase 2 (TG2), the target of the autoantibodies, deamidated gliadin peptides in positions that promoted their binding to HLA-DQ2/8 further enhanced the role of adaptive immunity [for review see 2, 3]. Yet, it has become increasingly clear that a highly specific adaptive response against gluten is not sufficient to trigger intestinal inflammation. Thus, only a subset of individuals bearing the at risk HLA molecules develop CD. Furthermore, humanized mice expressing both HLA-DQ8 on their antigen-presenting cells and the human CD4 co-receptor on their T cells developed a specific CD4+ response against gluten but no intestinal inflammation [4]. Notably however, when crossed on a NOD–/– background, HLA-DQ8 transgenic mice presented a skin disease similar to herpetiformis dermatitis and autoantibodies against transglutaminase [5]. These results point to the necessity of complementary mechanisms, possibly inherited, to trigger site-specific inflammation in CD. On the one hand, susceptibility to intestinal inflammation may depend on the possession of specific alleles for genes regulating the adaptive immune response, such as CTLA-4 [6] or of genes encoding cytokines produced by CD4+ T cells such as IL-2 and IL-21 [7]. On the other hand, several studies point to the role of nonspecific mechanisms related to innate immunity. A first clue was provided by the analysis of the mechanisms underlying the massive increase in intraepithelial lymphocytes (IELs), a hallmark of CD. A second set of data relies on the study of gluten peptides that seem to be toxic for patients despite the fact that they are not recognized by lamina propria CD4+ T cells. This chapter summarizes evidence that IEL activation depends on innate immune mechanisms, and discusses the capacity of gliadin peptides to elicit innate immune responses, before considering how innate and adaptive immune responses may interact to promote intestinal inflammation in CD.

The Role of Innate Immunity in IEL Activation

No Direct Evidence Supports Specific Recognition of Gluten by IEL in CD

Ferguson and Murray [8] were the first to demonstrate in 1971 that a massive increase in IEL is a hallmark of CD. They observed that IEL infiltration was maximal in active CD but remained high in many patients on a gluten-free diet (GFD). The contribution of IELs to villous atrophy CD was more recently suggested by several studies showing that: (i) CD8+ IELs were the main producer of IFN-γ in active CD [9]; (ii) CD IELs were enriched in cytolytic proteins (perforin, granzymes, FasL [10–13], and (iii) expression of the latter proteins was associated with increased epithelial apoptosis [10, 11]. Simultaneously, demonstration that malignant T-cell lymphomas, a rare but most severe complication of CD, take their origin in the IEL compartment indicated that IEL homeostasis was severely compromised in CD [14, 15].

Contrasting with conclusive evidence that CD4+ lamina propria T cells from patients are specifically stimulated by gluten-derived peptides, there is no strong indication that IEL expansion and activation are driven by direct recognition of gluten. Phenotypic analysis indicates that both CD8+ TCR-$\alpha\beta$ IELs and TCR-$\gamma\delta$ IELs CD8 positive or negative are increased in active CD. After a GFD, the numbers of TCR-$\alpha\beta$ IELs return to control levels while TCR-$\gamma\delta$ IELs remained elevated in most patients [16, 17]. The latter finding, consistent with the lack of known specificity of human TCR-$\gamma\delta$ IELs, was the first indication that IEL expansion cannot be entirely driven by direct recognition of gluten. Class I-restricted cross-presentation of gliadin peptides to cytotoxic CD8+ TCR-αβ lymphocytes has been demonstrated in vitro [18]. Yet, gliadin-specific T cells derived from culture of CD intestinal biopsies were exclusively CD4+ T cells, pleading also against specific gluten recognition by CD8+ TCR-αβ IELs. In contrast, recent evidence suggests that activation of IELs may be largely driven by nonspecific mechanisms related to innate immunity that involves the interplay between NK receptors and the proinflammatory and anti-apoptotic cytokine IL-15.

Parallel Upregulation of IL-15 in Enterocytes and NK Receptors on IELs in Active CD (fig. 1)
Analysis of human control IELs indicates that a significant proportion of T-IELs co-express NK receptors, and more particularly members of the lectin-like family, including CD161 expressed on approximately 60% normal IELs, CD94 present on 30% normal IELs [19] and NKG2D expressed in humans by the majority of normal IELs [20] as well as by peripheral CD8+ TCR-αβ and TCR-γδ lymphocytes. Active CD is associated with a marked increase in the proportion of CD94+ IEL cells (approximately 75%), an increase that is more particularly obvious in CD8+ TCR-αβ IELs (as the ratio of TCR-αβ/TCR-γδ IELs increases in active CD) [19]. In vitro, T-cell receptor stimulation and IL-15 (but none of the other cytokines tested) rapidly induced CD94 surface expression on control IELs, providing the first suggestion that IL-15 might be upregulated in CD [19]. It was then observed that IL-15 can also increase the level of NKG2D expression on control IELs [20], and that CD8 TCR-αβ IELs express more NKG2D in active CD patients than in controls [21].

Consistent with a role of IL-15 in the upregulation of CD94 and NKG2D on IELs in active CD, expression of IL-15 was found to be markedly increased in lamina propria mononuclear cells and most strikingly in the epithelium of active CD patients compared to controls [19, 22]. Increased production of IL-15 by epithelial cells was demonstrated by immunochemistry and more recently by Western blot [23]. Very small amounts of IL-15 were however detected in supernatants of enterocytes from CD patients [23], a finding consistent with other reports [24, 25] and our own data suggesting that the majority of IL-15 remains bound to the surface of enterocytes where it can be presented to IELs [22].

Central Role of IL-15 in Alterations of the Epithelial Compartment in CD (fig. 1)
IL-15 is a cytokine structurally related to IL-2 that shares with the latter cytokine the β and γ chains of their trimeric receptors. However IL-15 differs strikingly from IL-2 by its wide distribution (it can be produced by many cell types) as well as by its in vivo effects, largely directed toward NK and CD8 T cells. Analysis of IL-15–/– mice indicates that IL-15 is mandatory for the development and maintenance of murine NK cells and CD8αα IELs, as well as for the persistence of memory CD8 T cells. IL-15 is also a strong inducer of cytotoxic functions of NK cells and CD8 T cells [for review see 26, 27]. The preferential effect of IL-15 on these cell types is generally ascribed to their elevated expression of the β chain of the receptor compared to other lymphocyte subsets. Indeed the β and γ chains form a signaling module on lymphocytes that bind IL-15 with an intermediate affinity (Ka 10^{-9} M^{-1}) [28]. The third chain, RIL-15α, is ubiquitous and can bind IL-15 alone with a very high affinity (Ka 10^{-11} M^{-1}). While the trimeric receptor may be necessary to promote the generation of high avidity cytotoxic T cells [29], most studies suggest that IL-15 signaling on T lymphocytes occurs mainly via the βγ module recognizing soluble IL-15 or more likely IL-15 bound to RIL-15α. Indeed, IL-15 forms stable complexes with RIL-15α on cell surfaces which protect IL-15 from rapid clearance, present IL-15 in trans to neighboring NK and T cells and cause sustained IL-15 signal transduction in target cells [30].

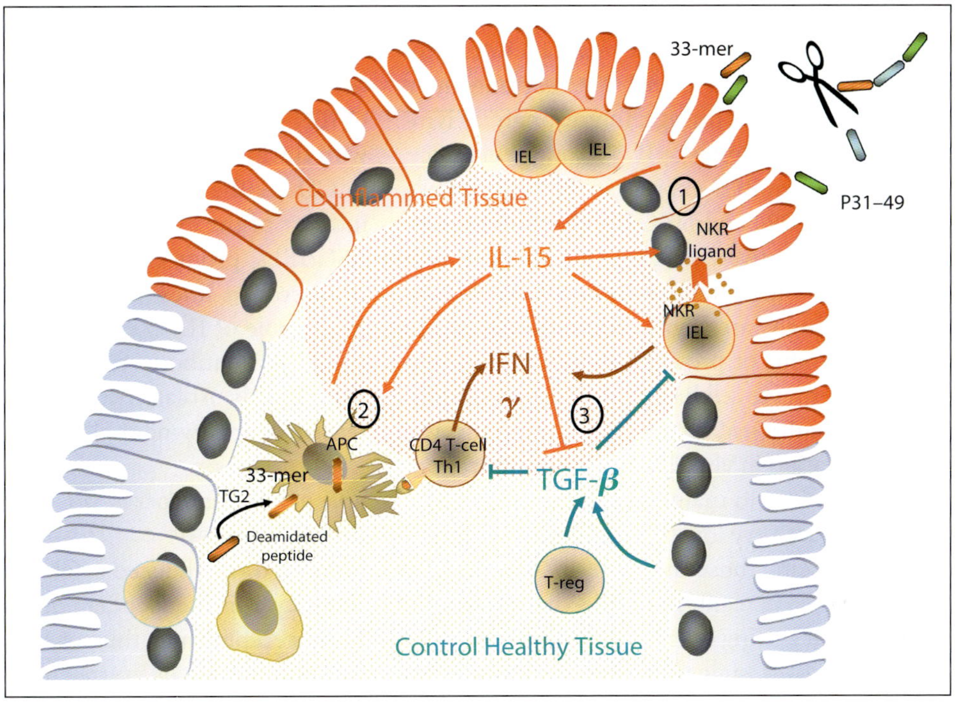

Fig. 1. The central role for IL-15 at the interface between innate and adaptive immunity in CD. IL-15 is synthesized both by epithelial cells and lamina propria mononuclear cells and can act on multiple targets. (1) In the epithelium, IL-15 has a direct action on IEL that promotes their survival and accumulation, stimulates their production of INF-γ and their cytotoxicity via innate immune NK receptors. IL-15 may also directly or indirectly promote the expression of epithelial ligands for these NK receptors. These combined effects of IL-15 result in an autoimmune attack of the epithelium and promote the emergence of lymphomas. (2) IL-15 can act directly on dendritic cells and stimulate their maturation and antigen presentation. This effect of IL-15 is thought to bolster the activation of gluten-specific CD4+ LPL [58]. (3) Finally, IL-15 can hamper local immunoregulation by blocking the Smad-3 pathway of TGF-β in both IEL and LPL. IL-15 can thus indirectly promote the release of Th1 cytokines and the cytotoxicity of intestinal lymphocytes.

The key contribution of IL-15 to the homeostasis NK and CD8 T cells is ascribed to its proliferative and potent anti-apoptotic effects, two properties that also explain the development of leukemias and lymphomas bearing CD8 and NK markers in transgenic mice overexpressing high levels of IL-15 [31]. Consistent with this in vivo observation in mice, in vitro experiments suggest that overexpression of IL-15 in CD plays a central role in the hyperplasia of IELs and the development of T lymphomas in CD. IL-15 is a potent inducer of the proliferation and survival of human IELs. This effect observed in normal IELs is even more conspicuous in the abnormal IELs that develop in patients with refractory clonal sprue (RCS) [22, 23]. RCS, now considered as a low grade intraepithelial T lymphoma, is a recurrent intermediary step between CD and high grade T-cell lymphoma [14, 32–34]. In RCS patients, the normal polyclonal (or oligoclonal) population of T IELs is progressively replaced by abnormal clonal IELs that retain a normal cytology and the

CD103 and CD7 markers but lack surface CD3-TCR complexes. However they contain intracytoplasmic CD3ε and a clonal Tγ rearrangement suggestive of a T-cell lineage. Interestingly, as lymphoma cells developing in IL-15 transgenic mice, clonal IELs from RCS express some NK markers, particularly CD94 and NKG2D, shared with normal T IELs in active CD [15, 35]. Moreover, RCS IELs express conspicuous levels of RIL-15 β chain and, accordingly, are highly responsive to IL-15 either exogenous or provided through co-culture with an enterocyte cell line, IL-15 being both necessary and sufficient to maintain their survival and proliferation in vitro [22]. The concentrations of IL-15 required to maintain the survival of RCS IEL in vitro are very low (0.1–0.2 ng/ml) and may correspond with those available in situ [23]. In fact, in situ, the percentage of IELs that are labeled by markers of cycling cells is very low in active CD as well as in RCS, suggesting that the main effect of IL-15 might be to prevent the normal elimination of activated IELs and to promote their accumulation [22]. IL-15-induced survival of RCS IELs that have initiated a malignant transformation (as attested by the presence of chromosomal abnormalities) may allow new transforming events and ultimately development of an aggressive lymphoma [36, 37]. Blocking IL-15 may thus be a therapeutic option in patients with RCS to prevent the evolution toward a high-grade T-cell lymphoma. Blockade of IL-15 might also inhibit epithelial lesions resulting from the cytotoxic attack of epithelium by RCS IELs.

Indeed, mice that overexpress IL-15 under the control of the gut epithelium-specific T3b promoter develop a severe small intestinal enteropathy associated with the accumulation of TCR-γδ and subsequently CD8+ TCR-αβ lymphocytes. Likely due to the use of a soluble version of IL-15 that can be efficiently secreted by epithelial cells, T-cell infiltration was most prominent in the lamina propria [38]. Yet this in vivo model provided the first convincing evidence that enterocyte-derived IL-15 can orchestrate epithelial lesions. In vitro data in IELs from controls, active CD and RCS patients indicate that IL-15 acts at several levels. First, IL-15 induces the production of IFN-γ by IELs [22, 23, 39], a finding consistent with the notion that the main producers of IFN-γ in CD are the IELs [9]. Second, IL-15 is a strong inducer of the cytotoxicity of normal T IELs and RSC IELs, promoting granzyme/perforin killing of enterocyte lines [22, 23]. Conforming with the in situ role of IL-15 in CD, adding a neutralizing anti-IL-15 antibody reduced the cytotoxicity of IELs freshly isolated from active CD and their release of granzyme B [23].

Role of NK Receptors in IEL Cytotoxicity in CD and RCS (fig. 1)

Notably, IL-15-induced cytotoxicity of IELs against enterocytes is independent of their expression of a T-cell receptor and thus of any specific recognition. Thus, it can be exerted by RCS IELs which do not express CD3-TCR complexes on their cell surface [22]. Subsequent studies demonstrated the implication of the NK receptors NKG2D and CD94. The role of NKG2D was demonstrated in active CD and in RCS [21, 35]. In both situations, expression of the ligand of NKG2D, MICA, a non-classical MHC class Ib, was markedly upregulated on epithelial cells and translocated on their surface. IELs from active CD killed cell lines that expressed MIC either spontaneously or after transfection [21]. Conversely, blockade of NKG2D and MICA with neutralizing antibodies prevented lysis of MIC+ enterocyte lines by RCS IELs [35]. A striking finding was that IL-15 could transform the co-signal given by NKG2D in unstimulated CD8+ TCR-αβ IELs into an autonomous signal (that bypassed the usual requirement for simultaneous T-cell receptor activation). The effect of IL-15 was ascribed to the upregulation of NKG2D and of DAP10, the adaptor molecule that recruits signaling molecules downstream NKG2D in T cells, as well as to the enhancement of the ERK pathway necessary for NKG2D-mediated cytotoxicity [21]. Moreover, adding IL-15 to intestinal organ cultures upregulated MICA expression in enterocytes [35], a finding consistent with the comparable inducing effect of IL-15 in human dendritic cells [40]. Altogether, these data suggest that, by simultaneously activating the NKG2D pathway in IELs and upregulating its ligand MICA on enterocytes, IL-15 can license an autoimmune attack on the epithelium by IELs in CD and RCS. The contribution of this mechanism to villous atrophy was recently demonstrated in vivo in a mouse model. Intraperitoneal injection of poly-IC, used to mimic stimulation of Toll receptor 3 by double-stranded RNA viruses, resulted in the rapid and transient induction of a small intestinal enteropathy associated with upregulation of IL-15 and Rae, the murine ligand of NKG2D in epithelial cells, and upregulation of NKG2D in IELs. Injection of antibodies neutralizing IL-15 or NKG2D markedly reduced the severity of the enteropathy [41]. Together with several reports indicating that IL-15 is induced by various intracellular pathogens, these data suggest that activation of the NKG2D/MIC or Rae pathway by IL-15 is a normal innate mechanism of defense of the epithelium that promotes the rapid elimination of infected cells. The rapid arrest of IL-15 synthesis after eviction of the pathogen avoids protracted epithelial damage. By contrast, in CD the chronic upregulation of IL-15 results in durable epithelial damage and chronic malabsorption.

NKG2D is not the only activating NK receptor able to promote T-cell receptor-independent cytotoxicity of IELs against enterocytes in CD. As mentioned above, CD94 is markedly upregulated in active CD. The function of CD94 as an NK receptor is dictated by its association with NKG2 molecules within heterodimers that can bind the same ligand, HLA-E, another non-classical MHC Ib molecule. CD94 can serve as an inhibitory receptor when associated with NKG2A, an adaptor molecule that recruits phosphatases via an ITIM motif present in its cytoplasmic tail. Upon binding to HLA-E, CD94/NKG2A delivers a negative signal that impairs the cytotoxicity of NK cells and negatively modulates T-cell receptor activation in memory CD8+ TCR-$\alpha\beta$ and TCR-$\gamma\delta$ lymphocytes. Notably, this heterodimer is expressed by the majority of CD94+ IELs in control intestines [19]. By contrast, the vast majority of CD94+ CD8+ TCR-$\alpha\beta$ IELs in CD do not express NKG2A, suggesting that this putative negative control imposed on IELs in the normal situation is removed in CD [19, 42]. On the contrary, in active CD, CD94 appears to associate on a substantial fraction of IELs (approximately 20%) with a distinct NKG2 isotype, NKG2C, that confers an activating function to the receptor [42]. Indeed NKG2C binds the adaptor molecule DAP12 which recruits a signaling cascade that promotes cell proliferation, IFN-γ secretion and cytotoxicity independent of any other signals. This signaling pathway is operative in CD94/NKG2C+ CD8+ TCR-$\alpha\beta$ IELs from active CD patients and can likely be triggered upon recognition of the ligand HLA-E, markedly upregulated on enterocytes in active CD and contribute to epithelial damage [42].

While the role of IL-15 in the induction of CD94 on IELs is established, the mechanism(s) that switch(es) off NKG2A expression and conversely induce(s) NKG2C are unclear. NKG2C is expressed at the surface of IELs in active CD but can be detected intracellularly in many IELs both in active CD and after GFD but not in controls, indicating persistent alterations of NKG2 regulation in CD. Study of the transcriptome of human NKG2C+ IEL clones showed significant upregulation of several genes belonging to the NK cluster on chromosome 19p13, suggesting that NK reprogramming might be a feature of CD8+ TCR-$\alpha\beta$ IELs in CD [42]. However recent reports in mice provide some hints concerning the mechanisms that may control expression of NK receptors in the intestine. Interestingly, NKG2A can be downmodulated by retinoic acid [43]. This derivative of vitamin A, electively produced by a subset of intestinal dendritic cells, plays an emerging key role in intestinal immune responses, controlling the homing of T and IgA cells, as well as the differentiation of regulatory T cells [for review see 44]. This additional effect of retinoic acid may be useful to promote the cytotoxic properties of IELs. Conversely, NKG2A is induced on CD8 T cells upon simultaneous stimulation by the T-cell receptor and TGF-β [45]. This cytokine is a potent inhibitor of lymphocyte activation and inflammation able in particular to re-control lymphocyte proliferation and survival, IFN-γ production and T-cell cytotoxicity [46]. Upregulation of NKG2A that possesses in its promoter a site for Smad3 [45], a transcription factor central for the anti-inflammatory effect of TGF-β [47], may participate to the down-modulating effect of TGF-β on cytotoxic T cells. In fact, TGF-β likely plays a more general role in the control of NK receptor expression. First, this cytokine downregulates NKG2D [48]. Furthermore, in mice with T cells deprived of TGF-β receptor II, there is a massive expansion of highly cytotoxic T cells that develop an NK-like program with high levels of CD94, NKG2, DAP12 and NKG2D parallel to the onset of generalized inflammation and fatal autoimmunity [49]. Our recent observation that IL-15 blocks the Smad3 pathway of TGF-β in IELs and lipoprotein lipase (LPL) of CD provides an additional mechanism through which IL-15 may promote activation of IEL and epithelial lesions in CD [50]. Indeed, the inhibitory effect of IL-15 on Smad3 implies activation of the JUN kinases, a pathway that blocks the down-modulating effect of TGF-β on NKG2D [51]. Finally, it is likely that the other NK receptors expressed by normal IELs (CD161) or upregulated in CD (NKP46, NKP30) may participate in the epithelial lesions. Yet the lack of currently identified ligands prevents delineation of their exact contribution.

Role of Gliadin Peptides in the Activation of Innate Immunity

The most ancient experimental approach to evaluate the toxicity of gluten-derived peptides is organ culture. It was shown that adding pepsin-trypsin digests of gluten (Frazer's fraction) to intestinal biopsies from CD patients on a GFD but not controls, resulted in damage to epithelial cells with decreased enterocyte height, distorted microvilli and decreased expression of brush border enzymes [52], changes associated in later studies with extensive epithelial apoptosis [53]. Conversely, epithelial morphology and expression of brush border enzymes, severely altered in biopsies of active CD patients, improved after a 48-hour culture in medium alone [54]. Using this technique, the group of de Ritis et al. [55] analyzed the toxicity of α-gliadins and suggested that the N-terminus contained several toxic fragments that could be released after digestion with chymotrypsin, including peptide 31–55 (p31–55). Toxicity of p31–55 was also observed in vivo after duodenal instillation of the peptide [56] and in organ culture with the shorter p31–43 [57]. In contrast p56–68 was not toxic in this setting. These results appeared quite paradoxical when p56–68 was found to be one dominant HLA-DQ2-restricted gliadin T-cell epitope, while p31–55 or p31–43 were not usual T-cell targets. Maiuri et al. [58] were the first to suggest that the latter peptide might induce an innate response in CD. Using organ culture, they observed that p31–43 induced early activation of CD3– (presumably macrophages and/or dendritic cells) but not CD3+ T lamina propria mononuclear cells. Thus p31–43 induced expression of IL-15, COX2, CD83, a marker of mature dendritic cells, and of CD25, an activation marker in CD3– cells. Adding this peptide also resulted in increased counts of CD8+and CD94+ IEL and epithelial apoptosis. In contrast to p31–43, two peptides corresponding to dominant T-cell epitopes (p56–68 and p68–75) had no effect alone but addition of p31–43 prior to the latter peptides induced activation of lamina propria CD3+ T cells attested by the expression of the activation markers CD25 and CD69 and enhanced epithelial damage. Finally, all the effects of p31–43 were blocked by a neutralizing anti-IL-15 antibody or an inhibitor of the P38-MAPkinase [58]. Comforting the hypothesis of a role of p31–43 in the induction of IL-15 in the intestine of CD patients, we observed that this peptide, like the Frazer gluten fraction, can stimulate the expression of MICA in organ culture of CD patients on a GFD but not controls, an effect blocked by an anti-IL-15 antibody [35].

More recent studies have tried to define the signal induced by p31–43. Again using organ culture, Maiuri et al. [59] observed that p31–43 induced rapid tyrosine phosphorylation and actin rearrangement in epithelial cells of CD patients on a GFD. This effect seemed to involve tissue transglutaminase 2 (TG-2) as it was blocked by an antibody directed against an epitope of this protein expressed at the surface of enterocytes. This putative role of TG-2 was independent of its enzymatic activity of trans- or deamidation, a function very essential to its role in the modification of T-cell epitopes requested for their efficient presentation by HLA-DQ molecules. While p31–43-induced changes were not observed in biopsies from control individuals, they were quite surprisingly reproduced in the T84 enterocyte line derived from a colic cancer [59]. The capacity of p31–43 to induce actin changes and tyrosine phosphorylation in different cell lines either of epithelial or fibroblast origin was also more recently reported by Barone et al. [60]. These authors suggested that the effects of p31–43 involved activation of the EGF receptor as they were similar to those induced by EGF and were blocked by inhibitors of the EGF pathway. In addition, pepsin trypsin digests of gliadin as well as p31–43 reproduced other effects of EGF in the cell lines, including ERK stimulation and entrance in the cell cycle after serum starvation. The authors suggested that gliadin peptides were not direct ligands of the EGF receptor but, rather, that they potentiated and prolonged EGF signaling by delaying its endocytosis and therefore its targeting and destruction in lysosomes. Accordingly, they observed that gliadin peptides delayed the elimination of fluorescent EGF from endocytic vesicles in cell lines but also in enterocytes in organ culture of biopsies from treated CD patients. The authors further documented a possible EGF-like effect of gliadin peptides in intestinal biopsies by showing that the pepsin-trypsin digest or p31–43 increased epithelial proliferation in organ culture of CD patients, an effect blocked by an anti-EGF receptor antibody. The latter effects were observed only in biopsies of CD patients but not controls, suggesting activation of the EGF pathway in CD patients [60]. The latter hypothesis is confirmed by data reported by Wijmenga [12th International Congress on Coeliac Disease, New York, 2006], who described increased in situ expression of EGF, a finding perhaps not unexpected given the lack of full recovery of villous architecture in many patients on a GFD.

Along the observation by Maiuri et al. [57] that p31–43 induced the activation and/or maturation of dendritic cells in organ cultures from CD patients on a GFD, several groups have observed that gliadin might stimulate murine and human macrophages and/or dendritic cells. Tuckova et al. [61] reported that crude gliadin or pepsin digests potentiate NO production in mouse peritoneal macrophages stimulated with IFN-γ. The effect of crude gliadin was observed in macrophages from C3H/HeJ mice unresponsive to lipopolysaccharide (LPS), pleading against LPS contamination. An enhancing effect of gliadin digests on iNOS and Cox2 activation by IFN-γ was also observed by de Stephano et al. [62] in the murine macrophage line Raw 264.7. In addition, gliadin or its pepsin-digest alone stimulated TNF, Rantes and IL-10 production in mouse peritoneal macrophages [63]. The use of synthetic peptides or of gliadin fractions separated by HPLC led Tuckova et al. [61, 63] to suggest the preponderant role of α-gliadin p19–30 and subsequently p246–259. Thomas et al. [64] also reported that peritoneal macrophages from

Balb/c mice stimulated by pepsin-trypsin digests of gliadin produced numerous proinflammatory cytokines. Curiously, they reproduced this effect both with p31–43 and with a large 33-mer peptide that has been defined as the paradigm of the gliadin peptides that activate adaptive immunity. These effects were not observed in macrophages from MyD88–/– mice suggesting an implication of Toll-like receptors [64]. That the same gliadin digests failed to induce NFkB activation in CHO cells transfected with Toll-like receptor 2 or 4 pleaded against an artifact linked to LPS contamination, although the sensitivity of the latter cells to LPS might be less than that of macrophages [64]. Using murine bone marrow-derived immature dendritic cells cultured in GM-CSF, Nikulina et al. [65] obtained distinct results but confirmed a stimulatory effect of gluten digests. They observed that chymotrypsin-treated wheat gluten induced dendritic cell maturation (as shown by increased expression of CD40, CD54, CD86 and MHC class II) and stimulated production of MIP-2, KC and, IL-1β (while little TNF and no IL-10 were produced). These effects were not blocked by polymixin B but were abolished by pretreatment with proteinase K and persisted in C3H/HeJ mice, pleading again against LPS contamination [65].

A stimulatory effect of gliadin peptides was more recently observed in human cells albeit with some discrepancies. Palova-Jelinkova et al. [66] initially reported that CD11cCD14– dendritic cells derived from adherent peripheral monocytes and cultured with GM-CSF increased their expression of CD80, CD83, CD86, and HLA-DR in the presence of pepsin digests from gliadin but not from ovalbumin or soya proteins. The same gliadin digests increased allo presentation and stimulated the production of IL-6, IL-8, and TNF but not of IL-12 via activation of NFkB and of several MAP kinases [66]. In a more recent article however, gliadin digests alone had no effect on the phenotypic maturation of the dendritic cells although they could synergize with IFN-γ [67]. Based on the analysis of IL-8 and TNF production, the latter work further suggested that gliadin digests might have a more pronounced effect on dendritic cells from CD patients (particularly if they were active) than from controls, and in HLA-DQ2+ than HLA-DQ2– healthy donors, but the mechanism(s) underlying these differences were not elucidated [67]. In a distinct study by Terazzano et al. [68], gliadin pepsin-trypsin digests had no effect on the phenotypic maturation in immature dendritic cells from controls but they stimulated expression of HLA-E, an effect ascribed to the homology of some α- and ω-gliadin-derived peptides with amino acid sequences that bind into the HLA-E peptide groove. It was suggested that binding of gliadin peptides stabilizes HLA-E and promotes its surface expression. A role of HLA-E distinct from the one described above in the activation of IELs was propounded as in vitro data indicated that increased expression of HLA-E protected dendritic cells against killing by CD94/NKG2A+ NK cells and promoted a dialogue with T cells resulting in enhanced IFN-γ production [68].

Interplay between Innate and Adaptive Immunity in CD

Mounting evidence indicates that intestinal damage in CD involves not only an adaptive response mediated by gliadin-specific lamina propria TH1 CD4 cells but also an innate-like cytotoxic response of IELs promoted by enterocyte-derived IL-15. Yet, the rules of the interplay between these two effector mechanisms are not delineated, inasmuch as the mechanisms that initiate IEL activation and/or IL-15 synthesis remain elusive.

The first question concerns the exact role of gluten (fig. 2). In contrast to its well-understood role in the adaptive response, its contribution to the induction of the innate response remains unclear. Our own attempts to demonstrate that

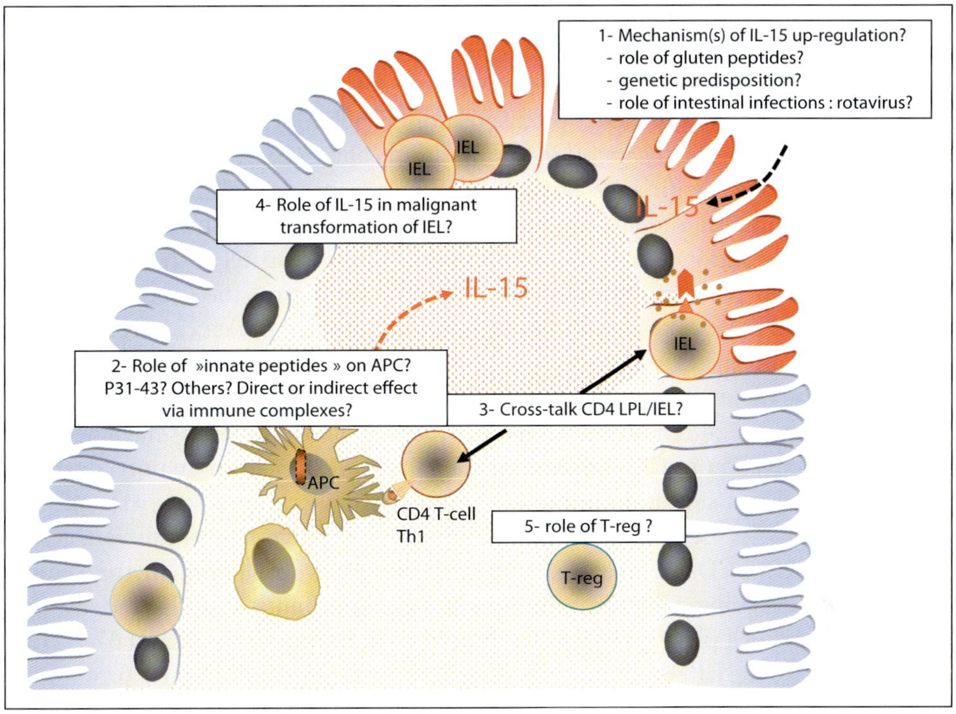

Fig. 2. Future questions on the role of innate immunity and IL-15 in CD. (1) Many clues suggest a central role for IL-15 but the mechanisms driving its upregulation remain to be deciphered. (2) Recent studies emphasize the possible role of gluten-derived peptides independent of their presentation by HLA molecules to CD4+ T cells. Yet the putative cellular targets and mechanism of action of these peptides remain to be elucidated. (3) Gluten-specific CD4+ LPL and IEL activated via innate-like mechanisms appear to be two complementary actors in the intestinal lesions caused by CD. Their putative cross-talk needs to be delineated. Among IELs, the contribution of CD8+ TCR-$\alpha\beta$ lymphocytes to epithelial destruction is now established. The role of TCR-$\gamma\delta$ IEL remains to be analyzed. (4) IL-15 promotes the survival of IEL either normal in CD or transformed in malignant refractory sprue. Which signaling pathways are activated? Are they therapeutic targets in clonal refractory sprue? (5) IL-15 can promote antigen-presentation and disrupt the regulatory pathway of TGF-β. Can IL-15 also interfere with a second key immunoregulatory pathway in intestine: the FoxP3 regulatory T cells? Via these combined effects, is IL-15 sufficient to drive the abnormal activation of Th1 gluten-specific CD4+ T cells?

p31–49 (used instead of p31–43) can signal into epithelial cell lines have been very disappointing and we have failed to demonstrate tyrosine phosphorylation and MAP kinase activation in several epithelial cell lines, including T84, Caco-2 and HT29 [unpublished results]. The capacity of gluten to signal into epithelial cells remains to be firmly established, notably by identifying how this peptide may bind the surface of epithelial cells. The impact of gluten on macrophage and/or dendritic cell activation may appear to be more convincingly demonstrated: thus, most of the studies discussed above used appropriate controls to eliminate artifacts, in particular those related to LPS contamination. By enhancing the maturation and activation of dendritic cells, gluten might indeed promote the adaptive response. Yet, the exact significance of this finding in the pathogenesis of CD is difficult to delineate and many questions remain unanswered on the nature of the peptides, on their mechanisms of action (is there a receptor?), on their dependence on a genetic predisposition. Observations that gluten peptides stimulate macrophages and dendritic cells not only in CD patients but also in mice and human controls plead against a genetic factor, but further studies are needed to define whether the putative mechanism(s) involved in these responses is(are) abnormally turned on in CD patients. To further increase the complexity, a recent puzzling observation suggests an alternative mechanism of macrophage activation in CD. Thus, Zanoni et al. [69] observed that a subset of anti-transglutaminase IgA antibodies isolated from the serum of patients with active CD cross-reacted with several proteins including the VP7 capsule protein of rotavirus, heat shock protein 60 and Toll receptor 4. Recognition of the latter receptor was associated with the capacity of the affinity-purified IgA to induce phenotypic maturation and secretion of proinflammatory cytokines while IgA purified along the same protocol from patients on a GFD had no effect [69]. Yet, this provocative observation needs to be substantiated by other observers.

A second question concerns the mechanisms that may promote IL-15 overproduction. A role of p31–43 in the induction of IL-15 in intestinal biopsies of patients has been suggested but needs to be substantiated by approaches less subjective than immunohistochemistry, and the mechanism of this putative effect will have to be elucidated. Current data indicate that upregulation of IL-15 in CD is induced at the post-translational level [22]. IL-15 translation is indeed tightly controlled by motifs present in the 5′ and 3′ untranslated regions (UTR) of the mRNA [for review see 27]. Interestingly, psoriasis, consistently associated with upregulation of IL-15 in skin, is genetically linked in Chinese patients to the 4q31.2 region which encodes IL-15. Moreover, a polymorphism in the mRNA 3′-UTR, which increased translation, was recently identified in these patients [70]. No association of CD with 4q31.2 has however been reported and limited data obtained in 4 patients with refractory sprue did not reveal a polymorphism in the 3′-UTR of IL-15 mRNA, and in particular not the polymorphism observed in psoriasis [22]. Alternatively, mechanisms that control IL-15 translation may be impaired in CD. Unfortunately, the signals that modulate the impact on the 5′ and 3′-UTR on IL-15 translation are not elucidated. Synthesis of IL-15 rapidly increases in response to many intracellular pathogens. Signals via Toll receptors and/or by type I interferons have been implicated but their role has been mainly described at the level of transcription [40, 41]. An alternative but not exclusive hypothesis is a role for signaling cascades implicated in the response to stress. This possibility is indicated by the impact of MAP kinases on the 5′ and 3′-UTR and thereby on the translation of many proinflammatory genes and oncogenes [71, 72]. Future studies are needed to delineate whether environmental and/or genetic factors modulating the host response to stress participate to the induction of IL-15 in CD (fig. 2).

The third question concerns the hierarchy of the adaptive and innate immune responses in the lamina propria and epithelium (fig. 2). HLA-DQ8 mice displayed strong CD4+ responses to gluten but developed no enteropathy and no increase in IELs [4]. This result is not surprising giving previous studies in transgenic mice which possess a large number of CD4+ T cells specific for a soluble antigen: in the latter mice, oral feeding with this antigen failed to induce any enteropathy except if the mice had previously been treated with an inhibitor of Cox enzymes, which is thought to impair local T-cell immunoregulation [73]. Impaired T-cell regulation in CD is indeed suggested by genetic studies showing in some populations linkages with the CTLA-4 gene [6], the ICAM-1 gene (with a polymorphism in the binding site for Mac-1, a receptor involved in the control of autoimmunity and IL-17 production)

[74, 75] and more recently with the 4q27 region which encodes the IL2 and IL-21 genes [7].

The role of the CD4 adaptive response in the activation of IELs is unclear. The production of IFN-γ may enhance HLA-E expression by enterocytes and thereby promote activation and cytotoxicity of CD94/NKG2C+ IELs (see above). Enhanced production of IL-21 has recently been observed in active CD [7]. This cytokine is produced by CD4+ T cells and has known synergistic effects with IL-15 [76]. IL-21 might thereby interact with IL-15 to promote IEL expansion and activation. Yet, the lack of IEL infiltration in many models of enteropathy associated with strong lamina propria CD4+ T-cell activation suggests that additional independent mechanism(s) initiate(s) IEL activation in CD. The early appearance of IEL infiltration in latent CD many years before the onset of villous atrophy [77] and, conversely, its persistence in many patients on a GFD suggest that the abnormal activation of the epithelial compartment is controlled by genetic factors. As already largely discussed, a primary defect in IL-15 regulation is an attractive albeit not demonstrated hypothesis. One attractive feature of this hypothesis is to provide a link between IEL and LPL activation. Thus enhanced production of IL-15 could initiate and sustain the activation of IELs as described above, but might also amplify the activation of CD4+ lamina propria T cells. First, IL-15 stimulates maturation and antigen-presentation by dendritic cells [78] and the number of mature antigen-presenting cells is increased in the mucosa of patients with active CD [79]. Second, IL-15 can impair local immunoregulation. Thus, Benahmed at al. [50] demonstrated that the Smad3 signaling pathway of TGF-β, central to the retro-control of intestinal inflammation [47], was inhibited by IL-15. Notably, mice lacking a TGF-β receptor II on their T cells develop severe autoimmunity associated with uncontrolled activation not only of highly cytotoxic CD8 T cells (see above) but also of CD4+ Th1 responses [49, 80]. Blocking the effect of IL-15 in organ cultures of patients with active CD simultaneously restored Smad3-dependent transcription and decreased IFN-γ transcription, indicating that inhibition of TGF-β signals by IL-15 promotes the local Th1 response in CD [50] (fig. 1).

Progressive accumulation of gliadin-specific CD4+ T cells in the lamina propria of patients exposed to gluten and of IELs in epithelium may finally reach a critical point in which local immunoregulation is overcome, resulting in intestinal inflammation that can only be interrupted by removing gluten. Intestinal infections by agents that induce IL-15 may precipitate this unfavorable outcome, a hypothesis supported by a recent prospective study showing that a high frequency of rotavirus infections increases the risk of CD autoimmunity in genetically predisposed children [81].

Conclusion

Intestinal damage in CD patients results from the activation of both an adaptive lamina propria CD4+ T-cell response and an innate-like cytotoxic response of IELs largely orchestrated by the cytokine IL-15. These responses driven by chronic exposure to gluten in CD patients are likely the pathological counterparts of normal acute intestinal responses to intracellular pathogens. While the interplay between genetics and gluten in the induction of the adaptive response is now well understood, further studies are needed to delineate the respective contributions of genetic and environmental factors, particularly gluten, in the induction of the innate response and IL-15 synthesis. It will also be necessary to define the hierarchy in lamina propria and intraepithelial activation. Animal models represent an useful tool to analyze these interactions and investigate the possible role of IL-15 as a link between the lamina propria and intraepithelial responses. Finally the central role of IL-15 in the disruption of intraepithelial homeostasis including the induction of an autoimmune cytolytic attack on the epithelium and emergence of lymphomas provides a potential therapeutic target in patients with severe forms of CD resistant to a GFD. Agents blocking IL-15 may be particularly useful in patients with RCF to prevent destruction of the epithelium, dissemination of the malignant cells, and the onset of an aggressive lymphoma.

Acknowledgments

INSERM U793 is supported by grants from INSERM, Association pour la Recherche contre le Cancer (ARC 3710), Ligue Nationale contre le Cancer, Fondation Princesse Grace, and the Association Française des Intolérants au Gluten. G.M. was supported by a fellowship from the Association pour la Recherche contre le Cancer. S.A. was supported by a fellowship from Sanofi-Aventis.

References

1 Sollid LM, Markussen G, Ek J, Gjerde H, Vardtal F, Thorsby E: Evidence for a primary association of celiac disease to a particular HLA-DQ α/β heterodimer. J Exp Med 1989;169:345–350.

2 Koning F, Schuppan D, Cerf-Bensussan N, Sollid LM: Pathomechanisms in celiac disease. Best Pract Res Clin Gastroenterol 2005;19:373–387.

3 Sollid L: Coeliac disease: dissecting a complex inflammatory disorder. Nat Rev Immunol 2002;9:647–655.

4 Black K, Murray J, David CS: HLA-DQ determines the response to exogenous wheat proteins: a model of gluten sensitivity in transgenic knockout mice. J Immunol 2002;169:5595–5600.

5 Marietta E, Black K, Camilleri M, Krause P, Rogers RS 3rd, David C, Pittelkow MR, Murray JA: A new model for dermatitis herpetiformis that uses HLA-DQ8 transgenic NOD mice. J Clin Invest 2004;114:1090–1097.

6 Djilali-Saiah I, Schmitz J, Harfouch-Hammoud E, Mougenot JF, Bach JF, Caillat-Zucman S: CTLA-4 gene polymorphism is associated with predisposition to coeliac disease. Gut 1998;43: 187–189.

7 van Heel DA, Franke L, Hunt KA, Gwilliam R, Zhernakova A, Inouye M, Wapenaar MC, Barnardo MC, Bethel G, Holmes GK, Feighery C, Jewell D, Kelleher D, Kumar P, Travis S, Walters JR, Sanders DS, Howdle P, Swift J, Playford RJ, McLaren WM, Mearin ML, Mulder CJ, McManus R, McGinnis R, Cardon LR, Deloukas P, Wijmenga C: A genome-wide association study for celiac disease identifies risk variants in the region harboring IL2 and IL21. Nat Genet 2007;39:827–829.

8 Ferguson A, Murray D: Quantitation of intraepithelial lymphocytes in human jejunum. Gut 1971;12:988–994.

9 Olaussen RW, Johansen FE, Lundin KE, Jahnsen J, Brandtzaeg P, Farstad IN: Interferon-gamma-secreting T cells localize to the epithelium in coeliac disease. Scand J Immunol 2002;56: 652–664.

10 Ciccocioppo R, Di Sabatino A, Parroni R, Muzi P, D'Alo S, Ventura T, Pistoia MA, Cifone MG, Corazza GR: Increased enterocyte apoptosis and Fas-Fas ligand system in celiac disease. Am J Clin Pathol 2001;115:494–503.

11 Di Sabatino A, Ciccocioppo R, D'Alo S, Parroni R, Millimaggi D, Cifone MG, Corazza GR: Intraepithelial and lamina propria lymphocytes show distinct patterns of apoptosis whereas both populations are active in Fas based cytotoxicity in coeliac disease. Gut 2001; 49:380–386.

12 Oberhuber G, Vogelsang H, Stolte M, Muthenthaler S, Kummer A, Radaszkiewicz T: Evidence that intestinal intraepithelial lymphocytes are activated cytotoxic T Cells In celiac disease but not in Giardiasis. Am J Pathol 1996;148:1351–1357.

13 Shiner M, Eran M, Freier S, Faber J, Branski D: Are intraepithelial lymphocytes in celiac mucosa responsible for inducing programmed cell death (apoptosis) in enterocytes? Histochemical demonstration of perforins in cytoplasmic granules of intraepithelial lymphocytes. J Pediatr Gastroenterol Nutr 1998;27:393–396.

14 Cellier C, Delabesse E, Helmer C, Patey N, Matuchansky C, Jabri B, Macintyre E, Cerf-Bensussan N, Brousse N: Refractory sprue, coeliac disease, and enteropathy-associated T-cell lymphoma. French Coeliac Disease Study Group. Lancet 2000;356:203–208.

15 Cellier C, Patey N, Mauvieux L, Jabri B, Delabesse E, Cervoni JP, Burtin ML, Guy-Grand D, Bouhnik Y, Modigliani R, Barbier JP, Macintyre E, Brousse N, Cerf-Bensussan N: Abnormal intestinal intraepithelial lymphocytes in refractory sprue. Gastroenterology 1998;114: 471–481.

16 Kutlu T, Brousse N, Rambaud C, Le Deist F, Schmitz J, Cerf-Bensussan N: Numbers of T cell receptor (TCR) a/b+ but not of TCR g/d+ intraepithelial lymphocytes correlate with the grade of villous atrophy in coeliac patients on a long term normal diet. Gut 1993;34:208–214.

17 Spencer J, Isaacson P, Diss T, McDonald T: Expression of disulfide-linked and non-disulfide-linked forms of the T cell receptor g/d heterodimer in human intraepithelial lymphocytes. Eur J Immunol 1989;19:1335–1338.

18 Gianfrani C, Troncone R, Mugione P, Cosentini E, De Pascale M, Faruolo C, Senger S, Terrazzano G, Southwood S, Auricchio S, Sette A: Celiac disease association with CD8(+) T cell responses: identification of a novel gliadin-derived HLA-A2-restricted epitope. J Immunol 2003;170: 2719–2726.

19 Jabri B, Patey de Serre N, Cellier C, Evans K, Gache C, Carvalho C, Mougenot J, Allez M, Jian R, Desreumaux P, Colombel J, Matuchansky C, Cugnenc H, Lopez-Botet M, Vivier E, Moretta A, Roberts AI, Ebert E, Guy-Grand D, Brousse N, Schmitz J, Cerf-Bensussan N: Selective expansion of intraepithelial lymphocytes expressing the HLA-E-specific natural killer receptor CD94 in celiac disease. Gastroenterology 2000;118: 867–879.

20 Roberts AI, Lee L, Schwarz E, Groh V, Spies T, Ebert EC, Jabri B: NKG2D receptors induced by IL-15 costimulate CD28-negative effector CTL in the tissue microenvironment. J Immunol 2001;167:5527–5530.

21 Meresse B, Chen Z, Ciszewski C, Tretiakova M, Bhagat G, Krausz TN, Raulet DH, Lanier LL, Groh V, Spies T, Ebert EC, Green PH, Jabri B: Coordinated induction by IL15 of a TCR-independent NKG2D signaling pathway converts CTL into lymphokine-activated killer cells in celiac disease. Immunity 2004;21:357–366.

22 Mention JJ, Ben Ahmed M, Begue B, Barbe U, Verkarre V, Asnafi V, Colombel JF, Cugnenc PH, Ruemmele FM, McIntyre E, Brousse N, Cellier C, Cerf-Bensussan N: Interleukin 15:a key to disrupted intraepithelial lymphocyte homeostasis and lymphomagenesis in celiac disease. Gastroenterology 2003; 125:730–745.

23 Di Sabatino A, Ciccocioppo R, Cupelli F, Cinque B, Millimaggi D, Clarkson MM, Paulli M, Cifone MG, Corazza GR: Epithelium derived interleukin 15 regulates intraepithelial lymphocyte Th1 cytokine production, cytotoxicity, and survival in coeliac disease. Gut 2006;55: 469–477.

24 Musso T, Calosso L, Zucca M, Millesimo M, Ravarino D, Giovarelli M, Malavasi F, Ponzi AN, Paus R, Bulfone-Paus S: Human monocytes constitutively express membrane-bound, biologically active, and interferon-gamma-upregulated interleukin-15. Blood 1999;93:3531–3539.

25 Ruckert R, Asadullah K, Seifert M, Budagian VM, Arnold R, Trombotto C, Paus R, Bulfone-Paus S: Inhibition of keratinocyte apoptosis by IL-15:a new parameter in the pathogenesis of psoriasis? J Immunol 2000;165:2240–2250.

26 Budagian V, Bulanova E, Paus R, Bulfone-Paus S: IL-15/IL-15 receptor biology: a guided tour through an expanding universe. Cytokine Growth Factor Rev 2006;17:259–280.

27 Fehniger TA, Caligiuri MA: Interleukin 15:biology and relevance to human disease. Blood 2001;97:14–32.

28 Giri JG, Ahdieh M, Eisenman J, Shanebeck K, Grabstein K, Kumaki S, Namen A, Park LS, Cosman D, Anderson D: Utilization of the beta and gamma chains of the IL-2 receptor by the novel cytokine IL-15. EMBO J 1994;13:2822–2830.

29 Oh S, Perera LP, Burke DS, Waldmann TA, Berzofsky JA: IL-15/IL-15Ralpha-mediated avidity maturation of memory CD8+ T cells. Proc Natl Acad Sci USA 2004;101:15154–15159.

30 Sato N, Patel HJ, Waldmann TA, Tagaya Y: The IL-15/IL-15Ralpha on cell surfaces enables sustained IL-15 activity and contributes to the long survival of CD8 memory T cells. Proc Natl Acad Sci USA 2007;104:588–593.

31 Fehniger T, Suzuki K, Ponnapan A, Van Deusen J, Cooper A, Florea S, Freud A, Robinson M, Durbin J, Caligiuri M: Fatal leukemia in interleukin15 transgenic mice follows early expansion in natural killer and memory phenotype CD8+ T cells. J Exp Med 2001;193:219–231.

32 Carbonnel F, Grollet-Bioul L, Brouet J, Teilhac M, Cosnes J, Angonin R, Deschaseaux M, Chatelet F, Gendre J, Sigaux F: Are complicated forms of celiac disease cryptic T-cell lymphomas? Blood 1998;92:3879–3886.

33 Cellier C, Cervoni JP, Patey N, Leborgne M, Marteau P, Landi B, Cerf-Bensussan N, Barbier JP, Brousse N: Gluten-free diet induces regression of T-cell activation in the rectal mucosa of patients with celiac disease. Am J Gastroenterol 1998;93:1527–1530.

34 Daum S, Cellier C, Mulder CJ: Refractory coeliac disease. Best Pract Res Clin Gastroenterol 2005;19: 413–424.

35 Hue S, Mention JJ, Monteiro RC, Zhang S, Cellier C, Schmitz J, Verkarre V, Fodil N, Bahram S, Cerf-Bensussan N, Caillat-Zucman S: A direct role for NKG2D/MICA interaction in villous atrophy during celiac disease. Immunity 2004;21:367–377.

36 Verkarre V, Romana SP, Cerf-Bensussan N: Gluten-free diet, chromosomal abnormalities, and cancer risk in coeliac disease. J Pediatr Gastroenterol Nutr 2004;38:140–142.

37 Verkarre V, Romana S-P, Cellier C, Asnafi V, Mention J, Barbe U, Nusbaum S, Hermine O, Macintyre E, Brousse N, Radford-Weiss I, Cerf-Bensussan N: Recurrent partial trisomy 1q22-q32 in clonal intraepithelial lymphocytes in refractory celiac sprue. Gastroenterology 2003;125:40–46.

38 Ohta N, Hiroi T, Kweon M, Kinoshita N, Jang M, Mashimo T, Miyazaki J, Kiyono H: IL-15-dependent activation-induced cell death-resistant Th1 type CD8alphabeta(+)NK1.1(+) T cells for the development of small intestinal inflammation. J Immunol 2002;169: 460–468.

39 Ebert E: Interleukin 15 is a potent stimulant of intraepithelial lymphocytes. Gastroenterology 1998;115: 1439–1445.

40 Jinushi M, Takehara T, Tatsumi T, Kanto T, Groh V, Spies T, Suzuki T, Miyagi T, Hayashi N: Autocrine/paracrine IL-15 that is required for type I IFN-mediated dendritic cell expression of MHC class I-related chain A and B is impaired in hepatitis C virus infection. J Immunol 2003;171:5423–5429.

41 Zhou R, Wei H, Sun R, Zhang J, Tian Z: NKG2D recognition mediates Toll-like receptor 3 signaling-induced breakdown of epithelial homeostasis in the small intestines of mice. Proc Natl Acad Sci USA 2007;104:7512–7515.

42 Meresse B, Curran SA, Ciszewski C, Orbelyan G, Setty M, Bhagat G, Lee L, Tretiakova M, Semrad C, Kistner E, Winchester RJ, Braud V, Lanier LL, Geraghty DE, Green PH, Guandalini S, Jabri B: Reprogramming of CTLs into natural killer-like cells in celiac disease. J Exp Med 2006;203:1343–1355.

43 Laouar A, Manocha M, Wan M, Yagita H, van Lier RA, Manjunath N: Cutting edge: distinct NK receptor profiles are imprinted on CD8 T cells in the mucosa and periphery during the same antigen challenge: role of tissue-specific factors. J Immunol 2007;178:652–656.

44 von Boehmer H: Oral tolerance: is it all retinoic acid? J Exp Med 2007;204: 1737–1739.

45 Gunturi A, Berg RE, Crossley E, Murray S, Forman J. The role of TCR stimulation and TGF-beta in controlling the expression of CD94/NKG2A receptors on CD8 T cells. Eur J Immunol 2005;35: 766–775.

46 Rubtsov YP, Rudensky AY: TGFbeta signalling in control of T-cell-mediated self-reactivity. Nat Rev Immunol 2007;7: 443–453.

47 Yang X, Letterio JJ, Lechleider RJ, Chen L, Hayman R, Gu H, Roberts AB, Deng C: Targeted disruption of SMAD3 results in impaired mucosal immunity and diminished T cell responsiveness to TGF-beta. EMBO J 1999;18:1280–1291.

48 Castriconi R, Cantoni C, Della Chiesa M, Vitale M, Marcenaro E, Conte R, Biassoni R, Bottino C, Moretta L, Moretta A: Transforming growth factor beta 1 inhibits expression of NKp30 and NKG2D receptors: consequences for the NK-mediated killing of dendritic cells. Proc Natl Acad Sci USA 2003. 100:4120–4125.

49 Marie JC, Liggitt D, Rudensky AY: Cellular mechanisms of fatal early-onset autoimmunity in mice with the T cell-specific targeting of transforming growth factor-beta receptor. Immunity 2006;25:441–454.

50 Benahmed M, Meresse B, Arnulf B, Barbe U, Mention JJ, Verkarre V, Allez M, Cellier C, Hermine O, Cerf-Bensussan N: Inhibition of TGF-beta signaling by interleukin-15 via phospho-c-jun upregulation: a new role for interleukin-15 in the loss of immune homeostasis in celiac disease. Gastroenterology 2007;132:994–1008.

51 Song H, Hur DY, Kim KE, Park H, Kim T, Kim CW, Bang S, Cho DH: IL-2/IL-18 prevent the down-modulation of NKG2D by TGF-beta in NK cells via the c-Jun N-terminal kinase (JNK) pathway. Cell Immunol 2006;242:39–45.

52 Falchuk ZM, Gebhard RL, Sessoms C, Strober W: An in vitro model of gluten-sensitive enteropathy. Effect of gliadin on intestinal epithelial cells of patients with gluten-sensitive enteropathy in organ culture. J Clin Invest 1974;53:487–500.

53 Maiuri L, Ciacci C, Raia V, Vacca L, Ricciardelli I, Raimondi F, Auricchio S, Quaratino S, Londei M: FAS engagement drives apoptosis of enterocytes of coeliac patients. Gut 2001;48:418–424.

54 Falchuk ZM, Nelson DL, Katz AJ, Bernardin JE, Kasarda DD, Hague NE, Strober W: Gluten-sensitive enteropathy. Influence of histocompatibility type on gluten sensitivity in vitro. J Clin Invest 1980;66:227–233.

55 de Ritis G, Auricchio S, Jones HW, Lew EJ, Bernardin JE, Kasarda DD: In vitro (organ culture) studies of the toxicity of specific A-gliadin peptides in celiac disease. Gastroenterology 1988;94:41–49.

56 Sturgess R, Day P, Ellis HJ, Lundin KE, Gjertsen HA, Kontakou M, Ciclitira PJ: Wheat peptide challenge in coeliac disease. Lancet 1994;343:758–761.

57 Maiuri L, Troncone R, Mayer M, Coletta S, Picarelli A, De Vincenzi M, Pavone V, Auricchio S: In vitro activities of A-gliadin-related synthetic peptides: damaging effect on the atrophic coeliac mucosa and activation of mucosal immune response in the treated coeliac mucosa. Scand J Gastroenterol 1996;31:247–253.

58 Maiuri L, Ciacci C, Ricciardelli I, Vacca L, Raia V, Auricchio S, Picard J, Osman M, Quaratino S, Londei M: Association between innate response to gliadin and activation of pathogenic T cells in coeliac disease. Lancet 2003;362:30–37.

59 Maiuri L, Ciacci C, Ricciardelli I, Vacca L, Raia V, Rispo A, Griffin M, Issekutz T, Quaratino S, Londei M: Unexpected Role of Surface Transglutaminase Type II in Celiac Disease. Gastroenterology 2005;129:1400–1413.

60 Barone MV, Gimigliano A, Castoria G, Paolella G, Maurano F, Paparo F, Maglio M, Nanayakkara M, Mineo A, Miele E, Troncone R, Auricchio S: Growth factor-like activity of gliadin, an alimentary protein: implications for celiac disease. Gut 2007;56:480–488.

61 Tuckova L, Flegelova Z, Tlaskalova-Hogenova H, Zidek Z: Activation of macrophages by food antigens: enhancing effect of gluten on nitric oxide and cytokine production. J Leukoc Biol 2000;67:312–318.

62 De Stefano D, Maiuri MC, Iovine B, Ialenti A, Bevilacqua MA, Carnuccio R: The role of NF-kappaB, IRF-1, and STAT-1alpha transcription factors in the iNOS gene induction by gliadin and IFN-gamma in RAW 264.7 macrophages. J Mol Med 2006;84:65–74.

63 Tuckova L, Novotna J, Novak P, Flegelova Z, Kveton T, Jelinkova L, Zidek Z, Man P, Tlaskalova-Hogenova H: Activation of macrophages by gliadin fragments: isolation and characterization of active peptide. J Leukoc Biol 2002;71:625–631.

64 Thomas KE, Sapone A, Fasano A, Vogel SN: Gliadin stimulation of murine macrophage inflammatory gene expression and intestinal permeability are MyD88-dependent: role of the innate immune response in Celiac disease. J Immunol 2006;176:2512–2521.

65 Nikulina M, Habich C, Flohe SB, Scott FW, Kolb H: Wheat gluten causes dendritic cell maturation and chemokine secretion. *J* Immunol 2004;173: 1925–1933.

66 Palova-Jelinkova L, Rozkova D, Pecharova B, Bartova J, Sediva A, Tlaskalova-Hogenova H, Spisek R, Tuckova L: Gliadin fragments induce phenotypic and functional maturation of human dendritic cells. J Immunol 2005;175:7038–7045.

67 Cinova J, Palova-Jelinkova L, Smythies LE, Cerna M, Pecharova B, Dvorak M, Fruhauf P, Tlaskalova-Hogenova H, Smith PD, Tuckova L: Gliadin peptides activate blood monocytes from patients with celiac disease. J Clin Immunol 2007;27:201–209.

68 Terrazzano G, Sica M, Gianfrani C, Mazzarella G, Maurano F, De Giulio B, de Saint-Mezard S, Zanzi D, Maiuri, L. Londei M, Jabri B, Troncone R, Auricchio S, Zappacosta S, Carbone E: Gliadin regulates the NK-dendritic cell cross-talk by HLA-E surface stabilization. J Immunol 2007;179:372–381.

69 Zanoni G, Navone R, Lunardi C, Tridente G, Bason C, Sivori S, Beri R, Dolcino M, Valletta E, Corrocher R, Puccetti A: In celiac disease, a subset of autoantibodies against transglutaminase binds toll-like receptor 4 and induces activation of monocytes. PLoS Med 2006;3:e358.

70 Zhang XJ, Yan KL, Wang ZM, Yang S, Zhang GL, Fan X, Xiao FL, Gao M, Cui Y, Wang PG, Sun LD, Zhang KY, Wang B, Wang DZ, Xu SJ, Huang W, Liu JJ: Polymorphisms in interleukin-15 gene on chromosome 4q31.2 are associated with psoriasis vulgaris in Chinese population. J Invest Dermatol 2007;127:2544–2551.

71 Dean JL, Sully G, Clark AR, Saklatvala J: The involvement of AU-rich element-binding proteins in p38 mitogen-activated protein kinase pathway-mediated mRNA stabilisation. Cell Signal 2004; 16:1113–1121.

72 Nikolcheva T, Pyronnet S, Chou SY, Sonenberg N, Song A, Clayberger C, Krensky AM: A translational rheostat for RFLAT-1 regulates RANTES expression in T lymphocytes. J Clin Invest 2002;110:119–126.

73 Newberry RD, Stenson WF, Lorenz RG: Cyclooxygenase-2-dependent arachidonic acid metabolites are essential modulators of the intestinal immune response to dietary antigen. Nat Med 1999;5:900–906.

74 Abel M, Cellier C, Kumar N, Cerf-Bensussan N, Schmitz J, Caillat-Zucman S: Adulthood-onset celiac disease is associated with intercellular adhesion molecule-1 (ICAM-1) gene polymorphism. Hum Immunol 2006;67:612–617.

75 Ehirchiou D, Xiong Y, Xu G, Chen W, Shi Y, Zhang L: CD11b facilitates the development of peripheral tolerance by suppressing Th17 differentiation. J Exp Med 2007;204:1519–1524.

76 Leonard WJ, Spolski R: Interleukin-21:a modulator of lymphoid proliferation, apoptosis and differentiation. Nat Rev Immunol 2005;5:688–698.

77 Mäki M, Holm K, Collin P, Savilahti E: Increase in g/d T cell receptor bearing lymphocytes in normal small bowel mucosa in latent celiac disease. Gut 1991;32:1412–1414.

78 Ohteki T, Suzue K, Maki C, Ota T, Koyasu S: Critical role of IL-15-IL15R for antigen-presenting cell functions in the innate immune response. Nat Immunol 2001;2:1138–1143.

79 Raki M, Tollefsen S, Molberg O, Lundin KE, Sollid LM, Jahnsen FL: A unique dendritic cell subset accumulates in the celiac lesion and efficiently activates gluten-reactive T cells. Gastroenterology 2006;131:428–438.

80 Li MO, Sanjabi S, Flavell RA: Transforming growth factor-beta controls development, homeostasis, and tolerance of T cells by regulatory T cell-dependent and -independent mechanisms. Immunity 2006;25:455–471.

81 Stene LC, Honeyman MC, Hoffenberg EJ, Haas JE, Sokol RJ, Emery L, Taki I, Norris JM, Erlich HA, Eisenbarth GS, Rewers M: Rotavirus infection frequency and risk of celiac disease autoimmunity in early childhood: a longitudinal study. Am J Gastroenterol 2006;101:2333–2340.

Dr. Nadine Cerf-Bensussan
INSERM U793, Faculté de Médecine, Université Paris Descartes
156, rue de Vaugirard
FR–75015 Paris (France)
Tel. +33 1 40 61 56 37, Fax +33 1 40 61 56 38, E-Mail cerf@necker.fr

Fasano A, Troncone R, Branski D (eds): Frontiers in Celiac Disease.
Pediatr Adolesc Med. Basel, Karger, 2008, vol 12, pp 82–88

Celiac Disease: Across the Threshold of Tolerance

Frits Koning

Department of Immunohematology and Blood Transfusion, Leiden University Medical Center, Leiden, The Netherlands

Abstract

Celiac disease (CD) is caused by an inflammatory T-cell response to gluten and gluten-like proteins present in wheat and related cereals. Gluten is a heterogeneous mix of proteins, most of which harbor multiple peptides that, after modification by the enzyme tissue transglutaminase, can strongly bind to the disease-predisposing HLA-DQ2 or HLA-DQ8 molecules. This can trigger polyclonal, gluten-specific T-cell responses in the lamina propria that are an essential component of the inflammatory process that leads to the characteristic symptoms associated with CD. Strikingly, however, most HLA-DQ2/8-positive individuals do not develop CD, indicating that strong regulatory mechanisms control the development of gluten-specific T-cell responses. Here I discuss the unique features of gluten and HLA-DQ2/8 and why this combination is so strongly associated with CD. Moreover, I discuss which events are required for the breaking of natural tolerance to gluten in susceptible individuals and how this can be reconciled with recent reports on the involvement of innate immunity in CD pathogenesis.

HLA-DQ2 and HLA-DQ8

It is well established that over 90% of celiac disease (CD) patients are HLA-DQ2 positive while the remainder is usually HLA-DQ8 positive [1, 2]. Like other HLA class II molecules, HLA-DQ2 and -DQ8 are expressed by professional antigen-presenting cells and meant to bind peptides derived from endocytosed proteins. Upon cell surface expression these class-II-peptide complexes can be detected by T cells.

As gluten is an exogenous protein, it is a logical assumption that uptake of gluten by antigen-presenting cells leads to the generation of HLA-DQ-gluten peptide complexes that can induce T-cell responses. In 1993, Lundin et al. [3] were the first to demonstrate that such T cells could be isolated from small-intestinal biopsies of CD patients. In a series of subsequent studies the gluten peptides that elicit these T-cell responses were identified [4–9].

Gluten

Gluten is a heterogeneous mix of water-insoluble proteins in wheat flour that gives dough its elastic properties. The major components are the glutenins and the gliadins, both representing complex protein families. In a single wheat variety, between 50 and 100 distinct gluten proteins can be present. Gluten owes its name to its high content of the amino acid glutamine, over 30%, a property that is strongly linked to its toxicity for CD patients (see below). Moreover, it contains a

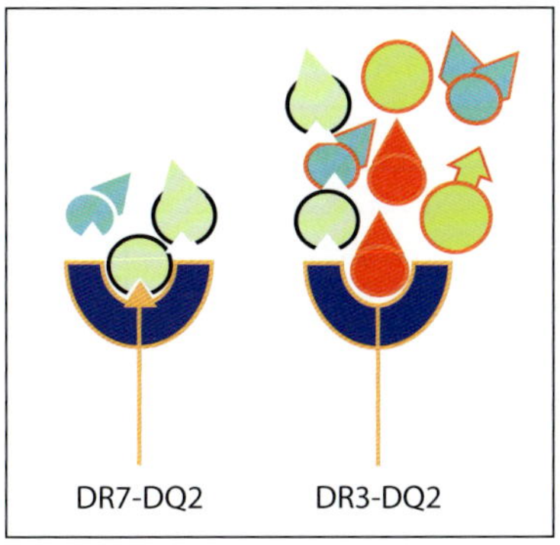

Fig. 1. The threshold of tolerance. The peptide-binding groove of the DR7-associated DQ2 molecule is slightly different from that of the DR3-associated DQ2 molecule. As a result, the DR7-DQ2 molecule can only bind a subset of the gluten peptides that can be bound by DR3-DQ2. This correlates with a high risk of disease development in the case of DR3-DQ2 and a very low risk for DR7-DQ2. This could be interpreted as a threshold of tolerance: tolerance is more easily maintained when gluten presentation levels are low.

high amount of the amino acid proline, which renders it resistant to degradation in the gastrointestinal tract [10]. As a result, gluten fragments persist in the gastrointestinal tract, and this is likely to further contribute to gluten toxicity. Finally, gluten is a commonly used protein in the food industry – the daily consumption of gluten is usually between 10 and 20 g. Thus, the exposure to gluten is high, a third factor contributing to the disease-inducing properties of gluten.

HLA-DQ, Gluten and Tissue Transglutaminase

Peptide binding to HLA is to a large extent dependent on the docking of side chains of amino acids in the bound peptide into pockets in the HLA molecule (fig. 1). In the case of HLA-DQ2 and -DQ8, it is well established that negatively charged amino acids are required for these interactions [11–13]. As gluten is virtually devoid of negatively charged amino acids, gluten peptides are therefore predicted to poorly bind to HLA-DQ2 and -DQ8, and this is indeed the case. This discrepancy was solved when it became clear that the enzyme tissue transglutaminase (tTG) can convert the abundant amino acid glutamine in gluten into glutamic acid. This introduces the negative charge(s) required for strong binding to HLA-DQ2/8 [14, 15].

The activity of tTG was found to be strongly dependent on the spacing between the amino acids glutamine (Q) and proline (P): while the glutamine in the sequence QP and QXXP (X is any amino acid) is not modified by tTG, it is in the sequence QXP [16]. As Q and P together make up approximately 50% of gluten, the sequences QP, QXP and QXXP are very common in gluten molecules. It is thus possible to make a highly accurate prediction of which glutamine residues in gluten will be modified. Together with the knowledge on the peptide-binding properties of HLA-DQ2, this can be used to predict which gluten-derived peptides are likely to have HLA-DQ2- or HLA-DQ8-binding properties and are thus probable targets for gluten-specific T cells in CD patients [16].

Several studies have now addressed the specificity of the gluten-specific T-cell response in CD [4–9]. This has revealed that polyclonal T-cell responses to multiple gluten peptides are almost invariably found in patients. The identified peptides are derived from all types of gliadins and glutenins, and most T-cell responses were found to be specific for tTG-modified peptides. Some peptides, in particular a proline-rich stretch in α-gliadin, appears to be immunodominant as responses to this peptide are observed in the large majority of patients while other peptides are less frequently recognized [7, 8, 10].

HLA-DQ2 Gene Dose Effect

It is well documented that the HLA-DQ2 gene dose has a major impact on the chance of disease development: HLA-DQ2 homozygous individuals have an at least 5 times higher risk of disease development compared to HLA-DQ2 heterozygous individuals [17]. This correlates with the fact that gluten-specific T cells respond more vigorously when gluten is presented by antigen-presenting cells from individuals that are homozygous for HLA-DQ2 compared to antigen-presenting cells that are from HLA-DQ2 heterozygous individuals [18]. Apparently, a double gene dose leads to a higher level of HLA-DQ2 expression. This in turn allows more efficient presentation of gluten peptides which leads to stronger T-cell responses and a higher risk of disease development. Quantity apparently matters.

There are other observations that also indicate that the level of gluten presentation is related to the probability of disease development. The DR3-DQ2 haplotype, for example, does predispose to CD while the DR7-DQ2 haplotype does not and a critical difference between these two DQ2 molecules is that while DR3-DQ2 can present a broad repertoire of gluten peptides, DR7-DQ2 can only present a subset of these [18].

Moreover, several studies have demonstrated that adult HLA-DQ2+ patients virtually all respond to a particular α-gliadin-derived peptide which has become known as the 33-mer [7, 8, 10]. This 33-amino-acid-long peptide is resistant to degradation in the gastrointestinal tract, a good substrate for tTG-mediated deamidation (table 1) and harbors several copies of immunogenic sequences that bind to HLA-DQ2 with relatively high affinity [10]. However, this is by no means the only gluten fragment that has these properties. A 26-amino-acid-long peptide has been identified in γ-gliadin that, similar to the 33-mer, is resistant to degradation, a substrate for tTG and harbors several immunogenic sequences [19]. Moreover, as gluten is a complex mixture of many related proteins, it comes as no surprise that database searches identified up to 60 gluten fragments that are predicted to have properties similar to that of the 33- and 26-mers [19], a number that closely matches an earlier prediction of the number of T-cell-stimulatory peptides in

Table 1. Characteristics of T-cell-stimulatory gluten peptides

Peptide	Sequence	Protein source	HLA-DQ
Glia-α2	PQPQLPYPQ	α-gliadin	DQ2
Glia-α9	PFPQPQLPY	α-gliadin	DQ2
Glia-α20	FRPQQPYPQ	α-gliadin	DQ2
Glia-γ2	FPQQPQQPF	γ-gliadin	DQ2
Glia-γ1	PQQSFPQQQ	γ-gliadin	DQ2
Glia-γ30	IIQPQQPAQ	γ-gliadin	DQ2
Glt-156	FSQQQQSPF	LMW glutenin	DQ2
Glt-17	FSQQQQQPL	LMW glutenin	DQ2
Glia-α	QGSFQPSQQ	α-gliadin	DQ8
Glt	QGYYPTSPQ	HMW glutenin	DQ8

Amino acids are indicated by the 1-letter code. Glutamine residues that are deamidated by tTG are underlined. LMW = Low-molecular-weight; HMW = high-molecular-weight.

gluten [16]. Clearly, their resistance to degradation allows such gluten peptides to persist in the gastrointestinal tract. Analogous to the HLA-DQ2 gene dose effect, this facilitates the generation of HLA-DQ-gluten peptide complexes and thus the likelihood of the development of a gluten-specific T-cell response.

Also, while the gluten-like proteins in barley and rye have been found to contain a broad repertoire of peptides that can be recognized by gluten-specific T cells, oats contains only a few of such peptides [16, 20]. As it is well established that barley and rye are harmful to CD patients, while oats is tolerated by many [21], this again argues that the level of exposure to T-cell-stimulatory gluten or gluten-like peptides plays an important role in CD development and/or severity of the disease-associated symptoms.

Finally, while a large number of HLA-DQ2-restricted gluten peptides have now been identified, only 2 HLA-DQ8-restricted peptides are known [4, 6], and it is tempting to speculate that this underlies the much stronger role of HLA-DQ2 in disease development compared to HLA-DQ8.

Altogether, it seems justified to conclude that the level of gluten presentation is an important factor influencing the likelihood of disease development.

Epitope Spreading versus Epitope Focussing

As mentioned, T-cell responses to the 33-mer are observed in virtually all adult patients, and this is therefore considered an immunodominant T-cell epitope. It is feasible, however, that the observed immunodominance may reflect an advanced stage in the development of the gluten-specific T-cell response and may not be indicative for the initiation of the disease. This is supported by our observation that in young children with CD, responses to the immunodominant peptide were only observed in about half of the children whereas these were found to have raised T cells against a diverse repertoire of other gliadin- and glutenin-derived peptides [9]. Moreover, we observed T-cell cross- reactivity towards homologous gliadin and glutenin peptides suggesting that this may play a role in the spreading of the gluten-specific T-cell response from gliadin to glutenin or vice versa [9]. Also, we found that T-cell responses to 3 peptides were independent of deamidation by tTG, an indication that native gluten peptides are immunogenic [9, 22].

Based on this we proposed that a gluten-specific T-cell response may be initiated by any of a relatively large number of immunogenic peptides derived from gliadin and glutenin. Both native and deamidated peptides may trigger such responses, and due to the ensuing tissue damage and the associated release of tTG deamidation of gluten is enhanced, generating more T-cell-stimulatory peptides and facilitating the generation of a polyclonal gluten-specific T-cell response. Cross-reactivity between glutenin and gliadin homologues may further contribute to the development of a diverse and spreading T-cell response. Over time, however, it is likely that the T-cell response will focus on those peptides that combine strong HLA-DQ2-binding properties with potent T-cell-stimulatory activity, such as the 33-mer. Thus, epitope spreading followed by epitope focussing is a model that reconciles the observations made in children and adults with CD [9].

Innate Immunity

More recently it has been reported that, next to adaptive responses, gluten appears to induce innate responses as well. This property has been particularly attributed to the so-called p31–43 peptide, a gluten peptide to which no adaptive immune responses have been found in the intestine of patients. Yet evidence has been presented that indicates that this peptide can facilitate a full-blown adaptive immune response and that it can induce MHC-class-I-related gene A expression on enterocytes (fig. 2), most likely through the induction of IL-15 [23–25]. On the other hand, no molecular mechanism through which this peptide would exert its activity has been identified. Perhaps more importantly, if gluten can directly stimulate the innate immune system, why can an overwhelming 99% of the general population eat wheat and related cereals without any sign of immune activation in the intestine? If we assume that the p31–43 does not have true innate stimulatory properties, why are biological effects observed with this peptide? In this respect it is important to note that gluten-specific antibodies, both of the IgG and IgA type, have been shown to be largely specific for the sequence QPFXXQXPY (in which X can be several amino acids) [26]. A very common variant of this sequence in gluten is QPFPPQLPY, a perfect match with the p31–43 peptide.

This raises the question if the effects of the p31–43 peptide can be attributed to the fact that it is the target of the humoral immune response against gluten. The p31–43 peptide is located just

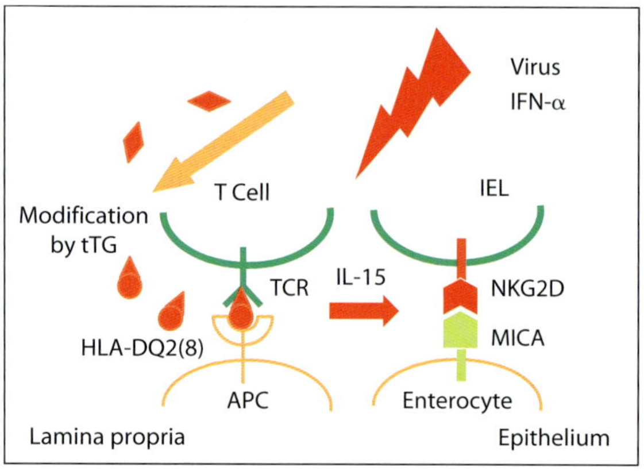

Fig. 2. The role of endogenous danger signals. When environmental insults like viral infections lead to the induction of endogenous danger signals (i.e. IFN-α), this could facilitate the generation of gluten-specific T-cell responses by induction of maturation of dendritic cells, upregulation of HLA-DQ expression and concomitant downregulation of anti-inflammatory processes that maintain mucosal tolerance. When a gluten-specific T-cell response has developed, this could result in local IL-15 production, driving the activation of intraepithelial lymphocytes (IEL) and upregulation of stress-associated ligands for NKG2 receptors (i.e. MICA, MHC-class-I-related gene A). TCR = T-cell receptor; APC = antigen-presenting cell.

C-terminal of the 33-mer, and it is thus feasible that gluten fragments are generated that contain both epitopes. Moreover, due to tTG activity the p31–43 epitope could be cross-linked to gluten fragments that harbor T-cell-stimulatory epitopes. Immune complexes may thus form that include both the p31–43 and T-cell-stimulatory epitopes. Under conditions of inflammation, due to a gluten-specific T-cell response in the lamina propria, the normal clearance of such complexes may be affected. Transport of such complexes over the epithelium, for example by dendritic cells monitoring the luminal content, would result in a wider availability of T-cell-stimulatory peptides in the lamina propria and thus enhance the inflammation. Although at present merely a hypothesis, such mechanisms would explain the observed effects of the p31–43 peptide. Moreover, this can be experimentally addressed.

Innate Events Required for Breaking Tolerance

While the recent work described above has demonstrated that a gluten-specific T-cell response is a crucial factor in CD development, it does not explain why only a small percentage of HLA-DQ2/8-positive individuals develop CD. What is pushing one individual over the edge while the other remains healthy? That question is unanswered but there are a number of interesting clues. One is that it is highly unlikely that an adaptive response to gluten can develop in the absence of innate immune activation. Another is that it appears that CD can develop at any age: more than 50% of diagnosed cases concern adults. Some of those may have had CD for a long time but many have led a normal life until symptoms developed. This either indicates development of CD at a much later age or worsening of (subclinical) symptoms leading to eventual diagnosis. One may thus say that some patients fail to establish tolerance to gluten – these are patients that develop CD upon gluten introduction into the diet – while others fail to maintain tolerance to gluten at a later age. Are these really two different processes or one and the same, only at different points in time?

It is clear that gluten is highly immunogenic, especially in the context of HLA-DQ2. In the intestine, however, food antigens are either ignored or responses to them are highly regulated in order to avoid deleterious reactions. Nevertheless, when pathogens gain access to the mucosa, local immune responses are required to clear the invaders. A primary effect of the infection will be the activation of the innate immune system, followed by an adaptive, pathogen-specific response. Given the immunogenic nature of gluten, and its virtual continuous presence, it is entirely feasible that under such conditions a local gluten-specific

T-cell-response may develop. Importantly, local inflammation would lead to IFN-γ production, and this is known to increase the expression of HLA molecules, including HLA-DQ, and thus increase the likelihood of the formation of HLA-DQ-gluten complexes. Depending on the duration and severity of the infection, the magnitude of the gluten-specific T-cell response may vary. In some instances it may become so strong that it can no longer be regulated upon eradication of the pathogen. Depending of the age this occurs, CD would develop in childhood or in adulthood. Another possibility is that in other instances the response is much weaker and can be controlled. Some memory T cells, however, may remain that can be reactivated upon a second insult, generating a larger pool of gluten-specific memory cells. When this pool slowly expands due to repeated (minor) insults, this could also lead to CD development at a later age.

In this scenario gluten-independent activation of the innate immune system facilitates the development of a gluten-specific adaptive response. While it is clear that CD development is also influenced by other factors, like the presence or absence of predisposing gene variants other than HLA-DQ, the above scenario would explain the development of CD upon IFN-α treatment in several patients [27–29]. It would also mean that any endogenous danger signal could potentially lead to CD development. Large and carefully executed multicenter studies will be required to test this hypothesis.

Concluding Remarks

CD is one of the best understood HLA-associated diseases. Through enzymatic modification a series of gluten peptides is generated that can bind to the disease predisposing HLA-DQ2 or -DQ8 molecules and trigger inflammatory T-cell responses. The challenge ahead is to understand which factors trigger disease in only a small subset of HLA-DQ2/8-positive individuals and determine disease severity and age of onset.

References

1 Sollid LM, Markussen G, Ek J, Gjerde H, Vartdal F, Thorsby E: Evidence for a primary association of coeliac disease to a particular HLA-DQ alpha/beta heterodimer. J Exp Med 1989;169: 345–350.

2 Spurkland A, Ingvarsson G, Falk ES, Knutsen I, Sollid LM, Thorsby E: Dermatitis herpetiformis and celiac disease are both primarily associated with the HLA-DQ (alpha 1*0501, beta 1*02) or the HLA-DQ (alpha 1*03, beta 1*0302) heterodimers. Tissue Antigens 1997;49:29–34.

3 Lundin KE, Scott H, Hansen T, Paulsen G, Halstensen TS, Fausa O, Thorsby E, Sollid LM: Gliadin-specific, HLA-DQ(α1*0501,β1*0201) restricted T cells isolated from the small intestinal mucosa of celiac disease patients. J Exp Med 1993;178:187–196.

4 van de Wal Y, Kooy Y, van Veelen P, Pena S, Mearin L, Molberg Ø, Lundin L, Mutis T, Benckhuijsen W, Drijfhout JW, Koning F: Small intestinal cells of celiac disease patients recognize a natural pepsin fragment of gliadin. Proc Natl Acad Sci USA 1998;95:10050–10054.

5 Sjostrom H, Lundin KEA, Molberg Ø, Korner R, McAdam S, Anthonsen D, Quarsten H, Noren O, Roepstorff P, Thorsby E, Sollid LM: Identification of a gliadin T cell epitope in coeliac disease: general importance of gliadin deamidation for intestinal T cell recognition. Scand J Immunol 1998;48:111–115.

6 van de Wal Y, Kooy YMC, van Veelen P, August SA, Drijfhout JW, Koning F: Glutenin is involved in the gluten-driven mucosal T cell response. Eur J Immunol 2000;29:3133–3139.

7 Arentz-Hansen H, Körner R, Molberg Ø, Quarsten H, Vader W, Kooy YMC, Lundin KEA, Koning F, Roepstorff P, Sollid LM, McAdam S: The intestinal T cell response to α-gliadin in adult celiac disease is focused on a single deamidated glutamine targeted by tissue transglutaminase. J Exp Med 2000; 191:603–612.

8 Anderson RP, Degano P, Godkin AJ, Jewell DP, Hill AV: In vivo antigen challenge in celiac disease identifies a single transglutaminase-modified peptide as the dominant A-gliadin T-cell epitope. Nat Med 2000;6:337–342.

9 Vader W, Kooy Y, van Veelen P, de Ru A, Harris D, Benckhuijsen W, Pena S, Mearin L, Drijfhout JW, Koning F: The gluten response in children with recent onset celiac disease: a highly diverse response towards multiple gliadin and glutenin derived peptides. Gastroenterology 2002;122:1729–1737.

10 Shan L, Molberg Ø, Parrot I, Hausch F, Filiz F, Gray GM, Sollid LM, Khosla C: Structural basis for gluten intolerance in celiac sprue. Science 2002;297: 2275–2279.
11 van de Wal Y, Kooy YMC, Drijfhout JW, Amons R, Koning F: Peptide binding characteristics of the coeliac disease-associated DQ(α1*0501,β1*0201) molecule. Immunogenetics 1996;44: 246–253.
12 Johansen BH, Vartdal F, Eriksen JA, Thorsby E, Sollid LM: Identification of a putative motif for binding of peptides to HLA-DQ2. Int Immunol 1996;8: 177–182.
13 Kwok WW, Domeier ME, Raymond FC, Byers P, Nepom GT: Allele-specific motifs characterize HLA-DQ interactions with a diabetes-associated peptide derived from glutamic acid decarboxylase. J Immunol 1996;156:2171–2177.
14 Molberg Ø, McAdam S, Körner R, Quarsten H, Kristiansen C, Madsen L, Fugger L, Scott H, Norén O, Roepstorff P, Lundin KEA, Sjöström H, Sollid LM: Tissue transglutaminase selectively modifies gliadin peptides that are recognized by gut derived T cells in celiac disease. Nat Med 1998;4:713–717.
15 van de Wal Y, Kooy YMC, van Veelen P, Peña AS, Mearin ML, Papadopoulos GK, Koning F: Selective deamidation by tissue transglutaminase strongly enhances gliadin-specific T cell reactivity. J Immunol 1998;161:1585–1588.
16 Vader W, de Ru A, van de Wal Y, Kooy Y, Benckhuijsen W, Mearin L, Drijfhout JW, van Veelen P, Koning F: Specificity of tissue transglutaminase explains cereal toxicity in celiac disease. J Exp Med 2002;195:643–649.
17 Mearin ML, Biemond I, Pena A., Polanco I, Vazquez C, Schreuder GT, de Vries RR, van Rood JJ: HLA-DR phenotypes in Spanish coeliac children: their contribution to the understanding of the genetics of the disease. Gut 1983;24:532–537.
18 Vader W, Stepniak D, Kooy Y, Mearin ML, Thompson A, Spaenij L, Koning F: The HLA-DQ2 gene dose effect in celiac disease is directly related to the magnitude and breadth of gluten-specific T-cell responses. Proc Natl Acad Sci USA 2003;100:12390–12395.
19 Shan L, Qiao SW, Arentz-Hansen H, Molberg O, Gray GM, Sollid LM, Khosla C: Identification and analysis of multivalent proteolytically resistant peptides from gluten: implications for celiac sprue. J Proteome Res 2005;4:1732–1741.
20 Vader W, Stepniak D, Bunnik EM, Kooy Y, de Haan W, Drijfhout JW, van Veelen PA, Koning F: Characterization of cereal toxicity for celiac disease patients based on protein homology in grains. Gastroenterology 2003;125: 1105–1113.
21 Janatuinen EK, Pikkarainen PH, Kemppainen TA, Kosma V-M, Järvinen RMK, Uusitupa MIJ, Julkunen RJK: A comparison of diets with and without oats in adults with celiac disease. N Engl J Med 1995;333:1033–1037.
22 Maiuri L, Ciacci C, Ricciardelli I, Vacca L, Raia V, Auricchio S, Picard J, Osman M, Quaratino S, Londei M: Association between innate response to gliadin and activation of pathogenic T cells in coeliac disease. Lancet 2003;362:30–37.
23 Maiuri L, Ciacci C, Auricchio S, Brown V, Quaratino S, Londei M: Interleukin 15 mediates epithelial changes in celiac disease. Gastroenterology 2000;119: 996–1006.
24 Hüe S, Mention J-J, Monteiro RC, Zhang SL, Cellier C, Schmitz J, Verkarre V, Fodil N, Bahram S, Cerf-Bensussan N, Caillat-Zucman S: A direct role for NKG2D/MICA interaction in villous atrophy during celiac disease. Immunity 2004;21:367–377.
25 Meresse B, Chen Z, Ciszewski C, Tretiakova M, Bhagat G, Krausz TN, Raulet DH, Lanier LL, Groh V, Spies T, Ebert EC, Green PH, Jabri B: Coordinated induction by IL15 of a TCR-independent NKG2D signaling pathway converts CTL into lymphokine-activated killer cells in celiac disease. Immunity 2004;21:357–366.
26 ten Dam M, van de Wal Y, Mearin ML, Kooy Y, Pena S, Drijfhout JW, Koning F, van Tol M: Anti-alpha-gliadin antibodies (AGA) in the serum of coeliac children and controls recognize an identical collection of linear epitopes of alpha-gliadin. Clin Exp Immunol 1998;114:189–195.
27 Bardella MT, Marino R, Meroni PL: Celiac disease during interferon treatment. Ann Intern Med 1999;131: 157–158.
28 Cammarota G, Cuoco L, Cianci R, Pandolfi F, Gasbarrini G: Onset of coeliac disease during treatment with interferon for chronic hepatitis C. Lancet 2000;356:1494–1495.
29 Monteleone G, Pender SLF, Alstead E, Hauer AC, Lionetti P, MacDonald TT: Role of interferon in promoting T helper cell type 1 responses in the small intestine in coeliac disease. Gut 2001;48:425–429.

Frits Koning, PhD
Department of Immunohematology and Blood Transfusion
Leiden University Medical Center, E3–Q
PO Box 9600
NL–2300 RC Leiden (The Netherlands)
Tel. +31 71 526 3827, Fax +31 71 526 5267, E-Mail f.koning@lumc.nl

Fasano A, Troncone R, Branski D (eds): Frontiers in Celiac Disease.
Pediatr Adolesc Med. Basel, Karger, 2008, vol 12, pp 89–98

The Role of the Intestinal Barrier Function in the Pathogenesis of Celiac Disease

Alessio Fasano[a] · Joerg D. Schulzke[b]

[a]Center for Celiac Research and Mucosal Biology Research Center, University of Maryland School of Medicine, Baltimore, Md., USA; [b]Medizinische Klinik I, Charité-Campus Benjamin Franklin, Berlin, Germany

Abstract

The primary functions of the gastrointestinal (GI) tract have traditionally been perceived to be limited to the digestion and absorption of nutrients and electrolytes, and to water homeostasis. A more attentive analysis of the anatomic and functional arrangement of the GI tract however suggests that another extremely important function of this organ is its ability to regulate the trafficking of macromolecules between the environment and the host through a barrier mechanism. The intestinal epithelial barrier controls the equilibrium between tolerance and immunity to non-self-antigens by regulating antigen trafficking both through the transcellular and paracellular pathways. When the finely tuned trafficking of macromolecules is deregulated in genetically susceptible individuals, autoimmune disorders can occur. Celiac disease is characterized by loss of intestinal barrier functions, and evidence is now accumulating suggesting a role of increased intestinal permeability in the early steps of the disease pathogenesis. This new paradigm subverts traditional theories underlying the development of autoimmunity, which are based on molecular mimicry and/or the bystander effect, and suggests that the celiac disease autoimmune process can be arrested if the interplay between genes and environmental triggers is prevented by reestablishing intestinal barrier function. Understanding the role of the intestinal barrier in the pathogenesis of celiac disease is an area of translational research that encompasses many fields and is currently receiving a great deal of attention. This chapter reviews the recent advance in intestinal mucosal biology involved in gliadin trafficking and possible alternative therapeutic approaches to correct the barrier defect typical of celiac disease.

The intestinal epithelium is the largest mucosal surface providing an interface between the external environment and the mammalian host, and its permeability depends on the regulation of intercellular tight junctions (TJs) as well as on the activity of transcellular transport via endocytosis. A century ago, TJs were conceptualized as secreted extracellular cement forming an absolute and unregulated barrier within the paracellular space. The contribution of the paracellular pathway of the gastrointestinal (GI) tract to the general economy of molecule trafficking between environment and host was therefore judged to be negligible. It is now apparent that TJs are extremely dynamic structures involved in developmental, physiological and pathological circumstances. Recently, particular attention has been placed on the role of TJ dysfunction in the pathogenesis of several diseases, particularly autoimmune diseases.

The Paracellular Pathway

The epithelial barrier function of the intestine is a complex result of numerous features acting in concert to tighten the mucosa against the unwanted entry of luminal noxious antigens and to prevent the loss of ions, water and other serum components from the circulation to the intestinal lumen. The main structure of this barrier function is the apical membrane of enterocytes connected to each other by a continuous network of TJs which tightens the lateral intercellular space between neighboring cells. Thus, the epithelial barrier can be differentiated into a trans- and paracellular pathway component. While in tighter epithelia like the large intestine (passive) transcellular transport accounts for almost the overall permeability of ions, leaky epithelia as the small intestine are characterized by a highly conductive paracellular pathway with a conductance contribution being higher than that of the transcellular pathway [1]. In addition, several other epithelial properties like mucus and glycocalyx covering the apical surface contribute to barrier function.

Depending on the specific intestinal segment under consideration, antigen uptake may depend upon other specialized structures/cells, such as M cells above Peyer's patches in the ileum. Whether or not epithelial apoptosis significantly contributes to the overall paracellular permeability is still a matter of debate. At least in semitight epithelia like the colon, a significant contribution has been directly shown by conductance scanning measurements [2]. In the colon, upregulation of the apoptotic rate to 12% changes the epithelium from a semitight to a leaky one [3].

Another barrier property which has only recently gained more attention is the transcellular uptake of antigens by endocytosis and subsequent transcytotic transport through the enterocytes to the basolateral compartment of the epithelium. This process is electrically silent and may be more relevant for the uptake of antigens than for the entry of ions (see detailed description below).

As far as the paracellular pathway is concerned, its permeability is mainly dependent on TJ competency, while the lateral intercellular space has only a limited contribution to the paracellular route [4].

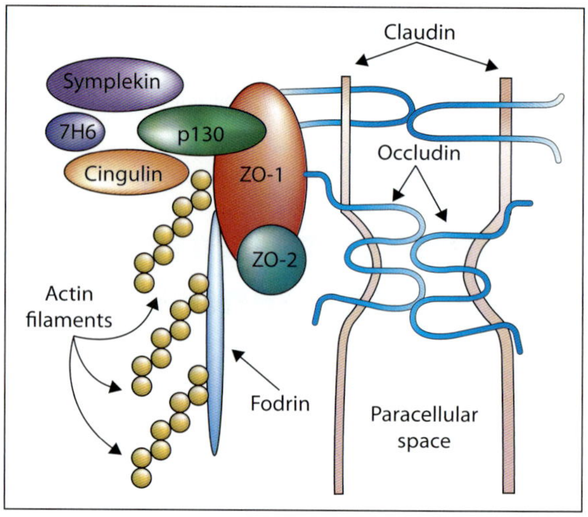

Fig. 1. Composition of intercellular TJs. The 3 key elements of intercellular TJs include: (1) the structural TJ proteins occludin and claudins, (2) the scaffold proteins ZO-1, ZO-2, fodrin, cingulin, symplekin, 7H6 and p130, and (3) the actin cytoskeleton.

Structure of Tight Junctions

Transmembrane TJ Proteins

To date, multiple proteins that make up the TJ strands have been identified (fig. 1) and include occludin [5] and members of the claudin family [6], a group of at least 20 tissue-specific proteins. The junctional adhesion molecule, a protein belonging to the immunoglobulin superfamily, has been described as an additional component of the TJ fibrils [7]. Junctional adhesion molecule reportedly binds to zonula occludin (ZO)-1, so aiding ZO-1 localization to the junctional complex [8]. Occludin cDNA analysis revealed that the predicted 504-amino-acid polypeptide (65 kDa) contains 4 transmembrane spanning domains with 2 extracellular loops and internal NH_2– and COOH– termini. Occludin expression levels and its distribution correlate with the number of TJ strands in a variety of epithelia [9]. The claudins are 20- to 27-kDa proteins that each contain 2 extracellular loops with variably charged amino acid residues among family members and short intracellular tails [9].

Cytoplasmic TJ Plaque Proteins

The cytoplasmic plaque of TJs includes multiple proteins that have been characterized at the molecular level, and several others that await further characterization. By interacting with each other and with cytoskeletal proteins, these scaffold elements (ZO-1, ZO-2, ZO-3, ZO-1-associated protein kinase) functionally couple integral membrane TJ proteins to actin microfilaments [10]. TJ plaque proteins also appear to be direct targets and effectors of different signaling pathways. The first described and best-characterized TJ plaque component is ZO-1, a 225-kDa multidomain protein. ZO-1 and ZO-2 associate with each other in heterodimers [6] in a detergent-stable complex with an uncharacterized 130-kDa protein (ZO-3). Most immunoelectron-microscopic studies have localized ZO-1 precisely beneath membrane contacts [11]. A number of TJ plaque proteins, including ZO-1 and ZO-2, possess one or more approximately 90-amino-acid PDZ domains that mediate protein-protein interactions with other PDZ-containing proteins (see below). These PDZ-containing proteins belong to the membrane-associated guanylate kinase family of proteins [12]. Several other peripheral membrane proteins have been localized to the TJ, including 7H6 [9], Rab 13 and 3b [13], $G\alpha_{i-2}$ [13, 14], protein kinase C [15], symplekin [16] and cingulin [17].

The Actin Cytoskeleton

To meet the many diverse physiological and pathological challenges to which epithelia are subjected, the TJ must be capable of rapid and coordinate responses that require the presence of a complex regulatory system. There is now a large body of evidence suggesting that structural and functional linkage exists between the actin cytoskeleton and the TJ complex of absorptive cells [18–20]. The actin cytoskeleton is composed of a complicated meshwork of microfilaments whose precise geometry is regulated by a large cadre of actin-binding proteins. The architecture of the peripheral actin cytoskeleton strategically localized to regulate the paracellular pathway appears to be critical for TJ function. Most of the peripheral actin is positioned under the apical junctional complex where myosin II and several actin-binding proteins, including α-catenin, vinculin, radixin and cingulin, have been identified [21].

The Transcellular Pathway

Another important route for antigens to cross the epithelium is transcellular uptake by transcytosis [22, 23]. Costaining experiments of endocytotic vesicle compartments have shown evidence for apical endocytosis being an initial step in transcytosis (fig. 2) [24]. However, little is known about the postendocytosis antigen modifications and release into the basolateral compartment. Finally, limited information is available on the regulation of transcytosis by proinflammatory signals; however, TNF-α and IFN-γ have been reported to have a stimulatory influence [25, 26].

Intestinal Permeability and Its Regulation

Specific regulation of the epithelial barrier function has been described via changes in epithelial TJ structure and function which has been shown to be relevant in intestinal inflammation and celiac disease [27–29]. Much work has been generated during the last decade to explain the mechanisms contributing to TJ disruption in response to proinflammatory cytokines like TNF-α and IFN-γ [30, 31] which are elevated in celiac disease. In acute sprue stages as Marsh IIIc, TJ strand architecture is altered in freeze fracture electron microscopy as a direct correlate of the barrier impairment [32]. A similar pattern and extent of TJ changes is also observed in epithelial

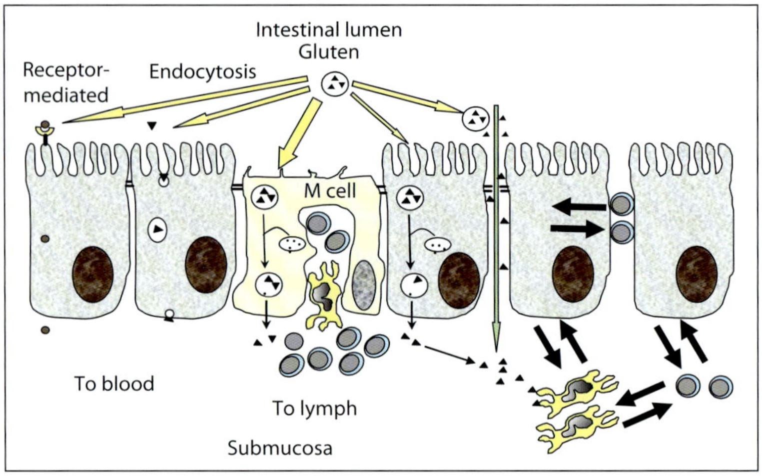

Fig. 2. Main pathways for the passage of macromolecules through the intestinal barrier. Intact macromolecules can be absorbed either via the transcellular or paracellular pathway. For the transcellular pathway, macromolecule uptake occurs by endocytosis, followed by fusion with lysosomes (phagolysosomes) with possible degradation of the macromolecules before being delivered in the submucosa. Conversely, macromolecules crossing through the paracellular pathway reach the submucosa unmodified.

cell models like HT-29/B6 after exposure to TNF-α and/or IFN-γ [33]. This is the complex result of several regulatory influences on the cellular TJ domain which comprises transcriptional regulation as well as cleavage and redistribution of TJ proteins off TJ strands.

In T84 cells, IFN-γ has been shown to cause redistribution of occludin, claudin-1, claudin-4 and junctional adhesion molecule A from the TJ [34]. This redistribution depends on endocytosis of TJ proteins. In contrast to calcium removal inducing clathrin-dependent endocytosis of tight and adherens junction proteins into a subapical cytoplasmic compartment [35], TJ protein internalization in response to IFN-γ is due to macropinocytosis [36] and leads to the formation of a vacuolar apical compartment, which is the result of a myosin-II-mediated cytoskeleton contraction, since it can be prevented by inhibition of rho-associated protein kinase but not by myosin light chain kinase. This indicates that rho/rho-associated protein kinase signaling is the underlying mechanism [37]. This is corroborated by experimental evidence from Crohn's disease, where pharmacological inhibition of rho kinase is able to prevent inflammation via nuclear factor κB inhibition [38]. The TNF-α-induced increase in epithelial permeability was associated with a nuclear-factor-κB-dependent increase in both transcription and activation of myosin light chain kinase in Caco-2 monolayers [39, 40]. In addition, there is also experimental evidence in epithelial cell models for a NFκB-independent barrier effect of TNFα by transcriptional activation of myosin light chain kinase via TNF receptor II leading to cytoskeletal tight junction dysregulation [41].

In addition, also the expression of TJ proteins is affected by proinflammatory cytokines as expected from the findings in celiac disease patients described above. The reduction in electrical resistance as a measure of barrier function in intestinal epithelial HT-29/B6 cell monolayers was accompanied by a decrease in occludin-specific mRNA after TNF-α treatment. Reporter gene analysis of the human occludin promoter showed its downregulation by TNF-α and IFN-γ, suggesting transcriptional regulation [42]. Furthermore, the pore-forming TJ protein claudin-2 is upregulated by TNF-α in HT-29/B6 monolayers, which is consistent with elevated claudin-2 levels in patients with active celiac disease [unpubl. data]. In T84 cells, TNF-α leads to the appearance of a 10-kDa claudin-2-specific fragment

[43]. The regulatory effect of the Th2-cytokine IL-13 is characterized by an elevation of claudin-2 expression [44].

Classical and Novel Theories of Autoimmune Pathogenesis

Classical Models of Autoimmune Diseases

Autoimmune diseases are the third most common category of diseases in the USA after cancer and heart disease; they affect approximately 5–8% of the population or 14–22 million persons. They can affect virtually every site in the body, including the GI tract. At least 15 diseases are the direct result of an autoimmune response, while circumstantial evidence links >80 conditions with autoimmunity.

Soon after autoimmune diseases had first been recognized more than a century ago, researchers began to associate them with viral and bacterial infections. A mechanism often called on to explain the association of infection with autoimmune disease is 'molecular mimicry', whereby antigens (or more properly, epitopes) of the microorganism are postulated to closely resemble self-antigens [45]. The induction of an immune response to the microbial antigen results in a cross-reaction with self-antigens and induction of autoimmunity. Once the process is activated, the autoimmune response becomes independent of continuous exposure to the environmental trigger and, therefore, the process is self-perpetuating and irreversible. Epitope-specific cross-reactivity between microbes and self-tissues has been shown in some animal models. Conversely, molecular mimicry in most human autoimmune diseases seems to be a factor in the progression of a preexisting subclinical autoimmune response, rather than in the initiation of autoimmunity by breaking tolerance [46].

Another theory suggests that microorganisms expose self-antigens to the immune system by directly damaging tissues during active infection. This mechanism has been referred to as the 'bystander effect' and occurs only when the new antigen is presented with the originally fed antigen [47]. Whether pathogens mimic self-antigens, release sequestered self-antigens or both, however, remains to be elucidated.

Recently, increased hygiene and a lack of exposure to various microorganisms are proposed to be responsible for the 'epidemic' of autoimmune diseases that has occurred over the past 30–40 years in industrialized countries [48]. The essence of the 'hygiene hypothesis', a fairly new school of thought, argues that the rising incidence of immune-mediated (including autoimmune) diseases is due, at least in part, to lifestyle and environmental changes that have made us too 'clean'. This hypothesis is supported by immunological data showing that the response to microbial antigens may induce Th1 cytokine expression that offsets the T-helper-2-polarized cytokine production in neonates. In the absence of microbes, the gut may be conducive to an exaggerated IgE production, atopy and atopic disease. Alternately, the absence of helminth infections eliminates the normal upregulation of Th2 in childhood, culminating in a more Th1-prone immune environment characteristic of autoimmune and inflammatory diseases. Regardless of whether autoimmune diseases are due to too much, or too little, exposure to microorganisms, it is now generally believed that adaptive immunity and imbalance between Th1 and Th2 responses are the key elements of the pathogenesis of the autoimmune process. Unfortunately, decades of research focused on these assumptions have not led to solutions for these devastating clinical problems.

A Paradigm Shift in the Pathogenesis of Autoimmune Diseases Involving Intestinal Barrier Dysfunction

A common denominator of autoimmune diseases is the presence of several preexisting conditions leading to an autoimmune process. The first is a genetic susceptibility for the host immune system to recognize, and potentially misinterpret, an environmental antigen presented within the GI tract. Second, the host must be exposed to the antigen. Finally, the antigen must be presented to the GI mucosal immune system following its paracellular passage (normally prevented by the TJ competency) from the intestinal lumen to the gut submucosa [49, 50]. In many cases, increased permeability appears to precede disease and causes an abnormality in antigen delivery that triggers the multiorgan process leading to the autoimmune response [51].

Therefore, the following hypothesis can be formulated to explain the pathogenesis of autoimmune diseases that encompasses the following 3 key points:

(1) Autoimmune diseases involve a miscommunication between innate and adaptive immunity.
(2) Molecular mimicry or bystander effects alone may not explain entirely the complex events involved in the pathogenesis of autoimmune diseases. Rather, the continuous stimulation by non-self-antigens (environmental triggers) appears necessary to perpetuate the process. This concept implies that the autoimmune response can be theoretically stopped and perhaps reversed if the interplay between autoimmune predisposing genes and trigger(s) is prevented or eliminated.
(3) In addition to genetic predisposition and the exposure to the triggering non-self-antigen, the third key element necessary to develop autoimmunity is the loss of the protective function of mucosal barriers that interface with the environment (mainly the GI mucosa).

Celiac Disease as Clinical Outcome of Impaired Intestinal Permeability

Epithelial TJs are seriously damaged in the small intestine of celiac disease patients when analyzed by freeze fracture electron microscopy which is compatible with a loss of barrier function [52, 53]. In control jejunum, TJ strand parameters, including strand count and meshwork depth, decline towards a lower complexity along the surface-to-crypt axis. This finding supports the general view of a more leaky crypt epithelium and a tighter villous epithelium under physiological conditions [52]. In active celiac disease, TJ strand count and meshwork depth are diminished, and these changes are more pronounced at the surface compared to the crypt (40% strand reduction from 5.0 to 3.0 at surface TJ) [52] (fig. 3). Thus, the hyperregenerative transformed mucosa typical of celiac disease is characterized by an inverted gradient of the morphological equivalent of tightness with a tighter crypt epithelium and a more leaky surface epithelium. Functionally, this was accompanied by a decrease in epithelial resistance as obtained by impedance spectroscopy from 20 $\pm$ 2 in control to 9 $\pm$ 1 $\Omega\cdot cm^2$ in active celiac disease [54]. This type of TJ change in celiac disease is specific for the sprue mucosa and is not secondary to diarrhea per se or to the hyperregenerative mucosal transformation, since it was not observed in the blind loop syndrome [55]. Furthermore, strand discontinuities were more frequent in celiac disease. While these structural changes are considered to be less

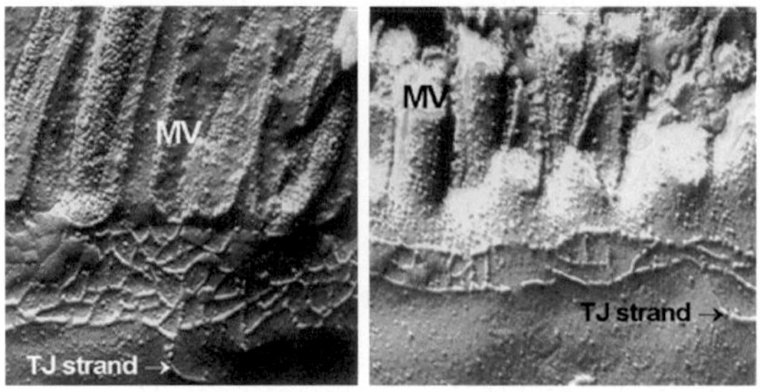

Control jejunum Celiac sprue

Fig. 3. TJ from the lower villus region of control jejunum and from the surface epithelium of acute celiac sprue. All electron micrographs are oriented so that microvilli (MV) are seen at the top. Magnification $\times$70,000.

important for ions, they enable the paracellular passage of macromolecules like gliadin which normally do not cross the epithelial barrier. Thus, strand discontinuities are a structural feature fitting the '2-stage model' criteria proposed by O'Mahony et al. [56]. Not everyone genetically predisposed to celiac disease is necessarily ill. Once the intestinal barrier is impaired, e.g. as the result of a GI infection, gliadin and its cleavage products can reach the submucosa and induce an immune response, leading to acute celiac disease. Subsequently, due to the inflammatory response, barrier function remains seriously impaired allowing gliadin in a vicious circle to be further taken up. This '2-stage model' gives an idea why patients can later on be without any symptoms, even when accidentally or purposely exposed to gluten. Taken together, these data suggest that the TJ defect in acute celiac disease is an important structural feature permitting increased passage of antigens including gluten into the submucosa.

Under gluten-free conditions, TJ parameters return to control values at the top of the villi, while strand counts are still slightly diminished in crypts [52]. Since the crypt base is the most conductive site along the surface-crypt axis, a decrease in TJ complexity is functionally most important at this location. However, symptom alleviation in celiac disease under gluten-free conditions stresses the importance of the restoration of strand discontinuities and of villous TJ properties in spite of the still altered crypt properties. In impedance spectroscopy, epithelial resistance was 20 ± 2 (control), 9 ± 1 (active celiac sprue) and 15 ± 1 $\Omega\cdot cm^2$ (gluten-free). Thus, the alteration in TJ structure towards a lower TJ complexity in celiac disease was paralleled by a decrease in epithelial resistance of 56% in patients during the acute phase of celiac disease and of 23% in patients on a gluten-free diet [54]. Thus, in patients on a gluten-free diet recovery was not complete, both morphologically and functionally. However, if these changes are related to a primary barrier defect or to 'minimal changes' secondary to exposure to traces of gluten (gluten cross-contamination) remains to be established.

So far, a molecular analysis of the TJ strands in celiac disease has not been performed. Preliminary analysis of immunoblot data suggests an upregulation of claudin-2, a pore-forming TJ protein, and a downregulation of claudin-4 [J.D. Schulzke, unpubl. data]. However, final data including TJ protein distribution studies by immunofluorescence microscopy are still urgently awaited.

So far direct experimental evidence for endocytosis to contribute to gliadin uptake in celiac disease is rather limited. Zimmer et al. [57, 58] have performed two studies based on electron microscopy, where gliadin was detected within the epithelial cells. With colocalization strategies to identify the intracellular route we found colocalization with rab5-green fluorescent protein in apical as well as basal early endosomes, where it regulates the fusion of clathrin-coated pits with early endosomes [24].

On the basis of these findings mucosal antigen uptake in acute celiac disease does most likely occur via both the transcellular and paracellular pathways. It is possible that during moderate activity of celiac disease transcytosis is the predominating route of antigen entry. Alternatively, minimal TJ alterations persisting under a gluten-free diet could also represent initial paracellular leaks in this respect. In more pronounced stages of celiac disease however, paracellular leakiness will most likely more and more overrule the transcellular uptake.

Correction of Intestinal Barrier Dysfunction as a Possible Alternative Treatment for Celiac Disease

If the postulated role of the intestinal barrier dysfunction in autoimmune pathogenesis is accepted, it is conceivable to hypothesize therapeutic regimens as an alternative to a gluten-free diet for the treatment of celiac disease. Zonulin inhibitors that would prevent the gliadin-induced, zonulin-mediated loss of intestinal barrier function could represent a potential therapeutic strategy. This approach has been extensively covered in the chapter by Paterson and Turner [this vol., pp. 157–171] and, therefore, it will not be further discussed here. The demonstration that celiac disease is characterized by impaired intestinal barrier function has introduced the concept of probiotic therapy: therapeutic application of potentially beneficial microorganisms, which act as probiotics. Probiotics have been postulated to exert several beneficial effects on gut mucosa, including the normalization of increased intestinal permeability [59–61].

Conclusions

The classical paradigm of autoimmune pathogenesis involving specific gene makeup and exposure to environmental triggers has recently been challenged by the addition of a third element, the loss of intestinal barrier function. Genetic predisposition, miscommunication between innate and adaptive immunity, exposure to environmental triggers and loss of the intestinal barrier function secondary to dysfunction of intercellular TJs seem to be all key ingredients involved in the pathogenesis of autoimmune diseases. This new theory implies that once the autoimmune process is activated, it is not autoperpetuating, rather can be modulated or even reversed by preventing the continuous interplay between genes and environment. Celiac disease represents a clinical model of this new paradigm. Indeed, removal of 1 (the environmental trigger gluten) of the 3 elements necessary for the autoimmune insult results in a complete resolution of the disease. Since TJ dysfunction allows the interaction between genes and environment, therapeutic strategies aimed at reestablishing the intestinal barrier function could offer alternative innovative, unexplored approaches for the treatment of celiac disease and, possibly, other autoimmune diseases in which intestinal barrier dysfunction has been demonstrated or hypothesized.

References

1 Boulpaep EL, Sackin H: Electrical analysis of intraepithelial barriers; in Bronner F, Kleinzeller A, Boulpaep EL (eds): Current Topics in Membranes and Transport. New York, Academic Press, 1980, vol 13, pp 169–197.

2 Gitter AH, Bendfeldt K, Schulzke JD, Fromm M: Leaks in the epithelial barrier caused by spontaneous and TNF-induced single-cell apoptosis. FASEB J 2000;14:1749–1753.

3 Bojarski C, Gitter AH, Bendfeldt K, Mankertz J, Schmitz H, Wagner S, Fromm M, Schulzke JD: Permeability of HT-29/B6 colonic epithelium as a function of apoptosis. J Physiol (Lond) 2001;535:541–552.

4 Kottra G, Fromter E: Tight-junction tightness of Necturus gall bladder epithelium is not regulated by cAMP or intracellular Ca^{2+}. II. Impedance measurements. Pflugers Arch 1993;425: 535–545.

5 Furuse M, Hirase M, Itoh M, Nagafuchi A, Yonemura S, Tsukita S, Tsukita S: Occludin: a novel integral membrane protein localizing at tight junctions. J Cell Biol 1993;123:1777–1788.

6 Furuse Mikio FK, Hiiragi T, Fujimoto K, Tsukita S: Claudin-1 and -2: novel integral membrane proteins localizing at tight junctions with no sequence similarity to occludin. J Cell Biol 1998; 141:1539–1550.

7 Martin-Padura I, Lostgalio S, Schneemann M, Williams L, Romano M, Fruscella P, Panzeri C, Stoppacciaro A, Ruco L, Vill A, Simmons D, Dejana E: Junctional adhesion molecule, a novel member of the immunoglobulin superfamily that distributes at intercellular junctions and modulates monocyte transmigration. J Biol Chem 1998;142:117–127.

8 Bazzoni G, Martinez-Estrada O, Orsenigo F, Cordenonsi M, Citi S, Dejana E: Interaction of junctional adhesion molecule with the tight junction components, ZO-1, cingulin, and occludin. J Biol Chem 2000;275:20520–20526.

9 Mitic LL, Van Itallie CM: Occludin and claudins: transmembrane proteins of the tight junction; in Cereijido M, Anderson JM (eds).Tight Junctions. Boca Raton, CRC Press, 2001, pp 213–230.

10 Citi S: The cytoplasmic plaque proteins of the tight junction; in Cereijido M, Anderson JM (eds): Tight Junctions. Boca Raton, CRC Press, 2001, pp 231–264.
11 Stevenson BR, Anderson JM, Bullivant S: The epithelial tight junction: structure, function and preliminary biochemical characterization. Mol Cell Biochem 1988;83:129–145.
12 Anderson JM: Cell signalling: MAGUK magic. Curr Biol 1996;6:382–384.
13 Zahraoui A, Joberty G, Arpin M, Fontaine JJ, Hellio R, Tavitian A, Louvard D: A small rab GTPase is distributed in cytoplasmic vesicles in nonpolarized cells but colocalized with the tight junction marker Zo-1 in polarized epithelial cells. J Cell Biol 1994; 124:101–115.
14 Denker BM, Saha C, Khawaja S, Nigam SK: Involvement of a heterotrimeric G protein a subunit in tight junction biogenesis. J Biol Chem 1996;271: 25750–25753.
15 Dodane V, Kachar B: Identification of isoforms of G proteins and PKC that colocalize with tight junctions. J Membr Biol 1996;149:199–209.
16 Keon BH, Schafer S, Kuhn C, Grund C, Franke WW: Symplekin, a novel type of tight junction plaque protein. J Cell Biol 1996;134:1003–1018.
17 Citi S, Sabannay H, Jakes R, Geiger B, Kendrich-Jones J: Cingulin, a new peripheral component of tight junctions. Nature (Lond) 1988;333:272–275.
18 Gumbiner B: Structure, biochemistry, and assembly of epithelial tight junctions. Am J Physiol 1987;253:C749–C758.
19 Madara JL, Barenberg D, Carlson S: Effects of cytochalasin D on occluding junctions of intestinal absorptive cells: further evidence that the cytoskeleton may influence paracellular permeability and junctional charge selectivity. J Cell Biol 1986;102:2125–2136.
20 Aijaz S, Balda MS, Matter K: Tight junctions: molecular architecture and function. Int Rev Cytol 2006;248:261–298.
21 Hecht F, et al: Expression of the catalytic domain of myosin light chain kinase increases paracellular permeability. Am J Physiol 1996;271:C1678–C1684.
22 Heyman M, Crain-Denoyelle AM, Desjeux JF: Endocytosis and processing of protein by isolated villus and crypt cells of the mouse small intestine. J Pediatr Gastroenterol Nutr 1989; 9:238–245.
23 Soderholm JD, Peterson KH, Olaison G, Franzen LE, Westrom B, Magnusson KE, Sjodahl R: Epithelial permeability to proteins in the noninflamed ileum of Crohn's disease? Gastroenterology 1999;117:65–72.
24 Schumann M, Richter JF, Wedell I, Moos V, Zimmermann-Kordmann M, Schneider T, Daum S, Zeitz M, Fromm M, Schulzke JD: Mechanisms of epithelial translocation of the alpha-2-gliadin-33mer in celiac sprue. Gut 2008, E-pub ahead of print.
25 Soderholm JD, Streutker C, Yang PC, Paterson C, Singh PK, McKay DM, Sherman PM, Croitoru K, Perdue MH: Increased epithelial uptake of protein antigens in the ileum of Crohn's disease mediated by tumour necrosis factor alpha. Gut 2004;53:1817–1824.
26 Terpend K, Boisgerault F, Blaton MA, Desjeux JF, Heyman M: Protein transport and processing by human HT29-19A intestinal cells: effect of IFN-γ. Gut 1998;42:538–545.
27 Bruewer M, Samarin S, Nusrat A: Inflammatory bowel disease and the apical junctional complex. Ann NY Acad Sci 2006;1072:242–252.
28 Clayburgh DR, Shen L, Turner JR: A porous defense: the leaky epithelial barrier in intestinal disease. Lab Invest 2004;84:282–291.
29 Laukoetter MG, Bruewer M, Nusrat A: Regulation of the intestinal epithelial barrier by the apical junctional complex. Curr Opin Gastroenterol 2006;22:85–89.
30 Hollander D: Crohn's disease, TNF-alpha, and the leaky gut: the chicken or the egg? Am J Gastroenterol 2002;97: 1867–1868.
31 Chiba H, Kojima T, Osanai M, Sawada N: The significance of IFN-γ-triggered internalization of tight-junction proteins in inflammatory bowel disease. Sci STKE 2006;2006:pe1.
32 Schulzke JD, Schulzke I, Fromm M, Riecken EO: Epithelial barrier and ion transport in coeliac sprue: electrical measurements on intestinal aspiration biopsy specimens. Gut 1995;37:777–782.
33 Schmitz H, Fromm M, Bentzel CJ, et al: Tumor necrosis factor-alpha (TNFalpha) regulates the epithelial barrier in the human intestinal cell line HT-29/B6. J Cell Sci 1999;112:137–146.
34 Bruewer M, Luegering A, Kucharzik T, et al: Proinflammatory cytokines disrupt epithelial barrier function by apoptosis-independent mechanisms. J Immunol 2003;171:6164–6172.
35 Ivanov AI, Nusrat A, Parkos CA: Endocytosis of epithelial apical junctional proteins by a clathrin-mediated pathway into a unique storage compartment. Mol Biol Cell 2004;15: 176–188.
36 Bruewer M, Utech M, Ivanov AI, et al: Interferon-γ induces internalization of epithelial tight junction proteins via a macropinocytosis-like process. Faseb J 2005;19:923–933.
37 Utech M, Ivanov AI, Samarin SN, et al: Mechanism of IFN-gamma-induced endocytosis of tight junction proteins: myosin II-dependent vacuolarization of the apical plasma membrane. Mol Biol Cell 2005;16:5040–5052.
38 Segain JP, Raingeard de la Bletiere D, Sauzeau V, et al: Rho kinase blockade prevents inflammation via nuclear factor kappa B inhibition: evidence in Crohn's disease and experimental colitis. Gastroenterology 2003;124:1180–1187.
39 Ma TY, Boivin MA, Ye D, et al: Mechanism of TNF-α modulation of Caco-2 intestinal epithelial tight junction barrier: role of myosin light-chain kinase protein expression. Am J Physiol Gastrointest Liver Physiol 2005; 288:G422–G430.
40 Ye D, Ma I, Ma TY: Molecular mechanism of tumor necrosis factor-alpha modulation of intestinal epithelial tight junction barrier. Am J Physiol Gastrointest Liver Physiol 2006;290: G496–G504.
41 Wang F, Schwarz BT, Graham WV, Wang Y, Su L, Clayburgh DR, Abraham C, Turner JR: IFN-γ-induced TNFR2 expression is required for TNF-dependent intestinal epithelial barrier dysfunction. Gastroenterology 2006;131: 1153–1163.
42 Mankertz J, Tavalali S, Schmitz H, et al: Expression from the human occludin promoter is affected by tumor necrosis factor alpha and interferon gamma. J Cell Sci 2000;113:2085–2090.
43 Willemsen LE, Hoetjes JP, van Deventer SJ, van Tol EA: Abrogation of IFN-gamma mediated epithelial barrier disruption by serine protease inhibition. Clin Exp Immunol 2005;142: 275–284.
44 Heller F, Florian P, Bojarski C, et al: Interleukin-13 is the key effector Th2 cytokine in ulcerative colitis that affects epithelial tight junctions, apoptosis, and cell restitution. Gastroenterology 2005; 129:550–564.

45 Perl A: Pathogenesis and spectrum of autoimmunity. Methods Mol Med 2004; 102:1–8.
46 Christen U, von Herrath MG: Induction, acceleration or prevention of autoimmunity by molecular mimicry. Mol Immunol 2004;40:1113–1120.
47 Miller A, Lider O, Weiner HL: Antigen-driven bystander suppression after oral administration of antigens. J Exp Med 1991;174:791–798.
48 Rook GA, Brunet LR: Microbes, immunoregulation, and the gut. Gut 2005;54:317–320.
49 Bjarnason I, et al: The G.U.T. of gut. Scand J Gastroenterol 2004;39:807–815.
50 Wendling D: Role of the intestine in the physiopathology of inflammatory rheumatism. Rev Rhum Mal Osteoartic 1992;59:389–392.
51 Watts T, et al: Role of the intestinal tight junction modulator zonulin in the pathogenesis of type I diabetes in BB diabetic-prone rats. Proc Natl Acad Sci USA 2005;102:2916–2921.
52 Schulzke JD, Bentzel CJ, Schulzke I, Riecken EO, Fromm M: Epithelial tight junction structure in the jejunum of children with acute and treated celiac sprue. Pediatr Res 1998;43:435–441.
53 Madara JL, Trier JS: Structural abnormalities of jejunal epithelial cell membranes in celiac sprue. Lab Invest 1980;43:254–261.
54 Schulzke JD, Schulzke I, Fromm M, Riecken EO: Epithelial barrier and ion transport in coeliac sprue: electrical measurements on intestinal aspiration biopsy specimens. Gut 1995;37:777–782.
55 Schulzke JD, Fromm M, Menge H, Riecken EO: Impaired intestinal Na- and Cl-transport in the blind loop syndrome of the rat. Gastroenterology 1987;92:693–698.
56 O'Mahony S, Vestey JP, Ferguson A: Similarities in intestinal humoral immunity in dermatitis herpetiformis without enteropathy and in coeliac disease. Lancet 1990;335:1487–1490.
57 Zimmer KP, Poremba C, Weber P, Ciclitira PJ, Harms E: Translocation of gliadin into HLA-DR antigen containing lysosomes in coeliac disease enterocytes. Gut 1995;36:703–709.
58 Zimmer KP, Naim H, Weber P, Ellis HJ, Ciclitira PJ: Targeting of gliadin peptides, CD8, alpha/beta-TCR, and gamma/delta-TCR to Golgi complexes and vacuoles within celiac disease enterocytes. FASEB J 1998;12:1349–1357.
59 Montalto M, et al: *Lactobacillus acidophilus* protects tight junctions from aspirin damage in HT-29 cells. Digestion 2004;69:225–228.
60 Rosenfeldt V, et al: Effect of probiotics on gastrointestinal symptoms and small intestinal permeability in children with atopic dermatitis. J Pediatr 2004;145:612–616.
61 Seehofer D, et al: Probiotics partly reverse increased bacterial translocation after simultaneous liver resection and colonic anastomosis in rats. J Surg Res 2004;117:262–271.

Prof. Alessio Fasano
Center for Celiac Research, Mucosal Biology Research Center
Health Science Facility II, Room S345, University of Maryland School of Medicine
Penn Street 20, Baltimore, MD 21201 (USA)
Tel. +1 410 706 5501, Fax +1 410 706 5508, E-Mail afasano@mbrc.umaryland.edu

Fasano A, Troncone R, Branski D (eds): Frontiers in Celiac Disease.
Pediatr Adolesc Med. Basel, Karger, 2008, vol 12, pp 99–106

Diagnosis of Coeliac Disease

Open Questions

Renata Auricchio · Riccardo Troncone

Department of Paediatrics and European Laboratory for the Investigation of Food-Induced Diseases, University Federico II, Naples, Italy

Abstract

In 1990, the European Society for Paediatric Gastroenterology, Hepatology and Nutrition revised its former diagnostic criteria for the diagnosis of coeliac disease (CD) and 2 requirements remain mandatory, the finding of villous atrophy and a full clinical remission after withdrawal of gluten from the diet. However, important changes that might have an impact on the diagnostic procedures for CD have occurred in recent years. Tests based on the detection of anti-endomysium antibodies, and subsequently of anti-tissue-transglutaminase (tTG), have been increasingly used as an initial screen for CD. The growing contribution of serology, together with the recognition of a wider spectrum of histological changes (see below), and the contribution by genetic tests demonstrate the necessity to move on to a revised diagnostic approach. The aim of this chapter is to analyse many open questions that remain concerning the diagnosis of CD: the role of serological and genetic tests that are questioning the same need of biopsy, the interpretation of minor histological changes, the management of special situations (selective IgA deficiency, potential CD), finally the possible implementation of new techniques (intestinal deposits of anti-tTG antibodies).

The Current Criteria of the European Society for Paediatric Gastroenterology, Hepatology and Nutrition

In 1990 [1], the European Society for Paediatric Gastroenterology, Hepatology and Nutrition (ESPGHAN) revised its former diagnostic criteria laid down in 1970. The 2 requirements mandatory for the diagnosis of coeliac disease (CD) remain: (1) the finding of villous atrophy with hyperplasia of the crypts and abnormal surface epithelium, while the patient is eating adequate amounts of gluten, and (2) a full clinical remission after withdrawal of gluten from the diet. The finding of circulating IgA antibodies to gliadin, reticulin and endomysium at the time of diagnosis, and their disappearance on a gluten-free diet, adds weight to the diagnosis. A control biopsy to verify the consequences of the gluten- free diet for the mucosal architecture is considered mandatory only in patients with an equivocal clinical response to the diet and in patients asymptomatic at first presentation (as is often the case in patients diagnosed during screening programmes, e.g. first-degree relatives of CD patients).

Gluten challenge is not considered mandatory, except under unusual circumstances. These include situations where there is doubt about the initial diagnosis, for example when no initial biopsy was done, or when the biopsy specimen was inadequate or not typical of CD. Gluten challenge should be discouraged before the age of 7 years and during the pubertal growth spurt.

Once decided, gluten challenge should always be performed under strict medical supervision. It should be preceded by an assessment of mucosal histology and performed with a standard dose of at least 10 g of gluten per day without disrupting established dietary habits. A further biopsy is taken when there is a noticeable clinical relapse or, in any event, after 3–6 months. Serological tests, IgA anti-gliadin (AGA), anti-endomysium (EMA) and anti-tissue-transglutaminase (tTG) antibodies, absorptive and permeability tests, more than clinical symptoms, can be of help in assessing the timing of the biopsy to shorten the duration of the challenge.

However, important changes that might have an impact on the diagnostic procedures for CD, have occurred in recent years. Tests based on the detection of EMA, and subsequently of anti-tTG antibodies, have been increasingly used as an initial screen for CD. Serological tests are largely responsible for the knowledge that CD is not a rare disease; moreover, with the notion of the relatively high prevalence of CD increasingly recognized, its spectrum of clinical presentations has broadened. The growing contribution of serology, together with the recognition of a wider spectrum of histological changes (see below), and the contribution by genetic tests demonstrate the necessity to move on to a revised diagnostic approach.

In fact, many open questions on CD diagnosis remain. The serological and genetic tests question the same need for biopsy, the interpretation of minor histological changes, the management of special situations and the possible implementation of new techniques.

Serological Tests

Over the last two decades serological tests have acquired a crucial role for the diagnosis of CD; EMA and, more recently, after the demonstration that tTG is the main auto-antigen recognized by EMA [2], anti-tTG antibodies have shown a great sensitivity and specificity for the diagnosis of CD [3]. The specificity is almost absolute also considering that subjects with positive serum EMA and normal histology have a high chance to develop enteropathy in the following years [4]. On the other hand, a note of caution comes from studies in adult patients indicating a lower sensitivity, particularly in subjects with milder forms of enteropathy [5]. In the last few years, after the first-generation tests based on the use of guinea pig antigen, most recent assays, based on the use of recombinant human enzyme as coating antigen in ELISA, have further improved the diagnostic efficacy. We can expect further improvement by the definition of the epitopes of tTG recognized by coeliac sera [6]. However, a series of technical problems common to other ELISA tests are still present, for example the correct definition of cut-off values. EMA and anti-tTG antibody tests have proved to correlate closely [7], even though some occasional patients remain negative for EMA despite being positive for anti-tTG antibodies, and vice versa. One explanation for this could be that EMA and anti-tTG ELISA test systems expose tTG antigenic epitopes in different ways.

Early diagnosis and treatment with a gluten-free diet reduce mortality and the prevalence of associated disorders in CD. A simple 'in the office' test of anti-tTG antibodies might be of great help in first-line screening for CD. Recent studies have evaluated the sensitivity and the specificity of commercial kits based on the rapid detection of IgA and IgG anti-human-tTG antibodies in one drop of whole blood. Results were compared with histology, conventional serum auto-antibody results and dietary adherence. All these studies concluded that the rapid test showed 97% of sensitivity and 97% of specificity for untreated coeliac patients, and identified all IgA-deficient patients. Coeliac auto-antibodies were detected also in 21% of treated patients, corresponding to dietary lapses [8–10].

IgA AGA by ELISA predates the previously described serological tests. Most of the data suggest that the specificity of the IgA AGA approximates 90%. However, far greater variation exists in estimates of the sensitivity of this test, although best estimates would place the sensitivity in the 85–90% range. Nonetheless, even if considering the sensitivity and the specificity of this test to be in the low 90% range, the use of IgA AGA would still not be attractive in the usual clinical practice owing to a very low positive predictive value and the existence of alternative serological tests with better diagnostic performance. Patients diagnosed below the age of 2 years seem to show an increased prevalence of EMA (and anti-tTG) negativity (in our experience they represent the 5% of diagnosis in this age group). For them the measurement of serum AGA is advised by most. Very recently antibodies against gliadin-derived deamidated peptides (D-AGA) have been assessed in the serum of CD patients at diagnosis and re-evaluated after 6 and 12 months of gluten-free diet; results have been compared to histology and to anti-tTG antibodies. Compared with conventional AGA, the peptide antibodies have a greater sensitivity, similar to anti-tTG antibodies, greater specificity, positive and negative predictive values, accuracy and likelihood ratios. The correlation between D-AGA and the severity of histological involvement showed a lower sensitivity of both forms of D-AGA in those patients with minor grades of enteropathy. At the same time D-AGA IgA seem to be more sensitive for detecting non-compliant patients [11].

Other auto-antibodies have been recognized in the serum of coeliac patients declining a gluten-free diet (calreticulin, actin, enolase). The only ones which have been explored for their potential diagnostic value are anti-actin auto-antibodies. Many studies suggest that they are a highly sensitive marker of the disrupted architecture of the intestinal epithelium of CD patients, with a potential relevance to diagnosis and follow-up [12]. However, this test has so far not found a place in the current diagnostic algorithm for CD.

Genetic Tests

The strongest association of CD is with the HLA class II D region markers, class I and class II region gene associations being secondary due to linkage disequilibrium. It has been suggested that the primary association of CD is with the DQ αβ-heterodimer encoded by the DQA1*05 and the DQB1*02 genes [13]. Such a DQ molecule has been found to be present in 95% or more of celiac patients compared with 20–30% of controls. The data available on DQ2-negative coeliac patients indicate that they almost invariably are HLA-DQ8 positive (DQA1*0301/DQB1*0302) [14]. A gene dosage effect has been suggested, and a molecular hypothesis for such a phenomenon has been proposed based on the impact of the number and quality of the HLA-DQ2 molecules on gluten peptide presentation to T cells [15]. The most likely mechanism to explain the association with HLA class II genes is, in fact, that the DQ molecule binds a peptide fragment of an antigen involved in the pathogenesis of CD to present it to T cells. From a diagnostic point of view, less than 2% of coeliac patients lack both HLA specificities; at the same time, approximately one third of the 'normal' population has one or the other marker; that means that the demonstration of being DQ2 and/or DQ8 positive has a strong negative predictive value, but a very weak positive predictive value for the diagnosis of CD. With these limitations the test may prove useful to exclude CD in subjects on a gluten-free diet, or in subjects belonging to an at-risk group (e.g. first-degree relatives, insulin-dependent diabetics, patients with Down syndrome) to avoid long-term follow-up. Simplified methods based on molecular typing of only the alleles associated with CD have been set up [16]. Other non-HLA genes could confer susceptibility to CD: considering the relevance of the immune response in the pathogenesis of the disease, candidate genes are those influencing the T-cell response. Among those, several reports imply involvement of the gene for the negative costimulatory molecule CTLA4 or a neighbouring gene [17]. A series of whole genome screening studies have been performed in CD [18]. The region that has most consistently been linked to CD is on the long arm of chromosome 5 (5q31–33) [19]. There is also evidence for susceptibility factors on the chromosomes 11q [18] and 19 [20].

At the moment, genetic analyses of these genes are not yet useful for the diagnosis of CD. In the future, it may be possible to assess the genetic risk of individuals to develop CD by combining DQ-DR HLA typing and the analysis of other non-HLA susceptibility genes. In fact, it has been demonstrated that patients with DQ2 have a different risk to develop the disease in relation to the linkage between DQ and DR. Five levels of genetic risk have been proposed [21]: group 1 with DR3/3 o DR3/7 (risk = 1), group 2 with DR5/7 (risk = 0.68), group 3 with DR3/X (risk = 0.23), group 4 with DR4/7, DR4/4, DR 7/7 (risk = 0.10), group 5 with other DR (risk = 0.02). A recent Italian study has demonstrated that a first-degree relative of a coeliac patient, who is DQ2 positive, has a different risk to develop the disease if he/she is DR3/3, DR3/7 or DR5/7 (20–40% of risk), half of the risk if he/she is DR3/X, and the risk decreases from 20 to 4% if he/she is DQ8 positive [22]. Based on these data, it is now possible to quantify the genetic risk of a first-degree relative of a coeliac patient at birth and envisage very precocious strategies to prevent the disease.

In conclusion, HLA testing is useful to rule out CD. Repeated antibody testing has been recommended to follow high-risk individuals such as close family members and patients who are affected by diseases associated with CD such as type 1 diabetes, Turner syndrome and Down syndrome. A negative test for the HLA risk alleles renders CD highly unlikely, and further serological testing of these individuals is unwarranted. It should be emphasized, however, that the use of HLA genotyping has limitations when the background frequencies of the HLA-DQ risk alleles in the test group are increased. This is clearly so for type 1 diabetes (associated with DQ2 and DQ8), Sjögren syndrome (associated with DQ2) and Graves disease (associated with DQ2). In accordance with this, a recent Italian study found that the distribution of the DQA1 and DQB1 alleles did not discriminate between the type 1 diabetes patients with or without CD and concluded that HLA typing is of limited use in this setting [23]. The family situation is a special case, and we argue that HLA testing is useful in this setting, because the presence of the risk factor is more directly linked with the disease risk.

Histology and Immunohistochemistry

A diagnosis of CD requires demonstration of characteristic histological changes in the small-intestinal mucosa, which are generally scored based on a system initially put forth by Marsh [24] and subsequently modified [25]. The histological changes in the small-intestinal mucosa can range from total to partial villous atrophy. In our Department, in the last 4 years 1,000 children underwent intestinal biopsies; 50% had a diagnosis of CD, with 92% of them presenting different degrees of villous atrophy at the histological examination. In fact, in some CD patients, only subtler changes of crypt lengthening with an increase in intra-epithelial lymphocytes (IELs), or simply an increase in IELs, may be present. In these cases, it is very important to consider also the serology and the HLA typing for a correct diagnosis. Analysis of multiple biopsies could be important and possibly to repeat the biopsy [26] taking multiple fragments from the distal duodenum and from the duodenal bulb [27]. Patchiness of the lesion has been reported, and in fact recent work suggests that different degrees of severity may be present; however, it is very unlikely that in the same individual completely normal fragments coexist with fragments showing some abnormality [26]. The site where to take a biopsy is still a matter of discussion. It is now accepted that patients with a positive CD serology and completely normal mucosa (no intra-epithelial infiltration) do exist (in our experience approx. 10% of all patients with a positive serology). Also in the latter cases the immunohistochemical analysis of jejunal mucosa may show abnormalities. Activation markers of cell-mediated immune response, such as increased expression of IL-2 receptor (CD25), of adhesion molecules (intercellular adhesion molecule 1) in the lamina propria and of HLA-DR in the crypts have been reported [28, 29]. The increased density of γδ-IELs seems to be a specific sign of CD [30]. Interestingly, although γδ-IELs tend to decrease on a gluten-free diet, the ratio γδ/CD3 remains high; it represents a useful marker of CD for patients on a gluten-free diet [31]. Unfortunately, γδ staining is possible only on frozen tissue and is then of limited value. The assessment of villous tip IEL correlates well with γδ density, and, being possible also on paraffin-embedded tissue, is of wider application [32].

Special Situations

Selective IgA Deficiency

Selective IgA deficiency, the commonest human immunodeficiency, is 10–15 times more common in patients with CD than in the general population, with a prevalence of 1.7–3% in patients with CD [33]. The importance of this association lies first in recognizing its existence and second in recognizing that, because the standard EMA and anti-tTG are IgA-based tests, patients with both CD and IgA deficiency cannot be reliably detected by these tests. In CD, IgA deficiency appears to result in higher titres of IgG EMA, IgG anti-tTG and IgG AGA, and it appears that the sensitivity of IgG EMA and IgG anti-tTG is close to 100% in IgA-deficient patients with CD. According to the last AGA review of diagnosis of CD [34], the prevalence of IgA deficiency is sufficiently low so that it is not necessary to consider the routine measurement of serum IgA levels along with IgA EMA and IgA anti-tTG as a first step toward CD diagnosis unless IgA deficiency is strongly suspected. In patients with a negative IgA EMA and IgA anti-tTG test, but in whom CD is still strongly suspected, measurement of serum IgA levels (and HLA typing) is reasonable as a next step. Alternatively, it is reasonable to proceed directly to the intestinal biopsy if the signs and symptoms suggest CD. However, in Italy, the National protocol for the diagnosis and the follow-up of CD advises the measurement of total IgA in all cases at the same time as the anti-tTG assessment.

Potential CD

A small percentage of subjects positive for CD antibodies (AGA, EMA and anti-tTG) have a small-intestinal mucosa without villous atrophy. Some of these patients have a Marsh 0 lesion (i.e. no intra-epithelial infiltration); yet, they show immunohistochemical signs of immune activation in the epithelium, in the lamina propria and in the crypts [31]. In a significant proportion of cases these subjects belong to at-risk groups. The titre of antibodies is often lower that that found in untreated CD patients with villous atrophy. In some cases fluctuating titres are noted, and it is not infrequent to see during the follow-up antibodies disappear from serum. There is no agreement on how to treat these patients. If symptomatic they are usually offered a trial with a gluten-free diet. Otherwise, most advise a very strict follow-up. In fact the natural history of these patients is still unknown, as well as the risks they are exposed to if left on a gluten-containing diet. A recent report [35] showing nutritional deficiencies also in patients with minor enteropathy, positive serology and 'right' genetics, resolving on a gluten-free diet, seems to indicate caution. Prospective studies are necessary.

New Diagnostic Tools

Intestinal Deposits of Anti-tTG Antibodies

While it has now been clearly shown that the site of production of EMA and anti-tTG antibodies is the gut mucosa [6, 36], and that their presence in the serum is possibly the result of their spillover, there is more than a working hypothesis that there are 'seronegative' subjects with the presence of such antibodies only in their intestinal secretions. In fact, already in the 90s it has been demonstrated that the presence of IgA and IgM AGA in the jejunal fluid can be a marker, together with a high IEL count, of latent gluten-sensitive enteropathy also in the absence of histological damage [37, 38].

A very recent study has demonstrated that autoantibodies (equivalent to EMA) targeted against transglutaminase 2 were deposited in the small-bowel mucosa of all CD patients with overt villous atrophy, regardless of serology, and further, these deposits were gluten dependent [39]. Thus, the detection of intestinal IgA deposits proved to be highly valuable in differentiating between CD and other causes of villous atrophy such as autoimmune enteropathy. Furthermore, a follow-up study showed that intestinal IgA deposits targeted against transglutaminase 2 are currently the best method to reveal early developing CD in 93% of subjects before the development of forthcoming villous atrophy [40]. Investigation of intestinal IgA deposits is a special method requiring frozen small-bowel biopsy specimens, which limits its utility. Nonetheless, this method should be available at least in specialized centres, since it is clearly beneficial in case where the conventional histology is not diagnostic.

Towards New Diagnostic Criteria?

In a situation where jejunal histology has lost specificity, and with the growing contribution by serology, and to a lesser extent by HLA, many propose to move to a new diagnostic approach mainly based on antibodies and genetics, the same definition of disease and the consequent need of a gluten-free diet which still awaits a definitive response. Although it should be unequivocally proved in large series, it is likely that patients with high titres of anti-tTG antibodies, HLA-DQ2 [8] and gluten-dependent symptoms have a villous atrophy. In these cases, the diagnosis could probably be established without the need for a biopsy. It is also quite clear that subjects with severe gluten-dependent enteropathy face a series of health risks, mainly nutritional; they probably have also a higher risk of developing auto-immunity, and, although less than previously thought, of presenting neoplastic complications.

Many recent studies mentioned in this chapter suggest that the ESPGHAN diagnostic criteria for CD diagnosis should be revised. Clinical response to a gluten-free diet does not always solve clinical problems, since patients without CD have also been shown to benefit from gluten-free dietary treatment. Secondly, it is currently recognized that many patients suffer from gluten-dependent symptoms and even CD complications such as osteoporosis before the development of villous atrophy [35]. These patients with potential or early developing CD do not fulfil the traditional ESPGHAN diagnostic criteria. On the other hand, it is important not to advise patients to adhere to a lifelong gluten-free diet without evidence. The contribution of the analysis of jejunal biopsies may still be very important; in particular, the study of the intestinal mucosa could prove decisive in the definition of the disease state. When CD is suspected but the histology is not diagnostic or when early developing CD is suspected, an increased density of $\gamma\delta+$ lymphocytes and villous tip IELs indicates CD. However, when there is any ambiguity in the diagnosis of CD in the presence of villous atrophy and further evidence is needed, intestinal transglutaminase-2-specific IgA deposits could be investigated.

In conclusion, until serological methods are improved and the genetic make-up of coeliac patients is better defined, it seems wise for a diagnosis of CD to still rely on a combined approach based of clinical criteria, histology, serology and genetics.

Acknowledgements

This work has been supported with grants from the Regione Campania.

References

1 Working Group of ESPGHAN: Revised criteria for diagnosis of celiac disease. Arch Dis Child 1990;65:909–911.

2 Dieterich W, Ehnis T, Bauer M, et al: Identification of tissue transglutaminase as the autoantigen of celiac disease. *Nat Med* 1997;3:797–801.

3 Sulkanen S, Halttunen T, Laurila K, et al: Tissue transglutaminase autoantibody enzyme-linked immunosorbent assay in detecting celiac disease. Gastroenterology 1998;115:1322–1328.

4 Collin P, Helin H, Maki M, Hallstrom O, Karvonen AL: Follow-up of patients positive in reticulin and gliadin antibody tests with normal small bowel biopsy findings. Scand J Gastroenterol 1993;28:595–598.

5 Rostami K, Kerckhaert J, Tiemessen R, von Blomberg ME, Mejer JWR, Mulder CJJ: Sensitivity of anti-endomysium and anti-gliadin antibodies in untreated coeliac disease: disappointing in clinical practice. Am J Gastroenterol 1999;94:888–894.

6 Marzari R, Sblattero D, Florian F, et al: Molecular dissection of the tissue transglutaminase autoantibody response in celiac disease. J Immunol 2001;166:4170–4176.

7 Troncone R, Maurano F, Rossi M, Micillo M, Greco L, Auricchio R, Salerno G, Salvatore F, Sacchetti L: IgA antibodies to tissue transglutaminase: an effective diagnostic test for celiac disease. J Pediatr 1999;134:166–171.

8 Korponay-Szabo IR, Raivio T, Laurila K, Opre J, Kiraly R, Kovacs JB, Kaukkinen K, Fesus L, Maki M: Celiac disease case finding and diet monitoring by point-of-care testing. *Aliment Pharmacol Ther* 2005;22:729–737.

9 Raivio T, Kaukkinen K, Nemes E, Laurila K, Collin P, Kovacs JB, Maki M, Korponay-Szabo IR: Self transglutaminse-based rapid celiac disease antibody detection by a lateral flow method. Aliment Pharmacol Ther 2006;24:147–154.

10 Nemec G, Ventura A, Stefano M, Di Leo G, Baldas V, Tommasini A, Ferrara F, Taddio A, Citta A, Sblattero D, Marzari R, Not T: Looking for celiac disease: diagnostic accuracy of two rapid commercial assays. Am J Gastroenterol 2006;101:1597–1600.

11 Sugai E, Vazquez H, Nachman F, Moreno ML, Mazure R, Smecuol E, Niveloni S, Cabane A, Kogan Z, Gomez JC, Maurino E, Bai JC: Accuracy of testing for antibodies to synthetic gliadin-related peptides in celiac disease. Clin Gastroenterol Hepatol 2006;4:1112–1117.

12 Pedreira S, Sugai E, Moreno ML, Vazquez H, Niveloni S, Smecuol E, Mazure R, Kogan Z, Maurino E, Bai JC: Significance of smooth muscle/antiactin autoantibodies in celiac disease. Acta Gastroenterol Latinoam 2005;35: 83–93.

13 Sollid ML, Markussen G, Ek J, et al: Evidence for a primary association of celiac disease to a particular HLA-DQ alpha/beta heterodimer. J Exp Med 1989;169:345–350.

14 Karell K, Louka AS, Moodie SJ, et al: HLA types in celiac disease patients not carrying the DQA1*05-DQB1*02 (DQ2) heterodimer: results from the European Genetics Cluster on celiac disease. Hum Immunol 2003;64:469–477.

15 Vader W, Stepniak D, Kooy Y, et al: The HLA-DQ2 gene dose effect in celiac disease is directly related to the magnitude and breadth of gluten-specific T cell responses. Proc Natl Acad Sci USA 2003;100:12390–12395.

16 Sacchetti L, Calcagno G, Ferrajolo A, Sarrantonio C, Troncone R, Micillo M, et al: Discrimination between celiac and other gastrointestinal disorders in childhood by rapid HLA typing. Clin Chem 1998;62:669–675.

17 Djilali-Saiah I, Schmitz J, Harfouch-Hammoud E, et al: CTLA-4 gene polymorphism is associated with predisposition to celiac disease. Gut 1998;43:187–189.

18 Babron MC, Nilsson S, Adamovic S, et al: Meta and pooled analysis of European coeliac disease data. Eur J Hum Genet 2003;11:828–834.

19 Greco L, Corazza G, Babron MC, et al: Genome search in celiac disease Am J Hum Genet 1998;62:669–675.

20 van Belzen MJ, Meijer JW, Sandkuijl LA, et al: A major non-HLA locus in celiac disease maps to chromosome 19. Gastroenterology 2003;125:1032–1041.

21 Margaritte-Jeannin P, Babron MC, Bourgey M, Louka As, Clot F, Percopo S, Coto I, Hugot JP, Ascher H, Sollid LM, Greco L, Clerget-Darpoux F: HLA-DQ relative risk for celiac disease in European populations: a study of the European Genetics Cluster on Celiac Disease. Tissue Antigens 2004;63: 562–567.

22 Bourgey M, Calcagno G, Tinto N, Gennarelli D, Margaritte-Jeannin P, Greco L, Limongelli MG, Esposito O, Marano C, Troncone R, Spampanato A, Clerget-Darpoux FF, Sacchetti L: HLA-related genetic risk for coeliac disease. Gut 2007;56:1054–1059.

23 Contreas G, Valletta E, Ulmi D, Cantoni S, Pinelli L: Screening of coeliac disease in north Italian children with type 1 diabetes: limited usefulness of HLA-DQ typing. Acta Paediatr 2004;93:628–632.

24 Marsh MN: Gluten, major histocompatibility complex, and the small intestine: a molecular and immunobiologic approach to the spectrum of gluten sensitivity ('celiac sprue') Gastroenterology 1992;102:330–354.

25 Oberhuber G, Granditsch G, Vogelsang H: The histopathology of celiac disease: time for standardized report scheme for pathologists. Eur J Gastroenterol Hepatol 1999;11: 1185–1194.

26 Ravelli A, Bolognini S, Gambarotti M, Villanacci V: Variabilitiy of histologic lesions in relation to biopsy site in gluten-sensitive enteropathy. Am J Gastroenterol 2005;100:177–185.

27 Bonamico M, Mariani P, Thanasi E, Ferri M, Nenna R, Tiberti C, Mora B, Mazzilli MC, Magliocca FM: Patchy villous atrophy of the duodenum in childhood celiac disease. J Pediatr Gastroenterol Nutr 2004;38:204–207.
28 Holm K, Savilahti E, Koskimies S, Lipsanen V, Maki M: Immunohistochemical changes in the jejunum of first-degree relatives of patients with celiac disease and the celiac marker DQ genes: HLA class II antigen expression, interleukin 2 receptor positive cells and dividing crypt cells. Gut 1994;35:55–60.
29 Kaukinen K, Maki M, Collin P: Immunohistochemical features in antiendomysium positive patients with normal villous architecture. Am J Gastroenterol 2006;101:675–676.
30 Spencer J, Isaacson PG, MacDonald TT, et al: Gamma/delta cells and the diagnosis of celiac disease. Clin Exp Immunol 1991;85:109–113.
31 Paparo F, Petrone E, Tosco A, Maglio M, Borrelli M, Salvati VM, Miele E, Greco L, Auricchio S, Troncone R: Clinical, HLA and small bowel immunohistochemical features of children with positive serum anti-endomysium antibodies and architecturally normal small intestinal mucosa. Am J Gastroenterol 2005;100:2294–2298.
32 Jarvinen TT, Collin P, Rasmussen M, Kyronpalo S, Maki M, Partanen J, Reunala T, Kaukinen K: Villous tip intraepithelial lymphocytes as markers of early-stage celiac disease. Scand J Gastroenterol 2004;39:428–433.
33 Cataldo F, Marino V, Bottaro G, Greco P, Ventura A: Celiac disease and selective immunoglobulin A deficiency. J Pediatr 1997;131:306–308.
34 Rostom A, Murray JA, Kagnoff MF: American Gastroenterological Association Institute technical review on the diagnosis and management of celiac disease. Gastroenterology 2006;131:1981–2002.
35 Kaukinen K, Maki M, Partanen J, Sievanen H, Collin P: Celiac disease without villous atrophy: revision of criteria called for. Dig Dis Sci 2001;46: 879–888.
36 Picarelli A, Maiuri L, Frate A, Greco M, Auricchio S, Londei M: Production of antiendomysial antibodies after in vitro gliadin challenge of small intestinal biopsy samples from patients with coeliac disease. Lancet 1996;348:1065–1067.
37 Arranz E, Ferguson A: Intestinal antibody pattern of celiac disease: occurrence in patients with normal jejunal biopsy histology. Gastroenterology 1993;104:1263–1272.
38 Wahnschaffe U, Urlich R, Riecken EO, Schulzke JD: Celiac disease-like abnormalities in a subgroup of patients with irritable bowel syndrome. Gastroenterology 2001;121:1329–1338.
39 Salmi T, Collin P, Korponay-Szabo IR, Laurila K, Partanen J, Huhtala H, Kiraly R, Lorand L, Reunala T, Maki M, Kaukinen K: Endomysial antibody-negative celiac disease: clinical characteristics and intestinal autoantibody deposits. Gut 2006;55:1746–1753.
40 Salmi T, Collin P, Jarvinen O, Haimila K, Partanen J, Laurila K, Korponay-Szabo IR, Huhtala H, Reunala T, Maki M, Kaukinen K: Immunoglobulin A autoantibodies against transglutaminase 2 in the small intestinal mucosa predict forthcoming celiac disease. Aliment Pharmacol Ther 2006;24:541–552.

Prof. Riccardo Troncone
Department of Paediatrics and European Laboratory for the Investigation of Food-Induced Diseases
University Federico II
Via Pansini 5, IT–80131 Naples (Italy)
Tel. +39 081 7463 383, Fax +39 081 5469 811, E-Mail troncone@unina.it

Fasano A, Troncone R, Branski D (eds): Frontiers in Celiac Disease.
Pediatr Adolesc Med. Basel, Karger, 2008, vol 12, pp 107–113

Current Guidelines for the Diagnosis and Treatment of Celiac Disease

Ricardo A. Caicedo · Ivor D. Hill

Department of Pediatrics, Wake Forest University School of Medicine, Winston-Salem, N.C., USA

Abstract

Evidence-based guidelines for the diagnosis and treatment of celiac disease (CD) have recently been published by the North American Society for Pediatric Gastroenterology, Hepatology and Nutrition. These recommend the diagnosis be confirmed with an intestinal biopsy in all cases before starting treatment. Serological tests for CD are useful for identifying those needing a biopsy to confirm the diagnosis. They may also be used to support the diagnosis and monitor compliance with treatment. For reasons of accuracy and costs, the transglutaminase antibody test is recommended for initial screening. Testing should be considered early in the evaluation of those with symptoms that are strongly associated with CD. Testing should be considered in those with less typical symptoms of CD when other causes have been excluded and in asymptomatic individuals with other conditions that are associated with an increased risk for CD. Treatment of CD requires strict adherence to a gluten-free diet for life. This entails eliminating all products derived from wheat, barley or rye.

Individuals with celiac disease (CD) must remain on a strict gluten-free diet (GFD) for life to ensure optimal health and well-being. Maintaining a strict GFD is difficult and has both financial and quality of life implications. Therefore it is essential to first confirm the diagnosis before starting treatment. Conversely, failure to identify and treat those with CD in a timely fashion has potential for adverse long-term health consequences. In an effort to improve care for those with CD, the North American Society for Pediatric Gastroenterology, Hepatology and Nutrition (NASPGHAN) recently published evidence-based guidelines for the diagnosis and treatment of CD in children [1]. This chapter will review the NASPGHAN guideline recommendations for the diagnosis, use of serological tests and treatment of CD.

Diagnosis

Confirmation of a diagnosis of CD still requires an intestinal biopsy in all cases. Initial diagnostic criteria were published by the European Society for Pediatric Gastroenterology and Nutrition in 1970 [2]. These required subjects to undergo a series of 3 intestinal biopsies over a period of 1 year or more. A subsequent review of a large series of children who had undergone this process revealed that in over 95% the 3-biopsy protocol was unnecessary. Based on this review, revised criteria for the diagnosis of CD were published in 1990 [3]. These state that in individuals over 2 years of age with symptoms suggestive of

CD, characteristic histological changes on small-intestinal biopsy and complete symptom resolution on a GFD, the diagnosis is considered confirmed. Serological tests for CD that revert from positive to negative after starting a GFD are supportive evidence for the diagnosis. In the very young child (under 2 years), and in some cases where the diagnosis remains in doubt, it may be necessary to use alternative strategies, including reverting to the 3-biopsy protocol, to confirm a diagnosis of CD.

Intestinal Biopsy and Histopathology

Small-intestinal biopsies are most commonly obtained by means of an endoscopic procedure. It is recommended that biopsies be obtained even if the macroscopic appearance of the duodenal mucosa is normal, as the described endoscopic features of CD are not reliable indicators of disease and may only be seen when there is severe villous atrophy. The mucosal changes may be patchy in distribution and vary in severity [4]. For this reason it is recommended to obtain multiple (4–6) biopsies [1]. Brunner's glands in the proximal duodenum may hamper interpretation of the histology, so it may be preferable to obtain biopsies from the more distal segments. A number of histological features have been described in CD (table 1). These can range from an increase in the number of intraepithelial lymphocytes in the early stages of the disease to complete villous atrophy in more advanced stages. A histological grading system described by Marsh [5] is commonly used in the assessment of biopsies for CD. According to this system, Marsh type 0 refers to normal histology, while a Marsh type 1 or infiltrative lesion is characterized only by an increase in the number of intraepithelial lymphocytes. The Marsh type 2 or hyperplastic lesion is characterized by hyperplasia of the crypts in addition to the increased intraepithelial lymphocytes. In the Marsh type 3 or destructive lesions there is additional variable degrees of villous atrophy (3a, 3b and 3c) while the type 4 or hypoplastic lesion represents the severest form of disease characterized by total villous atrophy and crypt hypoplasia. There is good evidence that Marsh type 3 lesions represent a distinctive feature of CD and can be used to confirm the diagnosis. There is less clear evidence that Marsh type 2 changes are distinctive for CD. In these cases additional supportive evidence, such as the presence of positive serological tests, is needed to confirm the diagnosis [6]. There is no evidence that Marsh type 1 changes are confined to CD, and in children this may represent a nonspecific finding. In individuals with only Marsh type 1 changes, additional strategies should be considered to confirm the diagnosis, including reverting to the older 3-biopsy protocol.

Table 1. Histological features of CD

Increased intraepithelial lymphocytes
Crypt elongation
Partial to total villous atrophy
Decreased villous:crypt ratio
Increased crypt mitotic index
Lamina propria lymphoplasmacytic infiltration
Decreased height of epithelial cells
Decreased number of goblet cells

Serological Tests for Celiac Disease

Serological tests are most frequently used to identify individuals who require an intestinal biopsy to confirm the diagnosis of CD. They may also be useful as supportive evidence in the diagnosis and for monitoring compliance with the GFD once the diagnosis has been confirmed. Commercially available tests include antigliadin IgG and IgA, antireticulin IgA, antiendomysium IgA (EMA) and anti-tissue-transglutaminase IgA (tTG). The antigliadin tests are relatively cheap and easy to perform but are associated with a high variability in sensitivity and specificity, and antigliadin antibodies are found in a number of other gastrointestinal diseases as well as healthy individuals. The antireticulin test is based on an immunofluorescent technique using rat liver or kidney as a substrate. This test is also associated with highly variable sensitivity and specificity. The EMA test is also based on an immunofluorescent technique using either monkey esophagus or human umbilical cord as a substrate. This assay is both highly sensitive and specific with many studies reporting figures of 95–100% for both parameters. The potential disadvantages of this test are that it is time consuming to perform and hence usually more expensive, and is operator dependent which may adversely affect its reliability. In addition there is evidence suggesting it is less reliable in children less than 2 years of age [1]. The tTG test initially used guinea pig protein but now predominantly uses human recombinant protein. Using the human recombinant protein, there is good evidence that the tTG test has sensitivities and specificities that are similar to those of the EMA test [7]. The tTG test is performed either by an ELISA or RIA technique and hence is quantitative and operator independent. Because both the EMA and tTG tests are based on an IgA antibody they cannot be used to identify individuals with CD who are IgA deficient. Selective IgA deficiency occurs in up to 3% of individuals with CD, and in these, alternative testing using IgG-based tests for EMA or tTG should be considered [8]. IgG-based tests for both EMA and tTG are not as readily available on a commercial basis.

Because of the variable and generally inferior accuracy of the antigliadin and antireticulin tests, these are no longer recommended for routine use to identify individuals with CD. Based on considerations of sensitivity and specificity, relative costs and ease of performance, the tTG assay is recommended as the initial test for CD [1]. Because selective IgA deficiency is more common in CD, consideration should be given to determining a serum IgA level at the same time so as to better interpret a negative tTG test. There is no evidence to show that use of a panel of serological tests for CD is better than a single tTG test and hence using a single tTG test is more cost effective [1, 7]. There have been recent reports of a new test based on the use of deamidated gliadin [9]. While the results suggest that this test may offer a useful alternative in the future, more data are needed before any recommendations can be made.

Limitations of Serological Tests

Although studies show that both EMA and tTG tests are highly sensitive and specific, these data were derived in a research setting and hence are likely to be less accurate in a clinical setting due to the lower pretest probability. In addition there is no standardization among the commercial laboratories performing the tests, and comparison of serological tests between different laboratories has demonstrated marked variability in results [10]. The tests also appear to be more accurate in those with more severe villous atrophy and less reliable in those with mild histological changes. Finally there are still relatively limited data on serological testing in children less than 5 years of age. For all these reasons, serological tests should not be relied on as the sole reason to either confirm or exclude a diagnosis of CD [1]. In individuals with clinical manifestations that are strongly suggestive of CD, an intestinal biopsy should be considered even if the serology is negative. Conversely the decision to treat with a GFD should not be based on the presence of positive serological tests alone.

Human Leukocyte Antigen Tests

HLA tests for the class II heterodimers, DQ2 and DQ8, are commercially available. These HLA haplotypes determine susceptibility to CD as over

Table 2. Clinical manifestations of CD

Gastrointestinal	Extraintestinal
Chronic diarrhea	Dermatitis herpetiformis
Failure to thrive in children	Dental enamel hypoplasia
Abdominal distention/gaseousness	Delayed puberty
Recurrent abdominal pain	Short stature
Nausea and vomiting	Iron deficiency anemia
Recurrent oral aphthous ulcers	Osteopenia
Hepatitis or hepatic steatosis	Recurrent spontaneous abortions
Constipation	Arthritis
	Alopecia
	Ataxia or polyneuropathy

95% of known cases are DQ2 positive with almost all the rest being DQ8 positive. However, approximately 30% of the general population in North America is also DQ2 positive. Thus, while the DQ2 or DQ8 genotype is considered necessary to develop CD, the presence of either one does not confirm the diagnosis. Conversely, the absence of both these HLA types has a negative predictive value of over 99% and virtually excludes the diagnosis of CD [11]. There are no studies to show that testing for these CD-specific HLA types is of any value in the initial screening for CD, and hence they are not recommended for this purpose. Conversely, these tests may be useful in select circumstances when the diagnosis remains uncertain despite an intestinal biopsy or as part of a long-term screening strategy for asymptomatic individuals who are at an increased risk for CD. In such cases a negative test would effectively exclude CD from further consideration.

Screening for Celiac Disease

Because CD is associated with intestinal damage, clinical manifestations are often related to the gastrointestinal tract. However, it is now known that the manifestations of CD are extremely variable (table 2) and up to 50% of newly diagnosed cases initially present with symptoms that are not related to the gastrointestinal tract [12, 13]. Furthermore, a number of asymptomatic individuals with characteristic changes of CD on small-intestinal biopsy have been identified during studies using serological tests to screen populations [13]. As a result of these studies a number of autoimmune and nonautoimmune conditions have been identified as strongly associated with CD (table 3). Physicians need to be aware of the variable clinical manifestations and the conditions that are associated with an increased risk for CD and consider a strategy of active case finding by use of serological tests in order to avoid delays in diagnosis.

Screening of Symptomatic Individuals

Many of the symptoms associated with CD listed in table 2 also occur with other common medical conditions, and hence serological tests for CD may not be necessary in the initial diagnostic workup of all such cases. In individuals with persistent diarrhea, particularly if accompanied by poor weight gain in children or weight loss at any age, CD should be an early consideration in the differential diagnosis. Other clinical manifestations for which there is good to reasonable evi-

Table 3. Conditions associated with an increased prevalence of CD

Autoimmune disorders
Type 1 diabetes
Autoimmune thyroiditis
Autoimmune hepatitis
Sjögren syndrome
Nonautoimmune disorders
First-degree relatives of CD patients
Down syndrome
Turner syndrome
Williams syndrome
Selective IgA deficiency

dence of a causal relationship with CD are dermatitis herpetiformis, dental enamel hypoplasia of the permanent teeth, anemia, short stature in children, delayed onset of puberty and osteoporosis [1]. It is recommended that serological tests for CD should be considered early in the diagnostic evaluation of such cases. In those with other gastrointestinal complaints such as recurrent abdominal pain, bloating, vomiting, constipation or hepatitis (elevated liver enzymes), serological tests for CD should be considered when no other cause for the symptoms can be identified. Similarly, for the other nongastrointestinal manifestations listed in table 2, tests for CD are recommended when other causes for the symptoms have been excluded.

Screening of Asymptomatic Individuals

Because of the strong association between CD and the conditions listed in table 3, it is believed that individuals who have these conditions should undergo testing for CD even if they are asymptomatic [1]. Those with positive serological tests are advised to undergo a small-intestinal biopsy and, if this demonstrates the characteristic findings of CD, they are advised to adhere to a strict GFD for life. This approach is based on the belief that early diagnosis and treatment of CD will prevent some of the adverse long-term health consequences associated with the disease. Those most commonly listed for untreated CD include a higher mortality rate, increased risk for malignancies (particularly intestinal lymphomas) and osteoporosis. In addition it has been suggested that prolonged exposure to gluten in susceptible individuals may increase their risk for developing other autoimmune disorders, and early diagnosis and treatment could prevent this happening. In children there is also concern that untreated CD could adversely affect growth and lead to permanent stunting if not corrected before puberty.

On the basis of standardized mortality rates, untreated CD is associated with excess mortality. However, this seems to be confined to those with severe symptomatic CD and did not apply to those with mild or no symptoms [14]. Similarly individuals with symptomatic CD who do not adhere to a GFD have an increased risk for intestinal malignancies. However, recent studies suggest that the relative risk for malignancies is much lower than originally estimated and in absolute terms intestinal lymphomas account for a very small number of all malignancies [15]. Furthermore, there are no data to show that asymptomatic individuals with CD are at an increased risk for malignancies. There is also clear evidence that many adults with CD will have a decreased bone mineralization and an increased risk for fractures [16]. There are some data to show that a few asymptomatic individuals with screening-identified CD have decreased bone mineralization but few data on the prevalence of this problem in asymptomatic cases, and no data to indicate that asymptomatic individuals with CD are at an increased risk for fractures. The evidence for early diagnosis and treatment of CD preventing the onset of other autoimmune disorders is relatively weak, and further prospective studies are needed before this can be used as a reason to justify screening asymptomatic individuals. Similarly the evidence for growth being adversely affected in asymptomatic children with CD is not conclusive and needs further study.

The NASPGHAN guidelines acknowledge that there are no studies to demonstrate any benefits of treating CD in asymptomatic individuals. Despite this, they recommend that all asymptomatic individuals who belong to a specific group at risk (table 3) should have serological testing beginning at the age of 3 years providing they are on an adequate gluten-containing diet [1]. With the exception of those with type 1 diabetes, these recommendations are also contained in the National Institutes of Health Consensus Conference statement on CD [6]. The reason given in the National Institutes of Health statement for excluding the type 1 diabetics is that there is insufficient evidence to show any benefit from treatment with a GFD in the short term. The benefits of screening asymptomatic individuals for CD have recently been questioned, particularly as they apply to those with type 1 diabetes and Down syndrome. The fact that compliance with the GFD in those with asymptomatic screening-identified CD is generally poor is further reason to question the value of testing those who are truly asymptomatic [17]. An alternative strategy has recently been offered by the American Gastroenterological Association in a position statement on CD [18]. In essence this calls for a heightened awareness of the conditions associated with an increased risk for CD and recommends that all symptomatic individuals with one of these conditions undergo serological testing.

Treatment

A strict GFD for life remains the only scientifically proven treatment for CD. In effect this excludes all forms of wheat, including spelt, kamut, triticale, semolina, farina, einkorn, bulgur and couscous, plus barley and rye from the diet. The potential harmful effect of gluten-reduced wheat starch is controversial. Malt is also to be avoided as it is a partial hydrolysate of barley protein. Previously oats were felt to be harmful but more recent evidence suggests that pure oats can be tolerated by most individuals with CD. There is still concern in recommending oats as the potential for contamination with wheat flour remains, so unless the purity of the oats can be guaranteed it is still recommended this grain be excluded from the diet [1].

There is evidence that even small amounts of gluten ingested on a regular basis can lead to mucosal damage in those predisposed to CD. The concept of a minimum allowable amount of gluten below which no harm will befall an individual with CD has been proposed by some. This had led to considerable debate over what level of gluten should be allowed to label a product as 'gluten free'. The proposed level of less than 20 parts per million recently suggested by the Food and Drug Administration in the USA has not been accepted by many with CD who believe that this level is still too high. In part the controversies surrounding this issue are the result of inaccurate gluten-detecting devices and the lack of good scientific data to show that there is a level below which no harm will occur in patients with CD.

Members of the Canadian and US dietetic associations have published evidence-based guidelines for the dietary treatment of CD [19]. These guidelines have been endorsed by the NASPGHAN, and continued dietitian involvement in the care of patients with CD is strongly recommended [1].

Following the diagnosis and initiation of treatment for CD, it is recommended that patients be followed regularly to monitor for resolution of symptoms, continued normal growth and development in children and maintenance of normal health and well-being. At each patient encounter, the importance of dietary compliance should be emphasized and the opportunity taken to educate the patient on the potential dangers of nonadherence to the diet. There is little evidence on how to most effectively monitor compliance. Serial testing using the serological tests for CD to demonstrate a progressive disappearance of the antibodies may provide indirect evidence that the patient is adhering to the diet. Similarly, a sudden rise in antibody levels from a previous negative or low level might indicate that the individual is knowingly or inadvertently ingesting gluten-containing products again. Once there is complete symptom resolution and individuals are clinically healthy, they can be followed on an annual basis.

References

1 Guideline for the diagnosis and treatment of celiac disease in children: recommendations of the North American Society for Pediatric Gastroenterology, Hepatology and Nutrition. J Pediatr Gastroenterol Nutr 2005;40:1–19.

2 Meuwisse G: Diagnostic criteria in coeliac disease. Acta Paediatr Scand 1970;59:461.

3 European Society of Paediatric Gastroenterology and Nutrition: Revised criteria for diagnosis of coeliac disease: report of the Working Group of the European Society of Paediatric Gastroenterology and Nutrition. Arch Dis Child 1990;65:909–911.

4 Bonamico M, Mariani P, Thanasi E, et al: Patchy villous atrophy of the duodenum in childhood celiac disease. J Pediatr Gastroenterol Nutr 2004;38:204–207.

5 Marsh MN: Gluten, major histocompatibility complex, and the small intestine: a molecular and immunobiologic approach to the spectrum of gluten sensitivity ('celiac sprue'). Gastroenterology 1992;102:330–354.

6 National Institutes of Health Consensus Development Conference statement on celiac disease. Gastroenterology 2004;128:S1–S9.

7 AGA Institute technical review on the diagnosis and management of celiac disease. Gastroenterology 2006;131: 1981–2002.

8 Meini A, Pillan NM, Villanacci V, Monafo V, Ugazio AG, Plebani A: Prevalence and diagnosis of celiac disease in IgA-deficient children. Ann Allergy Asthma Immunol 1996;77:333–336.

9 Sugai E, Vazquez H, Nachman F, Moreno ML, Mazure R, Smecuol E, Niveloni S, Cabanne A, Kogan Z, Gomez JC, Maurino E, Bai JC: Accuracy of testing for antibodies to synthetic gliadin-related peptides in celiac disease. Clin Gastroenterol Hepatol 2006;4:1112–1117.

10 Murray JA, Herlein J, Goeken J: Multicenter comparison of serologic tests for celiac disease in the USA. Gastroenterology 1997;112:A389.

11 Kaukinen K, Partanen J, Maki M, et al: HLA-DQ typing in the diagnosis of celiac disease. Am J Gastroenterol 2002; 97:695–699.

12 Dewar DH, Ciclitira PJ: Clinical features and diagnosis of celiac disease. Gastroenterology 2005;128:S19–S24.

13 Fasano A, Catassi C: Current approaches to diagnosis and treatment of celiac disease: an evolving spectrum. Gastroenterology 2001;120:636–651.

14 Corrao G, Corazza R, Bagnardi V, et al: Mortality in patients with coeliac disease and their relatives: a cohort study. Lancet 2001;358:356–361.

15 Catassi C, Fabiani E, Corrao G, et al: Risk of non-Hodgkin lymphoma in celiac disease. JAMA 2002;287:1413–1419.

16 Valdimarsson T, Lofman O, Toss G, Strom M: Reversal of osteopenia with diet in adult celiac disease. Gut 1996;38: 322–327.

17 Cranney A, Rostom A, Sy R, Dube C, Saloogee N, Garritty C, Moher D, Sampson M, Zhang L, Yazdi F, Mamaladze V, Pan I, MacNeil J: Consequences of testing for celiac disease. Gastroenterology 2005;128: S109–S120.

18 American Gastroenterological Association (AGA) Institute medical position statement on the diagnosis and management of celiac disease. Gastroenterology 2006;131:1977–1980.

19 Manual of Clinical Dietetics, ed 6. Chicago, American Dietetic Association, 2000.

Ivor D. Hill, MB, ChB, MD
Department of Pediatrics, Wake Forest University School of Medicine
Medical Center Boulevard
Winston-Salem, NC 27157 (USA)
Tel. +1 336 716 2328, Fax +1 336 716 9699, E-Mail ihill@wfubmc.edu

Fasano A, Troncone R, Branski D (eds): Frontiers in Celiac Disease.
Pediatr Adolesc Med. Basel, Karger, 2008, vol 12, pp 114–122

Current Therapy

M. Stern

University Children's Hospital, University of Tübingen, Tübingen, Germany

Abstract

A lifelong and strict gluten-free diet (GFD) can fully restore health and improve quality of life in patients with celiac disease and is therefore the basic line of treatment. However, in everyday practice more problems than expected remain: compliance is sometimes difficult to achieve and needs continuous educational and psychosocial support. Persisting symptoms and micronutrient deficiencies, in some cases obesity, are observed. A decreased quality of life has been described particularly in adult women on a GFD. Scientific progress in pathophysiology and also in gluten analysis (R5 ELISA system) has helped to improve evidence-based regulatory solutions for defining and controlling GFD at an international level. Alternative forms of therapy and prevention appear at the horizon today.

Celiac Disease – Hard to Treat and Impossible to Cure?

Celiac disease has rightly been said to be 'tricky to find, hard to treat, impossible to cure' (S. Lohiniemi). However, the situation has greatly improved in recent years due to the progress made both on the scientific and practical levels. New horizons have emerged, starting with celiac-active epitopes in cereal proteins, going beyond the definition of cereals detrimental to celiac patients, and culminating in the evidence-based control of a gluten-free diet (GFD). For practical purposes, and in discussions of celiac disease in the medical literature, 'the term gluten is used to refer to either gluten in wheat or, collectively, to the proteins (e.g. prolamines and glutelins) in just those grains that have been demonstrated to cause harmful health effects in individuals who have coeliac disease' [1]. The diagnosis celiac disease now covers a wide spectrum, which is reflected in therapy [2]. The GFD is, as a rule, indicated in all cases of classic as well as 'silent' celiac disease; however, it is not necessary in latent forms.

At present, the quality and efficacy of the GFD is subject to control both on the food and regulatory level and that of individual patients [2, 3]. The success of the GFD in celiac disease is, however, strongly dependent on compliance, the ascertainment of which is a difficult matter. The beneficial impact of the GFD clearly outweighs the potentially negative effects [4]. A recent report about a celiac cohort in Northern Ireland, which found evidence for a high risk of mortality at the time of diagnosis, has underscored the crucial importance of gluten-free nutrition for all celiac patients on a lifelong basis: the status of patients 1 year after diagnosis on a GFD showed that malignancy and risk of mortality in this cohort had decreased considerably [5]. The quality of life in celiac patients on a GFD has been an issue raised by different groups over the last few years, and investigations have revealed some unexpected as well as negative effects of the GFD.

From Celiac-Active Epitopes to Unacceptable Grains and vice versa

The subject of nutrition therapy for celiac disease has recently been reviewed in the USA [6–8]. Clinical Guidelines of the North American Society for Pediatric Gastroenterology, Hepatology and Nutrition consider dietary treatment for celiac disease (www.naspghan.org). These comprehensive guidelines stipulate the involvement of a registered dietician trained in working with celiac patients; in addition, the medical monitoring of celiac patients is mandatory. It is essential that the information provided to patients during dietary counseling promotes their motivation and education [8]. Since nutritional deficiencies relating to the inadequate intake of calories/proteins, iron, calcium, magnesium, zinc, vitamin D, vitamin B_{12}, folic acid, niacin, riboflavin and fiber may be present, testing is required and supplementation then needs to be introduced [6]. Obesity among celiac patients on a GFD could pose a practical problem. Cooperation with self-help groups and welfare institutions, such as national and international celiac societies, coupled with lifelong medical follow-up and psychosocial support are important aspects contributing to the success of nutrition therapy in celiac patients. The expense involved in such a therapeutic diet has been estimated to be 115% higher than in a normal control group comprising children and adults, and is a factor that further jeopardizes compliance. However, it was this very factor that led to a successful political campaign for GFD financially subsidized by governmental or health institutions in Finland and Italy.

Gluten is the rubbery wheat storage protein that remains when wheat dough is washed to remove starch. It is unique in terms of its amino acid composition and is high in glutamine and proline. The major protein fractions of gluten are gliadin (alcohol soluble) and glutenin (alcohol insoluble), with soluble gliadin containing monomeric proteins and insoluble glutenin containing aggregated proteins. The protein components and amino acid sequences of gliadin and glutenin are similar and repetitive. Wheat gliadins, rye secalins, barley hordeins and avenin from oats are also known as prolamines, i.e. proteins rich in proline. There is no evidence for a significant relationship between the storage proteins of maize, rice, millet or sorghum and these prolamines. A strong correlation was found between the specific chemical structure of prolamines and the activity of their peptide fragments in celiac disease [3]. Gliadins can be classified into 3 electrophoretical types, namely α, γ and ω. They can also be distinguished according to molecular weight: high, e.g. 67–88 kDa, as in high-molecular-weight glutenin; medium, 34–55 kDa as in ω-gliadin, and low, 28–39 kDa, as in α-gliadin, γ-gliadin or low-molecular-weight glutenin. The typically repetitive sequences found were PQQQF, PQQPFPQQ and QPQ PFPQQTYP (1-letter code for amino acids, P for proline and Q for glutamine). Through the organ culture experiment and also by means of in vivo instillation, specific peptides were shown to induce the celiac-disease-specific small-intestinal enteropathy [3].

Cereal proteins were found to contain several celiac-active 'toxic' epitopes that stimulate intestinal T cells in celiac patients. Differences were evident between individual patients (children as well as adults), and partial overlap was observed between the in vitro intestinal T-cell activity and in vitro/in vivo intestinal epithelial activity of these specific gluten peptides [9–11]. The 33-mer LQLQPFPQPQLPYPQPQLPYPQPQLPYPQP QPF is of particular importance. It is a gliadin

Table 1. Cereals in the GFD

Allowed grains	Forbidden grains
Amaranth	Wheat (all kinds of Triticum)
Buckwheat	Rye
Corn	Triticale
Millet	Barley
Quinoa	Kamut
Rice	(Oats)
Sorghum	
Tef	
Wild rice	

fragment with N-terminal amino acid positions 56–88 and is resistant to proteolytic breakdown. It contains overlapping T-cell epitopes, and its deamidated form is a potent T-cell stimulator which binds strongly to HLA-DQ2 [11]. This 33-mer is an immunodominant epitope. However, the peptide-specific T-cell response in celiac disease is marked by broad diversity. Active peptides have been found in various wheat varieties and also in barley, rye and oats [9, 12]. Celiac-active T-cell epitopes are present in gliadin as well as in glutenin [13]. In a recent clinical challenge study, the celiac activity of high-molecular weight glutenin was observed in 3 adult celiac patients [14].

These findings allow the categorization of grains into permissible and unacceptable (table 1). At present it is anticipated that investigations into T-cell epitopes will help to identify other grains for inclusion into the GFD, e.g. the Ethiopian cereal tef [15].

Oats represent a unique case in celiac disease and are conventionally not included in the GFD. Celiac-active T-cell epitopes are known to be present in avenin from oats [12]. However, clinical data from Scandinavia [16–18] have shown that oats are tolerated by many children and adults with celiac disease. No evidence of harmful effects was found by clinical, laboratory and small-intestinal investigations in 92 Finnish adult patients [16] even after 5 years of follow-up. The same was true for 93 Swedish children who were newly diagnosed as having celiac disease [17] and for 32 Finnish children with established celiac disease [18]. It must be mentioned, however, that several patients dropped out of the first two studies [16, 17]; besides this, long-term follow-up studies are not yet available.

A report on 19 adult celiac patients from Norway, who underwent a challenge with 15 g of oats per day for 12 weeks [19], showed that oats were well tolerated by the majority of patients. However, 1 patient developed subtotal villous atrophy and dramatic dermatitis, and improvement was achieved only by an oats-free diet. Evidence of clinical intolerance to oats [10] was observed in 2 other celiac patients whose intestinal immune response to an oats peptide was similar but not identical to that to wheat peptides.

Cross-contamination, predominantly by barley, is a further, major problem in a GFD which includes oats products. Although immunochemical detection is available (see below) and the technical possibilities for producing oats preparations free of contamination exist, the inclusion of oats in the diet of celiac patients remains controversial and continues to be an unresolved issue. Most national celiac societies, with the exception of Finland, reject oats in the GFD.

Compliance with and Effects of a Gluten-Free Diet

Prerequisites for compliance with a GFD are up-to-date information and proper motivation. Adherence to the diet is best accomplished when the patient understands its role in the alleviation of the symptoms he or she experiences. This was underscored in a study of 22 adolescents who, in comparison to a control group with classic symptoms, showed lower compliance after celiac disease had been detected by screening [20].

Noncompliance ranges from 7 to 55% in celiac patients as a whole and is related to factors such as age, sex, ethnicity, school grade, social class, education, celiac society membership and regular dietetic follow-up [21]. An unbalanced GFD could lead to excessive lipid and protein consumption and, consequently, to obesity [22]. Intensive medical and dietary support is necessary to prevent long-term complications and to achieve satisfactory dietary management [23]. The aim of such a management is not only to ensure compliance, but an adequate nutritional intake as well.

The short-term and long-term responses and alleviation of gastrointestinal symptoms serve as basic diagnostic criteria in celiac disease. However, their occurrence varies individually [24, 25]. The long-term positive effects of the GFD have been proven and even a few years on this diet, during childhood, led to sustained subjective and objective improvements as evidenced by symptom rating, laboratory data and small-intestinal histology [24–26]. Negative side effects, such as psychological burden and stress, induced by a GFD, were found to be more pronounced in women in comparison to men [24]. A broad spectrum of gastrointestinal and psychological symptoms were found in celiac patients on a GFD, and this was associated with a potentially negative impact on the quality of life. Nevertheless, the positive effects of the GFD can clearly be said to outweigh the negative side effects in the treatment of celiac disease.

Short- and long-term observations of celiac patients on a GFD revealed that histological recovery occurs gradually, may take more than 2 years and, in some cases, be incomplete. However, the extent or lack of histological recovery varied considerably in different groups of patients, with low recovery being mainly associated with poor compliance and, additionally, with age over 30 years [27–29]. From the clinical perspective, the treatment of celiac disease by means of a GFD is indicated in all classic cases and also in silent and atypical cases (table 2), but not, however, in latent celiac disease. The situation is further complicated by the fact that a symptomatic and histological response may also be evident in patients with borderline enteropathy (Marsh type 1–2) who do not meet the diagnostic criteria of the European Society for Pediatric Gastroenterology, Hepatology and Nutrition [30].

Table 2. Silent celiac disease – reasons for a GFD

Improvement of intestinal and extraintestinal symptoms
Mucosal recovery (villous architecture, inflammatory infiltration)
Catch-up growth (children and adolescents)
Prevention of
- deficiency symptoms (Fe, Ca, vitamin D, folic acid)
- refractory lesions
- autoimmune diseases
- malignant tumors (small-intestinal lymphoma)

Several other beneficial effects of the GFD have recently been reported, including changes in bone mineral density, improvements in neurological and psychological disorders such as depression, subsiding of severe liver disease, normalization of the serum lipoprotein profile, and the regulation of metabolic parameters in diabetic celiac patients. A detailed discussion of the impact of these changes would go beyond the scope of this chapter. At present, there is no reason to challenge the concept of the GFD as the basic treatment for patients with celiac disease even at a time when alternative therapy forms are being sought or introduced.

Evidence-Based Regulations and Control of Gluten-Free Food

Earlier methods for measuring gluten in food were neither specific nor sufficiently sensitive to detect low gluten levels; besides this, appropriate standards were missing and reproducibility was poor [3]. Today, the methods available for the measurement of gluten are reproducible, suitably sensitive and demonstrate high specificity. The international Prolamine Working Group introduced a gliadin preparation, serving as a basis for gluten analysis, which derived from 28 wheat cultivars representative of the three main European wheat-producing countries France, UK and Germany [31]. This gliadin preparation was developed and tested according to standard procedures. Immunochemical and physicochemical characterization of this material showed that no major gliadin components had been lost. Good results were found for solubility, homogeneity and stability, and its performance in enzyme immunoassays exhibited adequate reproducibility.

On the basis of this Prolamine Working Group gliadin material, the R5 ELISA method for gluten determination in food was established and described in a published report [32]. This sandwich ELISA method is based on a single monoclonal antibody (R5) against rye secalin. The antibody recognizes the sequence QQPFP as well as QQQFP, LQPFP and QLPFP [33]. Overlapping specificity was found for the known immunodominant prolamine epitopes. The test system recognizes gliadin, which is the analyte. By applying the multiplication factor of 2, results can be expressed as gluten (limit of detection = 3.2 mg/kg). Prior to the immunochemical procedure, samples had to be extracted by means of a cocktail solution which involved reducing 250 mM 2-mercaptoethanol and 2 M guanidine hydrochloride in a phosphate-buffered saline solution. This extraction procedure proved to be superior to simple extraction through 60% aqueous ethanol, e.g. in heated food samples. While the system does not react with maize, rice and oats, it was found suitable and sufficiently sensitive for wheat, rye and barley.

A collaborative R5 interlaboratory trial was carried out by the Prolamine Working Group [34]. Twelve coded samples were analyzed by 20 laboratories for this purpose. The R5 ELISA method was found to be robust, and repeatability and reproducibility data were acceptable. Investigations confirmed that the R5 method was well suited for the determination of gluten concentrations ranging from 20 to 200 mg/kg, a range which is currently under discussion by the Codex Alimentarius. The R5 now represents the state-of-the-art method for gluten analysis and, in 2006, the R5 ELISA for gluten analysis was endorsed by the Codex Alimentarius Committee on Methods of Analysis and Sampling as a type 1 method. However, certain difficulties still need to be resolved, such as those associated with matrix effects, or concerning the analysis of hydrolyzed products which require a separate competitive ELISA system. Such a system, based on the R5 antibody, is currently being developed. The subject of gluten analysis continues to be open to further development and methodological improvement.

Clinical investigations into gluten sensitivity are crucially important for the establishment of meaningful gluten analyses in scientific food control. Several studies have been conducted with the aim of addressing the difficult problem of determining the levels of gluten that would be tolerable in the GFD of celiac patients [3, 10, 35]. Preliminary studies revealed that 100 mg of gliadin per day exceeded a tolerable level as it induced celiac-specific histological lesions in children. Results of a more recent, long-term dietary survey of 76 adult celiac patients treated with either a wheat-starch-based or a naturally gluten-free diet revealed gluten contamination of up to 200 mg/kg in both dietary groups. The long-term mucosal recovery was good in both groups [36]. Other studies have also shown that, despite trace amounts of gluten, wheat-starch-derived gluten-free products were safe for celiac patients, and the authors concluded that a gluten threshold of 100 mg/kg of food 'can safely be set' [36]. The median daily flour consumption in this study was 80 g (range 10–300 g) leading to a median daily gluten intake of about 8 mg (range 1–30 mg).

A different approach was taken by another recent study of 39 Italian adults with biopsy-proven celiac disease [37]. These patients were randomized into three groups, in which either 0, 10 or 50 mg of gluten was ingested daily, over 90 days, via a capsule. A clinical relapse occurred in 1 of the patients challenged with 10 mg of gluten. Morphological investigations of villous height and crypt depth ratio provided evidence of improvement in the placebo group, no major changes in the 10-mg group and a decrease indicative of histological damage in the 50-mg group. It must, however, be mentioned that the baseline values in this study were not entirely normal and that mucosal improvement in the placebo group had not been anticipated. These findings as well as the low numbers of patients in each group (n = 13) make it difficult to draw general conclusions. The authors recommend a threshold of 20 mg/kg gluten, which needs to be viewed within the context of a relatively high consumption of gluten-free products in Italy (maximum = 500 g/day). This threshold includes a safety margin and assumes a level of exposure that is well below the 50 mg/ day applied in the study.

Data relating to the consumption of gluten-free products are rather controversial, and their great diversity can be attributed to the fact that they derive from different countries. A recent study [38] showed that the 50th percentile of the total amount of gluten-free products consumed per day ranged from 173 g in Spain to 265 g in Italy. This was more than in Finland [36]. Thus, at present, firm conclusions cannot be drawn for devising regulatory solutions.

The necessity for evidence-based regulations for gluten-free food has been emphasized by the Codex Alimentarius Committee on Nutrition and Food for Special Dietary Uses (CCNFSDU) [3] and also, more recently, by the European Food Safety Authority [39]. In addition, this matter was discussed in detail by the US Food and Drug Administration [1]. The CCNFSDU adopted the first Codex Standard on gluten-free food in 1981, in which cereals toxic to celiac patients were defined (wheat, rye, barley, oats and cross-bred varieties); a cutoff limit of 0.05 g Kjeldahl nitrogen per 100 g dry matter was set for gluten in raw materials used in the production of gluten-free food. Even though gluten analysis has now reached a highly developed stage (R5 ELISA), gluten analysis and the clinical investigation of the effects of gluten in celiac patients will obviously continue to be the focus of ongoing efforts in the scientific community. The recent CCNFSDU provisional clinical levels of 20 mg/kg of gluten for naturally gluten-free foods and 200 mg/kg for gluten-free products are a matter of debate. The same holds true for the question about whether oats should be excluded from the GFD (see above). Two main positions have emerged in the ongoing Codex discussions involving delegates from different countries: the first pertains to the single limit of 20 mg/kg for all foods considered gluten free, whereas the second relates to a 2-fold approach in which the limit for naturally gluten-free foods is set at 20 mg/kg and a cutoff of 100 mg/kg would be valid for products rendered gluten free, e.g. from wheat starch. Among the gluten-free products available in many European countries, those that are wheat starch based are widely consumed, particularly in the north. Studies in Finland concluded that a level of 100 mg/kg was safe and, therefore, acceptable (see above). One of the main objectives in establishing evidence-based limits and regulations is to ensure that celiac patients can make an informed choice by means of defined labeling and thereby adjust the intake of gluten individually.

Health-Related Quality of Life in Children and Adults with Celiac Disease

Health has physical, emotional and social dimensions. In order to recognize the value of each of these components to the well-being and daily life of celiac patients, the term 'health-related quality of life' was coined [40]. Psychological tools such as questionnaires, the 'well-being index' and personal interviews have been introduced into the care of celiac patients on a GFD in addition to the dietary surveys aimed at measuring the health-related quality of life and also for the purpose of evaluating the perceived burden of illness [41–43]. The data collected recently are remarkable und indicate that the objective and subjective findings in these patients do not match those of control groups, even in patients with good compliance. At the physical level, a higher number of gastrointestinal symptoms may be present, which persist despite therapy [24] (see above); however, this is not necessarily true in children [41]. The burden of illness appeared to be particularly high in adult women [40, 44] and low scores for general health and vitality were common among female patients. In contrast, the scores for male patients were either normal or, as in some cases, clearly better than controls. It must be stated here that these findings were not correlated with compliance. From these long-term results spanning a 10-year period, the authors concluded that other factors, beyond normalization of the intestinal mucosa, were highly relevant to the perceived health status of adult female celiac patients on a GFD. The short-term, preliminary results for the first year of treatment also indicated substantial improvements in the health-related quality of life [40].

The GFD also has an impact on lifestyle, such as when patients face difficulties in finding retailers of gluten-free food or when the decision to travel or eat at a restaurant must be overridden due to the risk of dietary transgression [45]. Celiac patients were shown to have high levels of psychophysiological reactiveness and alterations in personality that possibly interfere with proper adjustment to living with the disease [46]. They experience feelings of isolation, shame, fear of gluten contamination and anxiety resulting from the perception that they are a cause of inconvenience to others [47]. These feelings can lead to psychosocial conflicts and are indicative of a range of disturbances, manifesting in various degrees, which are related to celiac disease even if a given patient is on a gluten-free diet. The authors [47] concluded that it is crucial to take into account the psychological and social aspects of treatment in celiac patients. This in turn has reinforced the need to explore alternative forms of treatment.

Conclusions

The GFD is the basic therapy for celiac disease in childhood, adolescence and adulthood; this has been validated by recent and ongoing investigations. The introduction of the GFD must be based on the diagnostic spectrum of celiac disease, ranging from the classic to nonclassic forms. Information about the disorder must be offered throughout treatment with the aim of educating patients and providing psychosocial support, which in turn lead to better compliance. As shown above, the benefits of a GFD outweigh its potentially negative effects. However, normal levels for the health-related quality of life have yet to be achieved in celiac patients on a GFD, particularly in adult women, and the behavioral and emotional implications involved must be considered. Disease management by means of the GFD must include dietary control: it is certainly possible, both on the individual level of long-term follow-up of the patient and the food level by gluten analysis and control of gluten-free products in the laboratory. Regulatory solutions are currently being developed by institutions such as the Codex Alimentarius, the US Food and Drug Administration and the European Food Safety Authority. The questions relating to the inclusion in the GFD of oats or wheat-starch-based gluten-free products remain unresolved at present. Topics and open questions that need to be explored in future investigations are listed in table 3 and are rooted in the premise that lifelong adherence to a GFD cannot be taken for granted. Nevertheless, it is believed that a strict GFD 'can fully restore health and improve quality of life (...). Regular follow-up can help increase compliance and minimize complications' [8]. Future perspectives include alternative forms of therapy that are being conceived today and the development of the enormous potential that has been ascribed to primary preventative measures.

Table 3. Research topics

Improvement of gluten analysis
Long-term clinical studies as a basis of regulatory solutions
Long-term assessment of oats in the GFD
Psychosocial investigation of health-related quality of life
Factors to improve compliance and empowerment
Comparison of T-cell reactivity and clinical intestinal effects of gluten peptides
Search for additional allowed grains with acceptable baking quality for GFD
Nutritional research into micronutrient deficiencies and obesity in GFD
Development of alternative therapy forms targeted to genetic and molecular mechanisms in celiac disease

References

1 Shuren J: Food labelling: gluten-free labeling of foods. Fed Reg 2007;72:2795–2817.
2 Fasano A, Catassi C: Current approaches to diagnosis and treatment of celiac disease: an evolving spectrum. Gastroenterology 2001;120:636–651.
3 Stern M, Ciclitira P, van Eckert R, Feighery C, Janssen FW, Mendez E, Mothes T, Troncone R, Wieser H: Analysis and clinical effects of gluten in coeliac disease. Eur J Gastroenterol Hepatol 2001;13:741–747.
4 Rostom A, Murray JA, Kagnoff MF: American Gastroenterological Association (AGA) Institute technical review on the diagnosis and management of celiac disease. Gastroenterology 2006;131:1981–2002.
5 Anderson LA, McMillan SA, Watson RGP, Monaghan P, Gavin AT, Murray LJ: Malignancy and mortality in a population-based cohort of patients with coeliac disease or 'gluten sensitivity'. World J Gastroenterol 2007;13:146–151.
6 Kupper C: Dietary guidelines and implementation for coeliac disease. Gastroenterology 2005;128:S121–S127.
7 Schuppan D, Dennis MD, Kelly CP: Coeliac disease: epidemiology, pathogenesis, diagnosis, and nutritional management. Nutr Clin Car 2005;8: 54–69.
8 See J, Murray JA: GFD: the medical and nutrition management of coeliac disease. Nutr Clin Pract 2006;21:1–15.
9 Vader W, Kooy Y, van Veelen P, De Ru A, Harris D, Benckhuisen W, Pena S, Mearin L, Drijfhout JW, Koning F: The gluten response in children with celiac disease is directed toward multiple gliadin and glutenin peptides. Gastroenterology 2002;122:1729–1737.
10 Ciclitira PJ, Ellis HJ, Lundin KE: GFD – what is toxic? Best Pract Res Clin Gastroenterol 2005;19:359–371.
11 Qiao S-W, Bergseng E, Molberg Ø, Xia J, Fleckenstein B, Khosla C, Sollid LM: Antigen presentation to coeliac lesion-derived T cells of 33-mer gliadin peptide naturally formed by gastrointestinal digestion. J Immunol 2004;173: 1757–1762.
12 Vader LW, Stepniak DT, Bunnik EM, Kooy YMC, De Haan W, Drijfhout JW, Van Veelen PA, Koning F: Characterization of cereal toxicity for celiac disease patients based on protein homology in grains. Gastroenterology 2003;125:1105–1113.
13 Molberg Ø, Solheim Flæte N, Jensen T, Lundin KEA, Arentz-Hansen H, Anderson OD, Uhlen AK, Sollid LM: Intestinal T-cell responses to high-molecular-weight glutenins in celiac disease. Gastroenterology 2003;125: 337–344.
14 Ciclitira PJ, Dewar D, Ellis HJ, Engel W, Johnson M, Wieser W: Clinical toxicity of HMW glutenin subunits of wheat to patients with celiac disease; in Stern M (ed): Proceedings of the 19th Meeting of the Working Group on Prolamin Analysis and Toxicity, September 30 to October 3, 2004, Prague, Czech Republic. Zwickau, Verlag Wissenschaftliche Scripten, 2005, pp 147–149.
15 Spaenij-Dekking L, Kooy-Winkelaar Y, Koning F: The Ethiopian cereal tef in coeliac disease. New Engl J Med 2005; 353:1748–1749.
16 Janatuinen EK, Pikkarainen PK, Kemppainen TA, Kosma V-M, Järvinen RMK, Uusitupa MIJ, Julkunen RJK: A comparison of diets with and without oats in adults with celiac disease. N Engl J Med 1995;333:1033–1037.
17 Holm K, Mäki M, Vuolteenaho N, Mustalahti K, Ashorn M, Ruuska T, Kaukinen K: Oats in the treatment of childhood coeliac disease: a 2-year controlled trial and a long-term clinical follow-up study. Aliment Pharmacol Ther 2006;23:1463–1472.
18 Hogberg L, Laurin P, Fälth-Magnusson K, Grant C, Grodzinsky E, Jansson G, Ascher H, Browaldh L, Hammersjö JA, Lindberg E, Myrdal U, Stenhammer L: Oats to children with newly diagnosed coeliac disease: a randomised double blind study. Gut 2004;53:649–654.
19 Lundin KEA, Nilsen EM, Scott HG, Løberg EM, Gjøen A, Bratlie J, Skar V, Mendez E, Løvik A, Kett K: Oats induced villous atrophy in celiac disease. Gut 2003;52:649–652.
20 Fabiani E, Taccari LM, Ratsch IM, Di Giuseppe S, Coppa GV, Catassi C: Compliance with GFD in adolescents with screening-detected celiac disease: a 5-year follow-up study. J Pediatr 2000; 136:841–843.

21 Butterworth JR, Banfield LM, Iqbal TH, Cooper BT: Factors relating to compliance with a gluten-free diet in patients with coeliac disease: comparison of white Caucasian and South Asian patients. Clin Nutr 2004;23: 1127–1134.

22 Mariani P, Viti MG, Montuori M, La Vecchia A, Cipolletta E, Calvani L, Bonamico M: The gluten-free diet: a nutritional risk factor for adolescents with celiac disease? J Pediatr Gastroenterol Nutr 1998;27:519–523.

23 Hopman EGD, le Cessie S, von Blomberg BM, Mearin ML: Nutritional management of the gluten-free diet in young people with celiac disease in the Netherlands. J Pediatr Gastroenterol Nutr 2006;43:102–108.

24 Midhagen G, Haller C: High rate of gastrointestinal symptoms in celiac patients living on a gluten-free diet: controlled study. Am J Gastroenterol 2003;98:2023–2026.

25 Murray JA, Watson T, Clearman B, Mitros F: Effect of a gluten-free diet on gastrointestinal symptoms in celiac disease. Am J Clin Nutr 2004;79: 669–673.

26 Ciacci C, Iovino P, Amoruso D, Siniscalchi M, Tortora R, Di Gilio A, Fusco M, Mazzacca G: Grown-up coeliac children: the effects of only a few years on a gluten-free diet in childhood. Aliment Pharmacol Ther 2005; 21:421–429.

27 Wahab PJ, Meijer JWR, Mulder CJJ: Histologic follow-up of people with coeliac disease on a gluten-free diet. Am J Clin Pathol 2002;118:459–463.

28 Lee SK, Lo W, Memeo L, Rotterdam H, Green PH: Duodenal histology in patients with celiac disease after treatment with a gluten-free diet. Gastrointest Endosc 2003;57:187–191.

29 Tursi A, Brandimarte G, Giorgetti GM, Elisei W, Inchingolo CD, Monardo E, Aiello F: Endoscopic and histological findings in the duodenum of adults with celiac disease before and after changing to a gluten-free diet: a 2-year prospective study. Endoscopy 2006;38: 702–707.

30 Tursi A, Brandimarte G: The symptomatic and histologic response to a gluten-free diet in patients with borderline enteropathy. J Clin Gastroenterol 2003;36:13–17.

31 van Eckert R, Berghofer E, Ciclitira PJ, Chirdo F, Denery-Papini S, Ellis HJ, Ferranti P, Goodwin P, Immer U, Mamone G, Méndez E, Mothes T, Novalin S, Osman A, Rumbo M, Stern M, Thorell L, Whim A, Wieser H: Towards a new gliadin reference material – isolation and characterization. J Cer Sci 2006;43:331–341.

32 Valdés I, García E, Llorente M, Méndez E: Innovative approach to low-level gluten determination in foods using a novel sandwich enzyme-linked immunosorbent assay protocol. Eur J Gastroenterol 2003;15:465–474.

33 Kahlenberg F, Sanchez D, Lachmann I, Tuckova L, Tlaskova H, Méndez E, Mothes T: Monoclonal antibody R5 for detection of putatively coeliac-toxic gliadin peptides. Eur Food Res Technol 2006;22:78–82.

34 Méndez E, Vela C, Immer U, Janssen FW: Report of a collaborative trial to investigate the performance of the R5 enzyme- linked immunoassay to determine gliadin and gluten-free food. Eur J Gastroenterol Hepatol 2005;17: 1053–1063.

35 Hischenhuber C, Crevel R, Jarry B, Mäki M, Moneret-Vautrin DA, Romano A, Troncone R, Ward R: Review article: safe amounts of gluten for patients with wheat allergy or coeliac disease. Aliment Pharmacol Ther 2006;23:559–575.

36 Collin P, Thorell L, Kaukinen K, Mäki M: The safe threshold for gluten contamination in gluten-free products: can trace amounts be accepted in the treatment of coeliac disease? Aliment Pharmacol Ther 2004;29:1277–1283.

37 Catassi C, Fabiani E, Iacono G, D'Agate C, Francavilla R, Biagi F, Volta U, Accomando S, Picarelli A, De Vitis I, Pianelli G, Gesuita R, Carle F, Mandolesi A, Bearzi I, Fasano A: A prospective, double-blind, placebo-controlled trial to establish a safe gluten threshold for patients with celiac disease. Am J Clin Nutr 2007;85:160–166.

38 Gibert A, Espadaler M, Angel Canela M, Sanchez A, Vaque C, Rafecas M: Consumption of gluten-free products: should the threshold value for trace amounts of gluten be at 20, 100 or 200 ppm? Eur J Gastroenterol Hepatol 2006; 18:1187–1195.

39 NDA: Opinion of the Scientific Panel on Dietetic Products, Nutrition and Allergies on a request from the Commission relating to the evaluation of allergenic foods for labeling purposes. EFSA J 2004;32:1–197. www.efsa.eu.int/science/nda_opinions/catindex_en.html.HepHe.

40 Hallert C, Lohiniemi S: Quality of life of celiac patients living on a gluten-free diet. Nutrition 1999;15:795–797.

41 Kolsteren MM, Koopmann HM, Schalekamp G, Mearin ML: Health-related quality of life in children with celiac disease. J Pediatr 2001;138:593–595.

42 Roos S, Kärner A, Haller C: Psychological well-being of adult coeliac patients treated for 10 years. Dig Liver Dis 2006;38:177–180.

43 Häuser W, Gold J, Stallmach A, Caspary WF, Stein J: Development and validation of the Celiac Disease Questionnaire (CDQ), a disease-specific health-related quality of life measure for adult patients with celiac disease. J Clin Gastroenterol 2007;41:157–166.

44 Hallert C, Grännö C, Hultén S, Midhagen G, Ström M, Svensson H, Valdimarsson T: Living with coeliac disease: controlled study of the burden of illness. Scand J Gastroenterol 2002;37:39–42.

45 Zarkadas M, Cranney A, Case S, Molloy M, Switzer C, Graham D, Butzner JD, Rashid M, Warren RE, Burrows V: The impact of gluten-free diet on adults with celiac disease: results of a national survey. J Hum Nutr Dietet 2006;19:41–49.

46 De Rosa A, Troncone A, Vacca M, Ciacci C: Characteristics and quality of illness behavior in celiac disease. Psychosomatics 2004;45:336–342.

47 Sverker A, Hensing G, Hallert C: 'Controlled by food' – lived experiences of coeliac disease. J Hum Nutr Dietet 2005;18:171–180.

Prof. Dr. M. Stern
University Children's Hospital, University of Tübingen,
Hoppe-Seyler-Strasse 1
DE–72076 Tübingen (Germany)
Tel. +49 7071 298 3781, Fax +49 7071 29 5477, E-Mail martin.stern@med.uni-tuebingen.de

Fasano A, Troncone R, Branski D (eds): Frontiers in Celiac Disease.
Pediatr Adolesc Med. Basel, Karger, 2008, vol 12, pp 123–132

Update on the Management of Refractory Coeliac Disease

A. Al-toma · W.H.M. Verbeek · C.J.J. Mulder

Department of Gastroenterology, VU University Medical Centre, Amsterdam, The Netherlands

Abstract

Refractory coeliac disease (RCD) is being currently defined as persisting or recurring villous atrophy with crypt hyperplasia and increased intra-epithelial lymphocytes in spite of a strict gluten-free diet for more than 12 months or when severe persisting symptoms necessitate intervention independently of the duration of the dietary therapy. Two categories of RCD are being recognized: type I without aberrant T cells and type II with aberrant T cells detected by immunophenotyping of the intestinal mucosa. In contrast to patients with a high percentage of aberrant T cells, patients with RCD type I seem to profit from an immunosuppressive treatment. In cases of RCD II with persistent clinical symptoms and/or a high percentage of aberrant T cells in intestinal biopsies in spite of corticosteroid treatment, more aggressive therapeutic schemes should be considered. However, no therapy seems to be curative in RCD II. Cladribine seems to have some role in the management of these patients. High-dose chemotherapy followed by autologous stem cell transplantation has been used in patients resulting in a dramatic improvement in the clinical, laboratory, histopathological and immunological parameters.

Coeliac disease is a lifelong inflammatory condition of the gastro-intestinal tract that affects the small intestine in genetically susceptible individuals [1]. On small-bowel biopsy there is a characteristic, although not specific, mucosal lesion that impairs nutrient absorption by the involved bowel. Prompt improvement of nutrient absorption and healing of the characteristic intestinal mucosal lesion is seen upon withdrawal of dietary gluten.

Non-responsive coeliac disease can be described in terms of the clinical scenario of a lack of initial response to a prescribed gluten-free diet (GFD), or the recurrence of symptoms despite maintenance of a GFD in a patient who responded initially to the GFD [2]. Although clinical improvement is usually followed by histological improvement most of the time, on occasions there is evidence for histological improvement with persistence of clinical symptoms that could be related to other causes [3, 4]. Clinical improvement is usually evident within the first few weeks of starting GFD; however, it might take up to 2 years before a complete restoration of intestinal mucosa is evident [5].

Non-responsive coeliac disease is defined as a lack of initial response to a GFD, or the recurrence of symptoms despite adherence to diet in a patient who responded initially.

A specific definition of refractory coeliac disease (RCD) is missing in the literature. We define true RCD as persisting or recurring villous

Table 1. Diagnostic criteria

RCD I
Villous atrophy persisting or recurring despite strict adherence to a GFD
At least partial villous atrophy (Marsh 3A) according to the modified Marsh criteria
Excluding other causes of villous atrophy
When ≤10% aberrant T cells in intestinal biopsy
IEL phenotype is normal with the expression of surface CD3, CD8 and T-cell receptor
RCD II
The same as RCD I, in addition to the presence of ≥20% aberrant T cells in intestinal biopsy
The IELs have a normal morphology but exhibit an aberrant phenotype (normal expression of CD103 and CD7, down-regulation of surface CD3 to intracytoplasmic CD3, and the lack of surface T-cell markers CD4, CD8 and T-cell receptor)
Enteropathy-associated T-cell lymphoma has been confidently excluded

atrophy with crypt hyperplasia and increased intra-epithelial lymphocytes (IELs) in spite of a strict GFD for more than 12 months or when severe persisting symptoms necessitate intervention independently of the duration of the GFD [6]. RCD may not respond primarily or secondarily to GFD [7]. All other causes of malabsorption must be excluded, and additional features supporting the diagnosis of coeliac disease must be looked for, including the presence of antibodies in the untreated state and the presence of coeliac-related HLA-DQ markers.

Currently two categories of RCD are being recognized (table 1): type I without aberrant T cells and type II with aberrant T cells detected by immunophenotyping by flow-cytometric analysis or immunohistology of the intestinal mucosa [5]. Arbitrarily, based on our own experience, a percentage of aberrant cells, CD7+CD3– of CD103+ IELs or cytoplasmic CD3+ surface CD3– of CD103+ IELs, of ≤10% has been regarded as normal and more than 20% as definitively abnormal.

Pathogenesis of Refractory Coeliac Disease

Genetic and Environmental Factors

The environmental factor is mainly ingestion of gluten, while several genes contribute to the genetic predisposition [8]. The main genetic factors, as mentioned before, are given HLA-DQ genes, i.e. the genes encoding DQ2 or DQ8 in the HLA complex on 6p21. Approximately 95% of coeliacs have a DQ2 comprised of DQB1*302 and DQA1*03. A small number of individuals lacking either of those heterodimers have DQB1*02 or DQA1*05 alone [9, 10]. Gene dosage also affects coeliac disease susceptibility; individuals with the heterodimer comprised of DQB1*02 and DQA1*05 and most of the remaining 5% have a DQ8 heterodimer. Homozygous individuals who carry DQB1*02 and DQA1*05 in cis on both chromosomes have a greater risk of developing complicated forms of coeliac disease [11]. Non-HLA complex genes seem to contribute, but the nature and effects of these genes are less well known. The identification and knowledge of the function of additional genetic factors should improve the understanding of the actual pathogenesis of coeliac disease and lead to new diagnostic strategies in case finding and screening high-risk groups.

Diagnostic Approach to Refractory Coeliac Disease

Revision of the Initial Coeliac Disease

In a patient with villous atrophy refractory to a GFD, the first step requires reassessment of the initial diagnosis of coeliac disease, in order to exclude other diseases, such as giardiasis, tropical sprue, postinfectious diarrhoea, collagenous sprue, protein intolerance, tuberculosis (including atypical), AIDS, common variable immunodeficiency syndrome, Whipple's disease, radiation enteritis, immunoproliferative small-intestinal disease, Crohns' disease, eosinophilic gastroenteritis and autoimmune enteropathy.

The presence of circulating antigliadin, antiendomysium (EMA) or anti-tissue-transglutaminase (tTG) antibodies before the onset of the GFD, an HLA-DQ2 or -DQ8 status and an initial clinical and histological improvement after a strict GFD are strongly suggestive of coeliac disease. Regarding the histological features, an increased number of IELs (more than 30 lymphocytes/100 epithelial cells) is seen in almost all active coeliac disease patients [1].

Assessment of the Gluten-Free Diet

The most important cause for a non-responsive coeliac patient is failure to adhere to a GFD, which has been reported in up to 50% of adult coeliac patients [12]. The presence of persisting circulating EMA or anti-tTG antibodies is strongly suggestive of dietary mistakes [12]. However, the absence of circulating antibodies cannot rule out minor, inadvertent or voluntary, ingestion of gluten in the diet. On the other hand, persisting antibody titres may also be found in rare patients on a strict GFD with RCD and especially EMA [3]. Anti-tTG antibodies mostly return to normal within 2–3 months. A careful dietary inquiry performed by a dietician skilled in coeliac disease should be performed as the first line of investigation in a supposed RCD patient.

Exclude Other Causes of Diarrhoea with/without Villous Atrophy

In case of persisting diarrhoea despite demonstrable improvement in the histological lesion and exclusion of dietary mistakes, other associated disorders should be considered. Well-known causes responsible for symptoms mainly include microscopic colitis and more rarely intermittent pancreatic insufficiency in coeliac disease, secondary lactase deficiency, bacterial overgrowth, coexisting inflammatory bowel disease, irritable-bowel syndrome but also anal incontinence [4, 13]. Table 2 summarizes other causes of villous atrophy other than coeliac disease.

Table 2. Other causes than RCD for persisting villous atrophy (adapted from Daum et al. [6])

Mostly increased number of IELs
Giardiasis
Tropical sprue
Postinfectious diarrhoea
Collagenous sprue
Protein intolerance (cow's milk, soya)
Mostly normal number of IELs
Tuberculosis (including atypical)
AIDS
Common variable immunodeficiency syndrome
Whipple's disease
Radiation enteritis
Immunoproliferative small-intestinal disease
Crohn's disease
Eosinophilic gastro-enteritis
Autoimmune enteropathy

There are many other causes of villous atrophy besides coeliac disease. The clinical history should investigate longer stays near the equator for detection of tropical sprue. Small-bowel enteropathy seems to occur often in southern parts of Africa. Giardiasis should be excluded by immunofluorescence of stool samples and may be diagnosed by duodenal histology. Crohn's disease with involvement of the duodenum may mimic or even coexist with coeliac disease. The term 'collagenous sprue' should be used with caution, as this disease is not an established independent entity. A subepithelial matrix broader than 10–20 μm should point to the diagnosis of collagenous sprue. Deposition of excess of extracellular matrix underneath the basement membrane is an unspecific reaction, which can be seen in gluten-responsive coeliac disease, as well as in several other entities of RCD and also in enteropathy-associated T-cell lymphoma (EATL).

Collagenous-band-like structures regress to a large part in responsive coeliac disease. Autoimmune enteropathy is seen mainly in children and young adults, but may occur also in elderly patients. The histological picture often shows a diminished number of Paneth cells. The number of IELs is often normal, and patients present frequently with concurrent autoimmune diseases.

We have to realize that villous atrophy has also been reported in association with the presence of a thymoma, with protein intolerance, in conjunction with common variable immunodeficiency syndromes and eosinophilic enteritis. In common variable immunodeficiency, antibody testing for coeliac-disease-associated antibodies is not useful. Only histological and clinical improvement on a strict GFD may reveal underlying coeliac disease in single cases of common variable immunodeficiency.

Exclude Malignant Complications of Coeliac Disease
Unexplained weight loss, abdominal pain, fever and night sweating should alarm physicians of an overt EATL. Other markers for overt EATL may be positive stool blood tests, increased lactate dehydrogenase or β_2-microglobulin [14, 15].

In patients on GFD, EATL need not necessarily be accompanied by duodenal villous atrophy [16].

A high index of suspicion for an overt lymphoma should lead to an extensive workup including upper and lower endoscopy, ENT workup, CT scan of the thorax and abdomen with enteroclysis, video capsule enteroscopy and double balloon enteroscopy in order to obtain histological specimens. In some cases laparotomy, intra-operative enteroscopy and full-thickness biopsies are necessary, as the operative procedure may come to an earlier diagnosis which may be essential.

New advances in small-bowel imaging including CT scan and magnetic resonance enteroclysis can improve the diagnostic accuracy in these patients [17].

PET scan has been investigated in patients with EATL and RCD. In a prospective cohort of 8 EATL patients and 30 patients with RCD, Hadithi et al. [18] demonstrate that PET can visualize in all patients sites affected by EATL as confirmed on biopsy.

The diagnosis of overt T-cell lymphoma is based on histological and immunohistochemical features with mainly evidence of large or medium-size T-cell proliferation expressing a CD3+CD8+/– and CD103+ phenotype. The majority presents as CD3+CD8–CD30+ large-cell lymphoma; however, small-cell lymphomas are often CD3+CD8+CD30– [14, 15].

Diagnosis of small-bowel adenocarcinoma may even be more difficult than lymphoma. Especially tumours located in the jejunum and ileum, which are not reached by standard endoscopic techniques, require extensive investigations. Diagnosis may often be made only after operative procedures.

Obscure gastro-intestinal bleeding, obstructive symptoms, stenotic lesions on radiological examinations and video capsule enteroscopy retention should raise the suspicion of these malignancies (authors' own experience).

The Evolving Role of Double Balloon Enteroscopy
First described by Yamamoto et al. [19] in 2001, double balloon enteroscopy is a new endoscopic technique with the potential to allow complete visualization of the entire small bowel.

In a European retrospective study, enteroscopy was diagnostic in all patients suspected of having RCD [20].

Establishing the Diagnosis of Refractory Coeliac Disease

Finally, RCD is a diagnosis of exclusion, defined as a persisting villous atrophy that does not respond to a strict GFD (table 3). Demonstration of an aberrant clonal intra-epithelial T-cell population and/or

Table 3. Steps required to establish the diagnosis of RCD

Revision of the initial diagnosis of coeliac disease	The presence of antigliadin, EMA or anti-tTG antibodies before the institution of a GFD, an HLA-DQ2 or -DQ8 status and an initial clinical and histological improvement after a strict diet
Assessment of the diet	The presence of persisting EMA or anti-tTG antibodies is strongly suggestive of dietary mistakes
Exclude other causes of diarrhoea ± villous atrophy	See table 2
Exclude malignant complications of coeliac disease	EATL or small-bowel adenocarcinoma
Establish the diagnosis and differentiate RCD I from RCD II	Clinical behaviour, presence/absence of aberrant clonal intra-epithelial T-cell population and/or loss of antigen on IELs

loss of antigen on IELs seem to characterize this patient population at high risk for the development of overt lymphoma and differentiates RCD II from RCD I, which shows low or almost absent aberrant T cells. RCD II is also referred to as cryptic intestinal T-cell lymphoma (sprue-like intestinal T-cell lymphoma). Detection of a clonal T-cell population by testing for T-cell receptor (TCR) rearrangement is thought to be highly predictive of EATL development. However, oligo- or monoclonal IEL populations can be detected in the large majority of both RCD I and RCD II patients, also in patients who do not develop an EATL. Clonality is therefore of limited use in establishing the diagnosis of RCD and to predict the development of EATL.

Refractory Coeliac Disease Type I versus II

Clinical and Biological Behaviour

Patients with RCD I may represent an earlier stage of the disease than RCD II and the prognosis may be better, and the risk of developing an overt lymphoma is almost non-existent. In RCD I adherence to the GFD should be carefully investigated since a strict GFD may induce remission in some patients.

In RCD I, patients often develop concomitant autoimmune diseases, infectious and thromboembolic complications. Retrospective data from our patient population suggest that RCD I patients have a mortality rate which is not different from that of the general population (authors' own experience). The presence of mucosal ulcerations (ulcerative jejunitis) should alert the doctor for the possible presence of an early EATL [21].

RCD II is observed mostly in adults, and the mean age at diagnosis of RCD II is between 50 and 60 years but younger cases may be observed. Most of the patients develop severe malabsorption with weight loss, abdominal pain and diarrhoea. Some patients may also have skin lesions mimicking pyoderma gangraenosum or ulcerations mostly on the legs, arms and face, chronic chest or sinusoidal infections or unexplained fever. The link between coeliac disease and RCD II is usually suggested by the detection of circulating antigliadin, anti-EMA or anti-tTG antibodies before the initiation of the GFD in almost two thirds of patients, an HLA-DQ2 or -DQ8 status in almost all patients [11] and an initial response to GFD in about one third of patients with RCD II.

Endoscopic and Radiological Features

Usually in RCD I and II, the same pattern of villous atrophy is observed as in classical active coeliac disease. The finding of mucosal ulcerations, mostly in the jejunum, defines the clinical picture of ulcerative jejunitis [21]. In some cases of RCD II also stomach and/or colonic ulcerations may be found [22]. Enteroscopy using push, double balloon or video capsule methods should be performed in such patients with RCD II in order to search for overt lymphoma and ulcerative jejunitis. CT scan with magnetic resonance enteroclysis may be useful to exclude overt lymphoma and may demonstrate a mesenteric cavitation syndrome and hyposplenism (volume $<100\ cm^3$) in 30% of cases (authors' own experience). Enlarged mesenteric lymph nodes often accompany RCD, without necessarily being specific for a T-cell lymphoma. Staging investigations as recommended for non-Hodgkin lymphomas should be performed including bone marrow aspiration, CT scan of the thorax and abdomen, sonography of the neck as well as ENT workup especially in RCD II patients.

HLA-DQ Typing

Typing of HLA-DQA1* and -DQB1* alleles can be performed on whole-blood samples. In our immunology laboratory, this typing is being performed with a combined single-stranded conformation polymorphism/heteroduplex method by a semi-automated electrophoresis and gel staining method on the Phastsystem (Amersham-Pharmacia-Biotech, Uppsala, Sweden) [11].

We found a highly significant correlation between HLA-DQ2 homozygosity and the development of serious complications of coeliac disease, in particular RCD II and EATL [11]. The link between HLA-DQ2 homozygosity and development of RCD II and coeliac-disease-associated lymphoma of intra-epithelial origin thus suggests that the strength of the gluten-specific T-cell response in the lamina propria directly or indirectly influences the likelihood of RCD II and lymphoma development. It has been reported earlier by Vader et al. [23] that HLA-DQ2 homozygous antigen-presenting cells induce higher T-cell proliferation and cytokine secretion than HLA-DQ2/non-DQ2 heterozygous antigen-presenting cells. This may explain the strongly increased risk for disease development in HLA-DQ2 homozygous individuals. This would indicate that the adherence to a GFD is particularly important for coeliac disease patients who are homozygous for HLA-DQ2.

Small-Intestinal Biopsies

Upper gastro-intestinal endoscopy should be performed in all patients. At least 10 duodenal biopsies are to be taken for histological, immunohistochemical and flow-cytometric examination. Four to 6 biopsies are fixed and preserved in 10% formalin for histopathological and immunohistochemical evaluation. Three to 4 biopsies for TCR gene rearrangement studies are taken separately, preserved on Histocon and frozen at –20°C. For immunophenotypical evaluation 3–4 biopsies are taken and preserved in RPMI medium.

Immunophenotyping of Intra-Epithelial Lymphocytes

Lymphocytes and enterocytes are isolated from 3–4 small-intestinal biopsies. Intra-epithelial localization of lymphocytes is confirmed by surface expression of CD103 ($\alpha E\beta 7$-integrin, a gut-homing receptor for E-cadherin).

Arbitrarily, a percentage of aberrant cells, CD7+CD3– of CD103+ IELs or cytoplasmic CD3+ surface CD3– of CD103+ IELs, of $\leq 10\%$ has been regarded as normal and more than 20% as definitely abnormal.

T-Cell Receptor Gene Rearrangement Study

Clonality assessment for TCR-γ gene rearrangements is done using the Biomed-2 multiplex TCR-PCR protocol.

Detection of a clonal T-cell population by testing for TCR rearrangement is thought to be highly predictive of EATL development. However, oligo- or monoclonal IEL populations can be detected in the large majority of both RCD I and RCD II patients, also in patients who do not develop an EATL. Clonality is therefore of limited use in establishing the diagnosis of RCD and to predict the development of EATL [24, 25].

Refractory Coeliac Disease Type I versus II

In RCD I, histology of the small-bowel mucosa is in most cases indistinguishable from active untreated coeliac disease. The number of IELs may be lower than in RCD II and active coeliac disease although this has not been proven in prospective studies. The IEL phenotype is normal with the expression of surface CD3 associated with surface CD8 and TCR-β as in classical active coeliac disease. The number of CD8– and TCR-β+ IELs should exceed 50% of IELs, and a lower expression seems to be quite sensitive for differentiation from RCD II but not very specific.

In RCD II, an abnormal IEL clonal population may be observed in 80% of patients with RCD on small-intestinal biopsies. Although these IELs have a normal cytological feature, they exhibit an abnormal IEL phenotype with the expression of intracytoplasmic CD3e, surface CD103 and the lack of classical surface T-cell markers such as CD8, CD4 and TCR-αβ. Furthermore the abnormal IEL phenotype is associated with clonal TCR gene rearrangement. This abnormal IEL population usually represents more than 50% of the IELs and may also be observed in gastric and/or colonic epithelium in around two thirds of patients and may be found in the peripheral blood lymphocytes in one third. It may also be detected in skin lesions or in the chest in single patients, suggesting that RCD II is a diffuse gastro-intestinal disease.

The use of CD3 and CD8 on fixed biopsies is a very reliable method in order to assess the presence of this abnormal IEL phenotype, even retrospectively.

More recently, it has been shown on cell lines derived from clonal abnormal IELs that recurrent chromosomal abnormalities including a recurrent 1q trisomy may be found in these patients. The diagnostic yield of these cytogenetic features has not been evaluated so far. These chromosomal abnormalities, the clonality of the T-cell receptor gene and the loss of antigens on IELs, together with the frequent diffusion of the abnormal lymphocytes, indicate in spite of their normal cytology and low in situ proliferative capabilities that this clonal IEL population can be considered as a cryptic intra-epithelial lymphoma. This hypothesis is sustained by follow-up studies.

Medical Treatment Options

Treatment of Refractory Coeliac Disease I

In contrast to patients with a high percentage of aberrant T cells, patients with RCD I seem to profit from an immunosuppressive treatment. According to the data of Goerres et al. [26], azathioprine should be the first-line therapy after induction of clinical remission with corticosteroids. Dose and duration of treatment with azathioprine are not established.

In contrast to RCD II, long-term treatment with corticosteroids or locally acting budesonide may be considered only in patients who have contra-indications to other immunosuppressants.

Cyclosporine A, infliximab and tacrolimus have been reported to be effective in case reports, but further data are required particularly in the light of severe side effects [27]. These agents should only be considered in case of clinical deterioration despite corticosteroid therapy or intolerance to azathioprine. The intestinal absorption of cyclosporine A is worse than that of tacrolimus, which has to be considered in the acute treatment. Also parenteral administration of tacrolimus has to be considered. Close monitoring of renal function is inevitable.

Treatment with infliximab may induce prompt clinical and histological response but this effect has to be weighed against its possible acute allergic and chronic immunosuppressive side effects [28].

Treatment of Refractory Coeliac Disease II

RCD II is usually resistant to medical therapies. Response to corticosteroid treatment does not exclude underlying EATL, which has been shown in single cases. In case of RCD II with persistent clinical symptoms and/or a high percentage of aberrant T cells in intestinal biopsies in spite of a corticosteroid treatment, more aggressive therapeutic schemes should be considered.

However, no therapy seems to be curative in RCD II.

Some patients may benefit from azathioprine [26]. Caution is needed when instituting immunosuppressive therapy, as this may induce a high risk of progression to an overt lymphoma.

In most cases CHOP-like regimens have been applied, but also other agents used for nodal non-Hodgkin lymphoma may be applied. Maurino et al. [29] reported the results of treating 7 RCD II patients with azathioprine. Clinical and histological improvement was noted in 5 of 7 treated patients, although 3 patients died (1 from leukopenic fever and 2 died early). However, in their follow-up report on treating 13 patients with azathioprine, they reported a 46% mortality rate. A recent report on the anti-tumour-necrosis-factor agent infliximab for treatment of RCD has been published, but no data were provided on aberrant T cells (T flow cytometry or immunohistology) [30]. Recognizing that some patients with RCD II, and especially with ulcerative jejunitis, are suffering from a low-grade EATL, we treated a group of these patients with cytotoxic chemotherapy. Cladribine (2-chlorodeoxyadenosine, 2-CDA) is a synthetic purine nucleoside with cytotoxic activity. Cladribine is of proven value in the treatment of hairy cell leukaemia. Pathological cells in hairy cell leukaemia are CD103+ as in T cells in RCD II. In the last few years, clinical trials with 2-CDA have confirmed its effectiveness in selected autoimmune disorders. Seventeen patients received 2-CDA therapy [31]. This therapy was well tolerated without serious side effects. Six of 17 patients (35.8%) responded with clinical improvement, and another 6 had a significant decrease in aberrant T-cell percentages. Interestingly, one of our patients developed a complete clinical, immunological (aberrant T-cell percentage decreased from 70 to 15%) and histological recovery (Marsh classification 3C–1) and remained symptom free during more than 4 years of follow-up evaluation. Furthermore, ulcerative jejunitis, an endoscopic feature of RCD II, was seen to disappear in the 5 patients (29.4%) who had it initially, and interestingly none of these 5 patients thus far developed EATL. Seven patients (41.1%) developed EATL within 6–38 months after starting treatment and subsequently died despite multi-agent chemotherapy (cyclophosphamide, Adriamycin, vincristine and prednisone). Although EATL was excluded adequately at inclusion, 3 patients died of EATL within 5–7 months after therapy. Whether 2-CDA has accelerated the development of lymphoma cannot be concluded confidently. Few cases of secondary malignancies after 2-CDA through T-cell immunodepression have been reported. Thus, therapy with 2-CDA seems to have a role, although based on our data it is less than optimal in the treatment of RCD with aberrant T cells. It may be considered, however, as the only treatment thus far studied that showed significant reduction of aberrant T cells, seems to be well tolerated and may have beneficial long-term effects in a subgroup of patients showing significant reduction of the aberrant T-cell population.

Autologous Stem Cell Transplantation in Refractory Coeliac Disease II

In the last decade of the twentieth century, stem cell transplantation has become an increasingly accepted treatment option for patients with severe autoimmune diseases refractory to conventional treatment.

The application of this treatment option in gastroenterology has been explored in the last few years. We have tested the applicability of autologous stem cell transplantation in a selected group of refractory coeliacs with aberrant T cells [32].

Between March 2004 and March 2006, 7 patients were transplanted. EATL had been excluded by endoscopic examination, CT, body PET and bone marrow biopsy.

Stem cells were harvested from the peripheral blood after mobilization using granulocyte colony-stimulating factor. The conditioning regimen consisted of T-cell depletion with fludarabine and myeloablation with melphalan. On follow-up, our patients showed improvement in the small-intestinal histology, together with impressive clinical improvement as demonstrated by the disappearance of diarrhoea and abdominal pain, normalization of serum albumin, electrolytes and haemoglobin, increase in body mass index and improvement of the performance status. Two years after transplantation, our first patient is showing further improvement in his immunopathology status as demonstrated in a further decline in the percentage of aberrant T cells to 3% and histologically improved from Marsh 3A to Marsh 1. We propose that enhanced apoptosis of activated but aberrant T cells has led to this late but remarkable decline. Our most recent patient with clinically short-bowel syndrome is showing remarkable clinical, endoscopic and immunological improvement. Furthermore, the first 3 patients showed a significant increase in the percentage of CD8+ lymphocytes, which is seen as a marker of lymphocyte regeneration after autologous stem cell transplantation. Absence of a demonstrable improvement in the surface expression of CD8 on the IEL might be regarded as a poor prognostic indicator of response; this is only to be proved or disproved on a longer-term follow-up.

Although the short-term results in these patients are promising, the follow-up at present is too short to permit firm conclusions as to efficacy. The selection of patients for this treatment should be restricted to those patients with a substantial population of aberrant T cells, even after therapy with 2-CDA, who have a greater tendency to progress to highly lethal EATL.

Follow-Up and Overt Lymphoma in Refractory Coeliac Disease

RCD II is a serious disorder with a 5-year survival of less than 50%, and the most frequent cause of death is the occurrence of an overt T-cell lymphoma and recurrent infections. The presence of an abnormal clonal IEL population is significantly associated with a poor survival and a high risk of progression to overt lymphoma. The same clonal TCR gene rearrangement initially identified in patients with clonal RCD may be subsequently observed in lymphomatous specimens suggesting a continuum between RCD and high-grade lymphoma. The risk of developing an overt T-cell lymphoma in patients with RCD II seems to be favoured by immunosuppressive drugs.

Autologous stem cell transplantation in RCD II patients seems to be promising.

Whether a close monitoring with video capsule and/or PET scan is capable of detecting earlier lesions in RCD before the development of an overt lymphoma and results in a better outcome remains to be answered.

References

1 Working Group of the United European Gastroenterology Week in Amsterdam: When is a coeliac a coeliac? Eur J Gastroenterol 2001;13:1123–1128.

2 Schuppan D, Kelly CP, Krauss N: Monitoring non-responsive patients with celiac disease. Gastrointest Endosc Clin North Am 2006;16:593–603.

3 Wahab PJ, Crusius JB, Meijer J, Wand Mulder CJJ: Gluten challenge in borderline gluten-sensitive enteropathy. Am J Gastroenterol 2001;96:1464–1469.

4 Abdulkarim A, Burgart L, See J, Murray J: Etiology of nonresponsive celiac disease: results of a systematic approach. Am J Gastroenterol 2002;978:2016–2021.

5 Cellier C, Delabesse E, Helmer C, et al: Refractory sprue, coeliac disease, and enteropathy-associated T-cell lymphoma. Lancet 2000;356:203–208.

6 Daum S, Cellier C, Mulder CJ: Refractory coeliac disease. Best Pract Res Clin Gastroenterol 2005;19:413–424.

7 Marsh MN: Gluten, major histocompatibility complex and the small intestine: a molecular and immunobiologic approach to the spectrum of gluten sensitivity ('celiac sprue'). Gastroenterology 1992;102:330–354.
8 Van Belzen MJ, Meijer JW, Sandkuijl LA, et al: A major non-HLA locus in celiac disease maps to chromosome 19. Gastroenterology 2003;125:1032–1041.
9 Mazzarella G, Maglio M, Paparo F, et al: An immunodominant DQ8 restricted gliadin peptide activates small intestinal immune response in in vitro cultured mucosa from HLA-DQ8 positive but not HLA-DQ8 negative coeliac patients. Gut 2003;52:57–62.
10 Karell K, Louka AS, Moodie SJ, et al: European genetics cluster on celiac disease. HLA types in celiac disease patients not carrying the DQA1*05-DQB1*02 (DQ2) heterodimer: results from the European genetics cluster on celiac disease. Hum Immunol 2003;64: 469–477.
11 Al-Toma A, Goerres MS, Meijer JW, Pena AS, Crusius JB, Mulder CJ: Human leukocyte antigen-DQ2 homozygosity and the development of refractory celiac disease and enteropathy-associated T-cell lymphoma. Clin Gastroenterol Hepatol 2006;4:315–319.
12 Vahedi K, Mascart F, Mary JY, et al: Reliability of antitransglutaminase antibodies as predictors of gluten-free diet compliance in adult celiac disease. Am J Gastroenterol 2003;98:1079–1087.
13 Mulder CJ, Harkemar IM, Meijer JW, De Boer NK: Microscopic colitis. Rom J Gastroenterol 2004;13:113–117.
14 Chott A, Dragosics B, Radaszkiewicz T: Peripheral T-cell lymphomas of the intestine. Am J Pathol 1992;141: 1361–1371.
15 Daum S, Ullrich R, Heise W, et al: Intestinal non-Hodgkin's lymphoma: a multicenter prospective clinical study from the German Study Group on Intestinal non-Hodgkin's Lymphoma. J Clin Oncol 2003;21:2740–2746.
16 Schmitt-Gräff A, Hummel M, Zemlin M, et al: Intestinal T-cell lymphoma: a reassessment of cytomorphological features in relation to patterns of small bowel remodelling. Virchows Arch 1996; 429:27–36.
17 Tomei E, Diacinti D, Marini M, Mastropasqua M, Di Tola M, Sabbatella L, Picarelli A: Abdominal CT findings may suggest coeliac disease. Dig Liver Dis 2005;37:402–406.
18 Hadithi M, Mallant M, Oudejans J, et al: ^{18}F-FDG-PET-fluoro-deoxy-glucose positron emission tomography versus computed tomography for the detection of enteropathy-associated T-cell lymphoma in refractory celiac disease. J Nucl Med 2006;47:1622–1627.
19 Yamamoto H, Sekine Y, Sato Y, et al: Total enteroscopy with a nonsurgical steerable double-balloon method. Gastrointest Endosc 2001;53:216–220.
20 Ell C, May A, Nachbar L, et al: Push-and-pull enteroscopy in the small bowel using the double-balloon technique: results of a prospective European multicenter study. Endoscopy 2005;37:613–616.
21 Ashton-Key M, Diss T, Pan L, et al: Molecular analysis of T-cell clonality in ulcerative jejunitis and enteropathy-associated T-cell lymphoma. Am J Pathol 1997;151:493–498.
22 Verkarre V, Asnafi V, Lecomte T, et al: Refractory coeliac disease is a diffuse gastrointestinal disease. Gut 2003;52: 205–211.
23 Vader W, Stepniak D, Kooy Y, Mearin L, Thompson A, van Rood JJ, Spaenij L, Koning F: The HLA-DQ2 gene dose effect in celiac disease is directly related to the magnitude and breadth of gluten-specific T cell responses. Proc Natl Acad Sci USA 2003;100:12390–12395.
24 Bagdi E, Diss TC, Munson P, Isaacson PG: Mucosal intra-epithelial lymphocytes in enteropathy-associated T-cell lymphoma, ulcerative jejunitis, and refractory celiac disease constitute a neoplastic population. Blood 1999;94: 260–264.
25 Blumberg RS, Yockey CE, Gross GG, Ebert EC, Balk SP: Human intestinal intraepithelial lymphocytes are derived from a limited number of T cell clones that utilize multiple V beta T cell receptor genes. J Immunol 1993;150: 5144–5153.
26 Goerres MS, Meijer JW, Wahab PJ, et al: Azathioprine and prednisone combination therapy in refractory coeliac disease. Aliment Pharmacol Ther 2003; 18:487–494.
27 Wahab P, Crusius J, Meijer J, et al: Cyclosporin in the treatment of adults with refractory coeliac disease – an open pilot study. Aliment Pharmacol Ther 2000;14:767–774.
28 Gillet HR, Arnott IDR, McIntyre M, et al: Successful infliximab treatment for steroid-refractory celiac disease: a case report. Gastroenterology 2002;122: 800–805.
29 Maurino E, Niveloni S, Chernavsky A, et al: Azathioprine in refractory sprue: results from a prospective, open-label study. Am J Gastroenterol 2002;97: 2595–2602.
30 Turner SM, Moorghen M, Probert CS: Refractory coeliac disease: remission with infliximab and immunomodulators. Eur J Gastroenterol Hepatol 2005; 17:667–669.
31 Al-toma A, Goerres MS, Meijer JW, von Blomberg BM, Wahab PJ, Kerckhaert JA, Mulder CJ: Cladribine therapy in refractory celiac disease with aberrant T cells. Clin Gastroenterol Hepatol 2006;4:1322–1327, quiz 1300.
32 Al-toma A, Visser O, van Roessel HM, von Blomberg BME, Scholten PET, Ossenkoppele GJ, Huijgens PC, Mulder CJJ: Autologous hematopoietic stem cell transplantation in refractory celiac disease with aberrant T cells. Blood 2007;109:2243–2249.

Prof. C.J.J. Mulder
Department of Gastroenterology, VU University Medical Centre
PO Box 7057
NL–1005 MB Amsterdam (The Netherlands)
Tel. +31 20 4440 613, Fax +31 20 4440 554, E-Mail cjmulder@vumc.nl

Fasano A, Troncone R, Branski D (eds): Frontiers in Celiac Disease.
Pediatr Adolesc Med. Basel, Karger, 2008, vol 12, pp 133–138

The National Institutes of Health Consensus Conference Report

Mitchell B. Cohen[a] · John A. Barnard[b]

[a]Cincinnati Children's Hospital Medical Center and University of Cincinnati, Cincinnati, Ohio, and [b]Columbus Children's Hospital and Ohio State University, Columbus, Ohio, USA

Abstract

The National Institutes of Health (NIH) convened a Consensus Development Conference on Celiac Disease on June 28–30, 2004. The conclusions of this conference and the exhaustive literature review that preceded it are as follows. Celiac disease (CD) is an immune-mediated intestinal disorder affecting up to 1% of the US population. CD is underrecognized in part due to the varied manifestations of the disease. Sensitive and specific serological tests are available to aid in the diagnosis and screening of patients. Treatment of CD includes education and a lifelong gluten-free diet. The panel made recommendations regarding education of healthcare providers, standardized approaches to the testing for and diagnosis of CD and definition of a gluten-free diet. In addition, the panel urged greater collaboration among stakeholders, e.g. CD societies, CD interest groups, individuals with CD and healthcare providers to advance the research and treatment agendas.

The National Institutes of Health (NIH) convened a Consensus Development Conference on Celiac Disease on June 28–30, 2004 [1]. The impetus for this Conference was a number of new developments and controversies in celiac disease (CD):

- Recent data primarily in Europe, but also in the USA suggested that the prevalence of CD was much greater than previously estimated, possibly affecting up to 3 million Americans (1% of the US population), yet despite this recognition, CD was being considerably underrecognized.
- Recent identification of autoantigens that are involved in CD led to the development of new serological tests. However, the appropriate use of these tests remains controversial. These screening tests have identified many individuals with nonclassical CD, and there exists controversy regarding the approach to screening and treatment of these individuals.

The NIH Consensus Development program follows a rigorous and standardized approach to develop an unbiased, independent, state-of-the-science statement. Independent panels of health professionals and public representatives prepare reports based on: (1) the results of a systematic literature review prepared under contract with the Agency for Healthcare Research and Quality (AHRQ); (2) presentations by investigators working in areas relevant to the conference questions during a 2-day public session; (3) questions and statements from conference attendees during open discussion periods that are part of the public session, and (4) closed deliberations by the panel during the remainder of the second day and morning of the third. Panel members, including the authors, were chosen for their general expertise, but were not permitted to have specific expertise in CD to avoid bias. Panel members also included lay representatives. After weighing the scientific evidence, including the AHRQ report and data from 32 speakers, the panel drafted a statement to address the following key questions that were prepared in advance:

- How is CD diagnosed?
- How prevalent is CD?
- What are the manifestations and long-term consequences of CD?
- Who should be tested for CD?
- What is the management of CD?
- What are the recommendations for future research on CD and related conditions?

The consensus statement [1] reflects the panel's assessment of medical knowledge available at the time the statement was written. Thus, it provides a 'snapshot in time' of the state of knowledge on the conference topic.

Literature Review

Data contained in the AHRQ report [2] were reviewed in a 1-day executive meeting held approximately 4 weeks in advance of the Consensus Development Conference and were used as a resource during preparation of the consensus statement. The AHRQ report contained a series of systematic reviews on 5 areas of CD:

- Sensitivity and specificity of serological tests
- Prevalence and incidence of CD
- CD-associated lymphoma
- Consequences of testing for CD
- Interventions for the promotion and monitoring of adherence to a gluten-free diet

Staff at the National Library of Medicine performed a series of searches in support of the literature review of CD. Searches were run in the Medline® (1966 to October 2003) and Embase (1974 to December 2003) databases for each of the 5 areas of CD. Furthermore, for the objectives relating to consequences and adherence, PsycINFO (1840 forward), Agricola (1970 forward), CAB (1972 forward) and Sociological Abstracts (1963 forward) database searches were run in December 2003.

How Is Celiac Disease Diagnosed?

Out of 3,982 citations identified by the search strategy for the first review area, 60 studies fulfilled inclusion criteria. Data for the sensitivity and specificity of each serological marker were considered separately, and studies were further divided according to the age group of the study population. The results of this meta-analysis suggest that in the era of endomysial antibody (EMA) and tissue transglutaminase (tTG) antibody testing, antigliadin antibody testing in both children and adults is not helpful. The sensitivity and specificity of EMA and tTG are quite high (over 95% for sensitivity, and close to 100% for specificity), as are their positive and negative predictive values; however, the reported diagnostic parameters are taken from studies in which the prevalence of CD was, for the most part, much higher than that seen in the usual clinical practice. This would bias the performance of the test. The positive predictive values reported for these tests will certainly not be as high as that reported when these tests are used to screen the general population. The bulk of the evidence on the diagnostic characteristics of these tests was derived from studies that defined CD as having at least some degree of villous atrophy.

HLA-DQ2/DQ8 testing appears to be a useful adjunct in the diagnosis of CD. The test has high sensitivity (in excess of 90–95%); however, since approximately 30% of the general population and an even higher proportion of 'high-risk' subjects (e.g. diabetics and family members) also carry these markers, the specificity of this test is not ideal. The greatest diagnostic utility of this test appears to be its negative predictive value.

Based on the AHRQ report and the evidence presented in the conference presentations, the panel addressed the question 'How is CD diagnosed?' in the following manner:

- The single most important step in diagnosing CD is to first consider the disorder by recognizing its many clinical features.
- The best available tests are the IgA tTG and EMA test. Antigliadin antibody tests are not recommended. Serological testing for young children is less reliable although the cutoff age for this limitation is uncertain. The panel conservatively suggested 5 years of age.
- Biopsies of the proximal small bowel are indicated for disease confirmation as some degree of villous atrophy is required for the diagnosis of CD. A demonstration of normalized biopsy findings on a gluten-free diet is no longer considered necessary.
- When the diagnosis of CD is indeterminate, HLA testing may exclude CD by the absence of both DQ2 and DQ8 haplotypes.

How Prevalent Is Celiac Disease?

The literature search regarding the incidence and prevalence of CD contained a few excellent studies but the overall quality of reports of the included studies was found to be marginal to fair. For example, most of the studies did not report on whether the patients were consecutively enrolled, a factor that could contribute to selection bias. However, setting aside the quality of individual studies, the strength of the evidence is fairly good. Results also have to be interpreted in light of some of the limitations that have been identified regarding the diagnostic performance of the tests for CD. Nonetheless, the results of this report suggest that CD is a very common disorder with prevalence in the US general population that is likely close to 1:100 (1%). Several high-risk groups with a prevalence of CD greater than that of the general population were identified.

Based on this report and the evidence presented in the conference presentations, the panel addressed the question 'How prevalent is CD?' in the following manner:

- Population-based studies in the USA suggest a prevalence of CD between 0.5 and 1.0%. This includes both symptomatic and asymptomatic individuals.
- Certain populations have an increased risk including first- and perhaps second-degree family members of those with CD, people with type 1 diabetes mellitus (3–8%), Down syndrome (5–12%), Turner syndrome, Williams syndrome, selective IgA deficiency and autoimmune disorders.

What Are the Manifestations and Long-Term Consequences of Celiac Disease?

Based on the evidence presented in the conference presentations, the panel addressed the question 'What are the manifestations and long-term consequences of CD?' in the following manner:

- CD is a multisystem disorder with highly variable manifestations including any of the following gastrointestinal manifestations: diarrhea, weight loss, failure to grow in children, vomiting, abdominal pain, bloating, distention, anorexia and constipation. Classical CD presents with symptoms and sequelae of gastrointestinal malabsorption.
- It is also very common for CD to present with extraintestinal manifestations including: dermatitis herpetiformis (a sine qua non of CD), iron deficiency anemia, unexplained short stature, delayed puberty, infertility, recurrent fetal loss, osteoporosis, vitamin deficiencies, fatigue, protein calorie malnutrition, recurrent aphthous stomatitis, elevated transaminases, dental enamel hypoplasia, autoimmune thyroiditis and a variety of neuropsychiatric conditions. Without classical gastrointestinal symptoms, these represent 'atypical' symptoms

although patients with atypical disease probably outnumber those with classical disease.
- 'Silent' CD refers to individuals with no symptoms and a positive screening test or villous atrophy found on small-intestinal biopsy. Latent CD is defined as a positive serological test with a normal biopsy. These patients may later develop symptoms and histological changes of CD.

Malignancy/Lymphoma
The AHRQ report identified 379 references resulting from the literature search on CD and lymphoma. Eight cohort studies and one case-control study were selected for data extraction and were found to be of good quality. There is a strong association between CD and gastrointestinal lymphoma, especially non-Hodgkin lymphoma. A delay in the diagnosis of CD, and perhaps diagnosis of CD in adulthood as opposed to in childhood, may be associated with poorer outcome in persons with lymphoma. It has been suggested that adherence to a gluten-free diet for 5 years reduces the risk of lymphoma in celiac patients.

Based on this report and the evidence presented in the conference presentations, the panel addressed the part of the question relating to the consequences and complications of CD.
- Most complications of CD generally occur after many years of disease. Inadequate adherence to a gluten-free diet can result in any of the manifestations of CD described above.
- Non-Hodgkin lymphoma is more common in persons with CD, but it is still rare. There is no established approach to screen for small-intestinal lymphoma. There is also an increased risk of small-intestinal adenocarcinoma in patients with CD.

Who Should Be Tested for Celiac Disease?

Out of 1,199 citations that were identified by the search strategy for the fourth AHRQ report question, 35 articles satisfied the screening criteria. Based on this report and the evidence presented in the conference presentations, the panel addressed an additional question 'Who should be tested for CD?' in the following manner:
- Individuals with suggestive gastrointestinal symptoms should be tested.
- Individuals with unexplained, persistent hepatic transaminase elevations, short stature, delayed puberty, iron deficiency anemia, recurrent fetal loss and infertility should be tested. Individuals with biopsy proven dermatitis herpetiformis almost certainly have CD.
- There is inadequate evidence of benefit to recommend screening the general population at this time.
- Although patients with CD often present with osteoporosis, data do not support cost-effective screening of this population.
- While individuals with type 1 diabetes have a higher risk for CD, the panel concluded there was insufficient evidence of a documented health benefit to recommend screening asymptomatic individuals with type 1 diabetes at this time. This conclusion was contested by celiac experts in the final plenary session, and other expert analyses have concluded differently [3]. Diabetics with suggestive symptoms, including unexplained hypoglycemia, should be tested. In its research recommendations, the panel felt that celiac screening in diabetes was an important area for further exploration.
- Patients with Down syndrome and Williams syndrome who are unable to describe their symptoms accurately should also be screened.

What Is the Management of Celiac Disease?

For the fifth question, out of 502 citations identified by the search strategy, 20 studies met level 3 inclusion criteria. Based on this report and the evidence presented in the conference presentations, the panel addressed the question 'What is the management of CD?' in the following manner:

- The management of CD is a gluten-free diet for life
- The strict definition of a gluten-free diet is complicated by the lack of an accurate method to detect gluten in food products and the lack of scientific evidence for what constitutes a safe amount of gluten ingestion
- The following are the 6 key elements for management that form an acrostic for CELIAC:
  - **C**onsultation with a skilled dietician
  - **E**ducation about the disease
  - **L**ifelong adherence to a gluten-free diet
  - **I**dentification and treatment of nutritional deficiencies
  - **A**ccess to an advocacy group
  - **C**ontinuous, long-term follow-up by a multidisciplinary team

What Are the Recommendations for Future Research on Celiac Disease and Related Conditions?

Based on the literature review and presentations, the panel recommended the following future research agenda:

- Conduct a cohort study to determine the natural history of untreated CD, especially 'silent' CD
- Determine the response to gluten peptides in DQ2+/DQ8+ individuals without CD; determine which factors prevent disease
- Identify which factors are involved in the induction of CD in genetically susceptible individuals
- Develop an animal model(s) of CD that can be used to dissect pathogenic mechanisms
- Determine prevalence of CD in ethnic groups in the USA
- Research on prevention of CD, e.g. timing of introduction of cereals in infants coupled to assessment of immune response (B cell and T cell) to glutens
- Define the relationship between CD and autoimmune and neuropsychiatric disorders
- Identify non-HLA genetic modifiers that influence severity or phenotype of CD
- Develop noninvasive methodology to detect and quantify the activity of CD
- Define the minimum safe exposure threshold of gluten in the diet relative to CD
- Develop alternatives to a gluten-free diet
- Analyze the performance and cost-effectiveness of serological testing for CD in the general population
- Conduct research into screening methods for adenocarcinoma and lymphoma
- Analyze the benefit of screening high-risk groups relevant to clinically important outcomes, e.g. individuals with type 1 diabetes mellitus
- Investigate the health-economic consequences of CD
- Identify and validate serological assays for CD diagnosis in young children
- Investigate the quality of life of individuals with CD

The panel also recommended education of physicians, dieticians, nurses and the public about CD by a trans-NIH initiative, to be led by the National Institute of Diabetes and Digestive and Kidney Diseases, in association with the Centers for Disease Control and Prevention. As a result of this initiative, a CD brochure was produced by the National Digestive Diseases Information Clearinghouse which is available via the web (http://digestive.niddk.nih.gov/ddiseases/pubs/celiac/index.htm).

References

1 National Institutes of Health Consensus Development Conference statement on celiac disease, June 28–30, 2004. Gastroenterology 2005; 128:S1–S9.

2 Rostom A, Dubé C, Cranney A, et al: Celiac disease: summary, evidence report/technology assessment No 104. AHRQ Publ No 04-E029-1, June 2004. Rockville, Agency for Healthcare Research and Quality, 2004. http://www.ahrq.gov/clinic/epcsums/celiacsum.htm.

3 Guideline for the diagnosis and treatment of celiac disease in children: recommendations of the North American Society of Pediatric Gastroenterology, Hepatology and Nutrition. JPGN 2005; 40:1–19.

Mitchell B. Cohen, MD
Gastroenterology, Hepatology and Nutrition
Cincinnati Children's Hospital Medical Center
3333 Burnet Avenue, Cincinnati, OH 45229 (USA)
Tel. +1 513 636 3008, Fax +1 513 636 5581, E-Mail mitchell.cohen@cchmc.org

Fasano A, Troncone R, Branski D (eds): Frontiers in Celiac Disease.
Pediatr Adolesc Med. Basel, Karger, 2008, vol 12, pp 139–147

Beyond Coeliac Disease Toxicity

Detoxified and Non-Toxic Grains

Luud J.W.J. Gilissen · Ingrid M. van der Meer · Marinus J.M. Smulders

Plant Research International, Wageningen, The Netherlands

Abstract

Coeliac disease (CD) is a food-related problem. Increasing knowledge about the diversity in CD toxicity of individual wheat species and varieties, and of the individual gluten proteins enables the food industry to increasingly take responsibility in the production of CD-safe foods. Several strategies to obtain CD-safe wheat material including selection, breeding and genetic modification are elaborated from recent examples. Attention is also given to the rapidly increasing interest by the CD population in oats as a safe replacer of wheat, rye and barley.

A common start of many publications on coeliac disease (CD) is to refer to the disease as an autoimmune disorder of the small intestine in genetically susceptible individuals caused by an abnormal immune response to dietary gluten that can only be treated by a strict and lifelong adherence to a gluten-free diet. Isn't there any space to escape?

First of all, the disease is an intolerance to gluten, and as such the disease mainly occurs in countries in which wheat is the major staple food. In these countries, breastfeeding was found to be beneficial in case of gluten introduction into the diet of babies with CD. Also, a gradual introduction into the baby diet of low amounts of gluten might help the immune system to cope with the immunogenic activity of gluten and to prevent or strongly decrease the development and expression of CD [1]. Other possibilities to fight CD involve the possible application of enzymes (endopeptidases) that are able to specifically break down gluten proteins and destroy their CD-toxic fragments, even under physiological conditions in the stomach. In addition, interference at the molecular level of the immune system has been suggested, e.g. through blocking of the binding of CD-toxic gluten fragments to their receptors [2]. These last two strategies are at the level of reducing the symptoms by interfering with the physiological process when CD is already diagnosed, whereas the first two strategies are focused on preventing induction of CD.

While research found such possibilities that need however further testing and implementation into society to force back the CD problem, we see at the same time a rapid increase in the consumption of wheat- and gluten-containing foods, not only in developed countries, but also in countries where rice, maize or sorghum are the traditional staple foods. This change is related to the westernization (McDonaldization) process where consumption of (gluten-containing) fast foods is rapidly taking over the traditional eating habits and food consumption patterns. This process occurs in countries with a rapidly growing economy, including China, India and several South-American economies. This change will certainly have consequences for the growth of the CD problem in these countries and worldwide.

CD becomes more and more a food-related problem with an increasing responsibility for the food-producing sector. This makes it necessary to also consider possibilities for reducing or eliminating the CD toxicity of foods, starting from the primary products, the cereals wheat, barley and rye. Generally, two strategies can be followed. The first strategy is directed towards elimination of intrinsic CD-toxic factors from gluten proteins in cereals that are now toxic for CD patients. The second strategy relates to the use of alternative grain species that do not contain toxic gluten; here the main issue is to avoid cross-contamination by CD-toxic cereals during production processes of foods (bakery products) from alternative grains. These strategies will be elaborated below, but we will start with describing the malefactor and its complex appearance: gluten.

What Is Gluten?

Gluten proteins are part of the storage proteins in wheat grains, next to other storage proteins, the albumins (that are soluble in water) and the globulins (that are soluble in salt solution). Gluten is the water-insoluble, alcohol-soluble protein fraction that makes up the majority of the total seed protein of wheat. Generally, in gluten two types of proteins are distinguished, glutenins and gliadins, with several subtypes (high- and low-molecular-weight glutenins; α-, γ- and ω-gliadins). The genetics of gluten is as complex as the wheat taxon itself. The general bread wheat varieties have a hexaploid genome composition, whereas the pasta (durum) wheats are tetraploids. Bread wheat *(Triticum aestivum)* contains 3 separated genomes (A, B and D) resulting from an interspecific hybridization of the diploid species *T. tauschii* (providing the D genome) with a tetraploid durum type wheat *(T. turgidum)* containing the A and B genomes. This hybridization occurred 10,000 years ago, early in the development of agriculture at the end of the last ice age. The tetraploid is much older, originating from hybridization between *T. urartu* (A genome) and *T. speltoides* (B genome). The genetics of gluten shows, for example, an estimated gene copy number for α-gliadins ranging from 25 to even 150 [3]. These genes are present in tandem repeats on the homoeologous chromosomes. The other gluten gene families are also coded by 3 homoeologous loci, but the gene copy number per locus is lower. In barley and rye, similar proteins occur. The B and D hordeins in barley and the high-molecular-weight secalins in rye correspond to the wheat glutenins, whereas the γ- and C hordeins in barley and the γ- and ω-secalins are comparable to wheat gliadins. Collectively, these alcohol-soluble proteins in these cereals are called prolamines, especially in reference to their industrial applications. With regard to CD, the term 'gluten' refers to any of the prolamines of wheat, barley and rye, or cereals in general.

Gluten proteins have very specific characteristics, due to the occurrence of repetitive domains, their high content of proline and glutamine, and the presence of several cystein residues with their specific SH (sulphide) groups. Through polymerization by disulphide bridges, glutenins form extended elastic molecular networks, to which the gliadins adhere and provide the viscosity through water binding. These characteristics make wheat gluten a highly useful and versatile protein with numerous applications in the food industry, especially in bread making and as a binder. With regard to baking, the highly elastic and viscous gluten network is responsible for keeping the carbon dioxide in the dough, thus giving it volume. However, the corresponding proteins in barley and rye have less visco-elastic

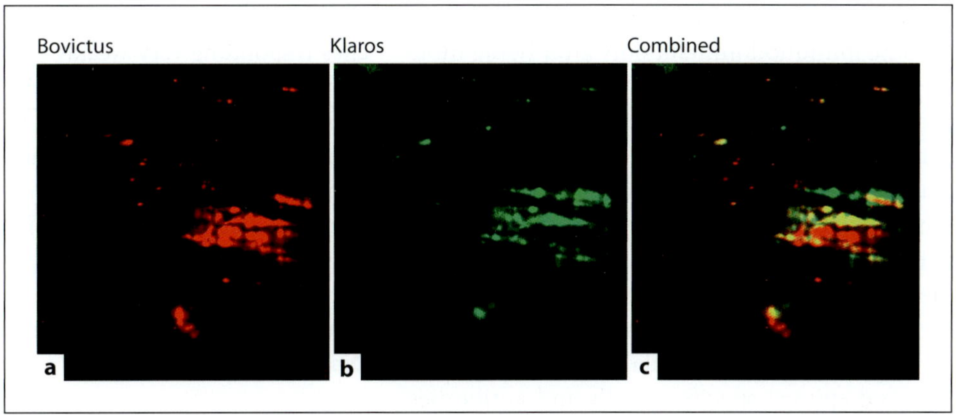

Fig. 1. Two-dimensional difference in gel electrophoresis of gluten protein extracts isolated from modern wheat cultivars Bovictus (**a**) and Klaros (**b**). Protein extracts have been labelled with 2 different fluorescent dyes and run on the same protein gel. **c** Overlap of the 2 scanned images, which shows that some proteins are present in both cultivars (yellow spots) whereas other proteins are only expressed in Bovictus (red spots) or in Klaros (green spots) [Van den Broeck et al., manuscript in preparation].

properties (compare for example rye bread to wheat bread).

Are All Glutens Coeliac Disease Toxic?

As described above, gluten proteins are the products of large gluten gene families. Not all these genes will be expressed equally in a given wheat variety. Some might be considered pseudogenes since they contain stop codons and may not be expressed at all [3], and the degree of expression of the other gluten genes is different as can be easily concluded from 2-dimensional electrophoresis as shown in figure 1 [Van den Broeck et al., manuscript in preparation]. During the development of the wheat kernel, not all gluten genes are expressed. Gene expression is regulated by natural gene silencing, and the degree of silencing differs between the different gene families [4, 5]. In the tetraploid and hexaploid wheat species, gene expression is also regulated by mutual interaction of the 3 different genomes [6]. Furthermore, soil quality (fertility) and climate effects are influencing the protein quantity in the kernel. Together, these phenomena result in differences of gluten composition among species and varieties (fig. 1).

Major and minor differences at the amino acid level make the individual gluten proteins specific in the context of the development of CD. The sensitivity to proteolytic enzymes is different among these proteins and largely depends on the number and position of the proline residues, as gastric and pancreatic proteases lack postproline cleaving activity. Generally, oligopeptides are the ultimate gluten degradation products. Recent research suggests that different gluten peptides are involved in the disease process in a different manner. Two types of biological activity are distinguished. Some gluten peptides are defined as 'toxic' because of their ability to induce damage to the intestinal mucosa of CD patients [7]. Other peptides are called 'immunogenic' as they stimulate HLA-DQ2- or -DQ8-restricted T cells. Within the latter category, several epitopes are known to be 'immunodominant', i.e. they cause a strong reaction in generally all patients. In addition, various peptides have been identified that become immunodominant only after being modified by tissue transglutaminase, a process that occurs naturally during digestion of gluten in the damaged intestine of CD patients. These peptides may thus reinforce the disease response [8, 9]. No other (plant) food protein types are known containing similar sequences. As far as known today, the gluten proteins from wheat, barley and rye are the only proteins able to induce CD.

Currently, using molecular sequence information and epitope-specific T cells and antibodies, the heterogeneity of epitope occurrence has been shown at the protein level and at the plant variety and species level [3, 10–13]. Van Herpen et al. [3] isolated α-gliadin gene sequences from several diploid wheat species as representatives of the 3 genomes in hexaploid bread wheat. The genes could be assigned clearly to 3 groups, representing the A, B and D genome, on the basis of sequence similarity and average length of the polyglutamine repeats. The genes from these genomes also showed their specificity in the presence of 4 T-cell-stimulatory peptide sequences as well. By sequence similarity, α-gliadins of hexaploid bread wheat from the public database could be assigned directly to 3 similar groups. The A genome sequences of the diploid species *T. monococcum* and those of bread wheat assigned to chromosome 6A invariably contained only 2 epitopes (Glia-α2 and Glia-α20). Most intact genes of the B genome and homologous sequences of chromosome 6B of bread wheat did not contain any canonical epitope sequence. In contrast, sequences from *T. tauschii* (D genome) and those from chromosome 6D of bread wheat contained all the 4 T-cell epitopes, and many of these genes individually included all 4 epitopes. This indicates that the 3 genomes contribute differently to the epitope content and suggests large differences in CD toxicity among wheat varieties [3].

Identification of 16 different diploid, tetraploid and hexaploid wheat species and varieties revealed a great variation in CD toxicity in T-cell and monoclonal antibody assays, with some species and varieties responding very weakly and some others very strongly [12]. In summary, these data indicate the presence of large variation of CD toxicity among wheat species and varieties. This opens possibilities to produce non- or less toxic wheat varieties through selection, breeding and genetic modification.

How to Obtain Wheat That Is Safe for Coeliac Disease Patients?

Basically, detoxified wheat can be obtained by several routes using selection, breeding and genetic modification. Selection is based on the assumption (depicted in fig. 2) that genetic diversity increases from modern cultivars to wild ancestral species and that concomitantly also the chances of finding non-toxic plants will increase. However, it must be considered that, inversely, the agricultural productivity and food-industrial applicability will decrease, and the time required to rebuild a highly productive bread wheat variety from such more primitive germplasms will also increase accordingly. The selection and breeding strategies can be carried out at several levels: (1) selection from the currently used pool of modern wheat varieties of those varieties that have a reduced level or are free of CD epitopes; (2) selection within all bread wheat varieties and landraces as available from gene banks; these selections can be used directly or improved by breeding combinations of favourable genotypes; (3) reconstruction of a bread wheat variety through breeding starting from selected low CD-toxic tetraploid durum wheat varieties, with a selected low CD-toxic D genome species; (4) building a new bread wheat starting from selected diploid lines that are completely free of CD epitopes; (5) a different strategy involving the use of genetic modifications, especially to eliminate CD-epitope-containing gluten proteins from existing varieties using RNA interference. In all strategies, the success will depend on the comprehensiveness of our knowledge of immunodominant

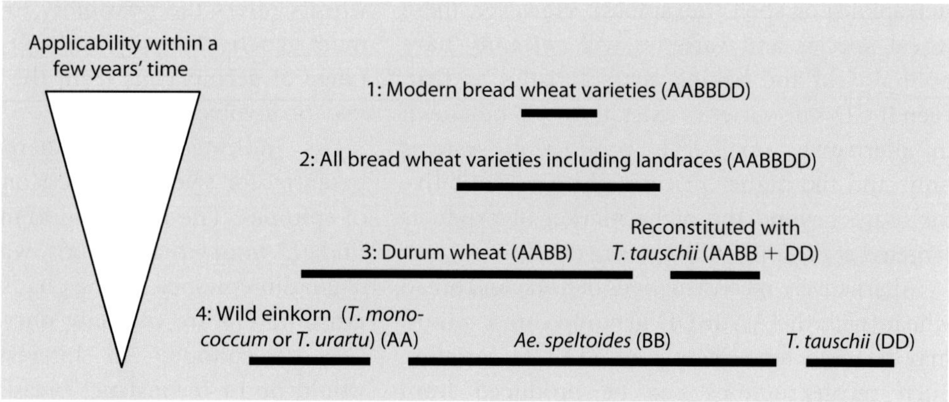

Fig. 2. Hypothetical distribution of genetic variation within wheat (as indicated by the width of the black bar underlining the different depicted wheat varieties or species), used to develop various strategies to search for wheat varieties safe for CD patients. The triangle represents the decrease in food technological applicability and the agronomic value from 1 to 4. *Ae.* = *Aegilops.*

T-cell epitopes. Epitopes that have been identified can now be detected by gluten-specific T-cell clones, with monoclonal antibodies and with specific DNA tests.

The feasibility of the first two selection strategies depends on whether sufficient genetic variation is present among varieties. Molberg et al. [14] and Spaenij-Dekking et al. [12] demonstrated in T-cell and antibody-based assays that large variation appears to exist in the amount of CD4 T-cell-stimulatory peptides present in α- and γ-gliadins and glutenins within the genus *Triticum*. Spaenij-Dekking et al. [12] tested 6 hexaploid bread wheat varieties of which 2 were modern commercially available varieties. The variation among the 6 varieties for the various epitopes tested was promising, but in order to find 1 or more varieties with low levels for all epitopes, if existing, still many more varieties need to be tested. Logistically, large-scale testing may be a problem with T-cell tests, but it is feasible when using antibody assays. We are currently carrying out large-scale screenings of modern bread wheat varieties [Van den Broeck et al., in preparation]. In order to enhance the screening efficiency, the set-up of the screening is sequential: only those varieties from a large screening population that do not contain the dominant toxic α-gliadin epitopes Glia-α9 and Glia-α20 [15] are included in the next round for screening γ-gliadin epitopes, and in further rounds for glutenin epitopes.

If 1 or several commercially available varieties can be selected, the cultivation by farmers and the use in the commodity chain is relatively straightforward, as regular production methods will lead to good yield, and usage characteristics will be within the normal range. Such varieties might then become widely used for the production of CD-safe bread and other foods. Here, another problem may rise that is related to the normal practice of wheat flour production with regard to mixing of several varieties to meet the standard bread-making quality. It is expected that the collection of CD-safe varieties may be too narrow to obtain such standard quality characteristics. If within the commercial varieties not sufficient variation will be found, the genetic diversity with regard to CD safety can be tested in alternative wheats, such as einkorn (diploid), emmer (tetraploid) or spelt (hexaploid). However, these wheat species and varieties will certainly have poorer yield and baking characteristics so that, even if CD-safe varieties exist, they will be grown in alternative, small-scale production systems only, and the higher price might be prohibitive for usage beyond the niche market of products targeted at patients with a severe condition.

Alternatively, reconstructions of hexaploid bread wheat (with the AABBDD genome composition) may be used for selection of CD-safe varieties. Such reconstructions can be produced from tetraploid *T. turgidum* (e.g. emmer wheat, with the AABB genome) and *T. tauschii* (DD). Such synthetic hexaploids thus mimic the original polyploidization that led to bread wheat, which occurred some 10,000 years ago. Currently, over 100 of such reconstructions with high variation especially in the DD genome composition are available (http://www.cimmyt.org/english/wps/news/wild_wht.htm). Molberg et al. [14], Spaenij-Dekking et al. [12] and Van Herpen et al. [3] showed that the T-cell-stimulatory epitopes were not randomly distributed across the 3 genomes, with the D genome containing most of the epitopes. Notably, *T. tauschii* (DD) lines contain and express α-gliadin genes with a 33-mer that includes 2 epitopes. Epitope DQ2-αII (Glia-α2) was not found in A and B genome sequences [3] or proteins, and T cells did not recognize it in 33 *T. monococcum* (AA) and 18 tetraploid (AABB) accessions [14]. Epitope DQ2-αI (Glia-α9) was present in DNA sequences from a *T. monococcum* (A genome) accession [3] but not in *T. speltoides* and *T. longissima* (BB genome). A T-cell clone of Molberg et al. [14] did detect a signal in α-gliadin protein of *T. monococcum*, as well as in 9 out of 14 tetraploid durum and emmer wheat accessions. For γ-gliadin and low-molecular-weight glutenin epitopes, the differences between species were not so striking, but there were significant differences among accessions within each of the species [12, 14]. Combining these different genomes in reconstructions of hexaploid bread wheats offers the possibility to introduce much more genetic diversity, and CD safety, as a broad range of germplasms from the ancestral species may be involved.

As indicated above, there seems enough potential for selecting accessions with low levels of epitopes. The most important step may be to find *T. tauschii* accessions with low levels of α-gliadin epitopes, as the gliadin genes on chromosome 6D are the only ones that feature the Glia-α2 epitope. An interesting experiment would be to reconstruct bread wheat with a *T. tauschii* line harbouring a large deletion on chromosome 6S, which, as Molberg et al. [14] have shown, can eliminate the toxic peptides, and to determine its bread-making quality. Such materials may be used to select and breed wheat varieties suitable for consumption by CD patients, contributing to a well-balanced diet and an increase in their quality of life.

Finally, one may attempt to eliminate the production of gluten proteins with T-cell-stimulatory epitopes using genetic modification. Such a strategy may face considerable public opposition to genetically modified (GM) crops, notably by consumers in some European countries. However, while the majority of European consumers currently rejects the 'green' agricultural genetic modification, they are positive about 'red' medical genetic modification, which is considered to be more necessary, and thereby more acceptable, than food-related applications [16]. Extending medical applications into the agricultural domain, Schenk et al. [submitted] found that hay fever patients indeed perceived greater 'benefits' as compared to non-patients in the (hypothetical) case of GM birch trees that produce non-allergenic pollen. Apparently, the perceived 'benefits' increased with an increasing impact of allergic complaints on quality of life. This suggests that CD patients may appreciate and endorse GM-plus but CD-minus wheat much more than the average consumer.

Eliminating T-cell-stimulatory epitopes in wheat gluten is, however, not a simple task, as the

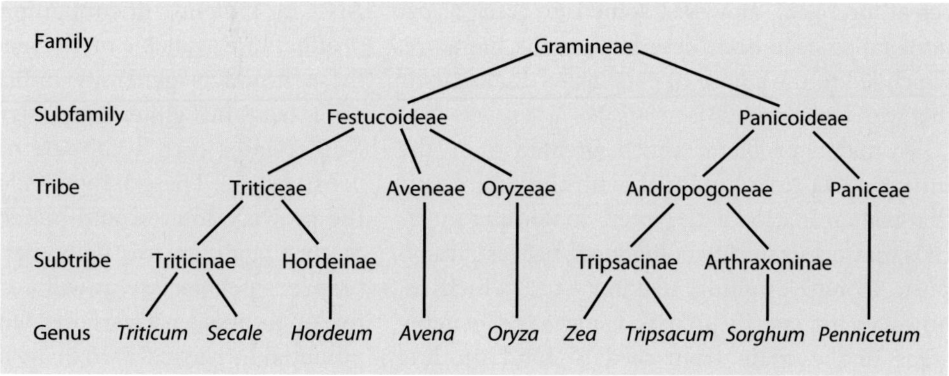

Fig. 3. Cereal prolamine evolution and homology revealed by sequence analysis [20].

composition of these storage proteins, with high levels of proline and glutamine, leads to many different but related peptides that may have high affinity to HLA-DQ2. Elimination of all gluten is not feasible either, as these proteins form the basis of the unique baking and other food-industrial quality characteristics. However, we are currently exploiting the strategy of eliminating specifically α-gliadins that contain intact epitopes using RNAi. RNAi has been shown to enable elimination of the allergen Mal d 1 in transgenic apples [17, 18], and Wieser et al. [19] have demonstrated that it is possible to eliminate all α-gliadins in bread wheat with such an approach. The consequences for bread making appeared to be relatively small.

What about Other Grains?

Wheat, rye and barley are very closely related species that are even intercrossable, with the man-made new species *Triticale*, an interspecific cross between wheat *(Triticum)* and rye *(Secale)*, as a prominent example. Most closely related to this Triticeae family is oats (Aveneae family), followed by tef (Chlorideae), rice (Oryzeae) and finger millet (ragi, Festucaceae). More distantly related are maize (Trypsacinae), sorghum (Andropogoneae) and millet (Paniceae; fig. 3). In the seeds of all these species, similar prolamine proteins can be detected. Table 1 shows the relative amounts of prolamines in seed proteins in various cereals. Due to the generally high content of the amino acids glutamine and proline and the low content of lysine in the prolamines of wheat, rye and barley, the nutritional value of these cereals is relatively low. In contrast, rice and oats have relatively low prolamine contents, but oat prolamine has the highest lysine content (>4% of the total prolamine content) and has several other, widely documented nutritional and health-promoting qualities, e.g. because of their β-glucan and fatty acid composition. These prolamines are generally non-toxic to CD patients and are therefore, especially in Scandinavian countries, promoted and even allowed as a good alternative

Table 1. Prolamine content of seed protein and the relative content of lysine of different cereals [21]

Cereal	Prolamine % of total seed protein	Lysine % of prolamine
Rice	8	3.5
Oats	12	4.2
Barley	40	3.5
Wheat	45	3.1
Maize	50	1.6
Sorghum	60	2.1

cereal food [22]. However, some rare cases of oat intolerance have been described in the literature, which led to the advice to patients to discuss their diet with clinicians [23].

A major problem, much greater than the intrinsic CD-toxic potential, with these cereals is that contamination with gluten-containing materials may occur during cultivation, harvest, transport, storage, milling, baking etc., which is, however, not specific to oats. Generally, the many steps in the chain from seed to food product often take place at separate locations. Reliable control and traceability systems are required to guarantee absence of contamination. Such a contamination-free oat chain has been proven to be a realistic option, as it has been practiced for at least 7 years in Sweden by Lantmännen AS-Factor. This company claims a maximum contamination of 20 ppm prolamine from wheat, rye or barley in their products. This standard equals the naturally gluten-free food situation [24, 25]. Also in Finland, uncontaminated CD-safe oat products are available on the market. The label on these products generally indicates 'made from pure oat and gluten-free ingredients'. In The Netherlands, such a CD-safe oat chain is under construction. These activities clearly demonstrate the growing interest and patient's acceptance of oat in the gluten-free daily diet [26, 27]. From a breeder's perspective, it will be possible to select for, or to breed oat varieties with absence of the potential intrinsic CD toxicity, in a much simpler manner as compared to wheat. In this way, the oat story seems rapidly coming to a happy end.

Acknowledgements

Thanks are due to the Celiac Diseases Consortium, an Innovative Cluster approved by the Netherlands Genomics Initiative and partly funded by the Dutch Government (BSIK03009).

References

1 Farrell RJ: Infant gluten and celiac disease – too early, too late, too much, too many questions. JAMA 2005;293: 2410–2412.

2 Stepniak D, Koning F: Celiac disease – sandwiched between innate and adaptive immunity. Hum Immunol 2006;67: 460–468.

3 Van Herpen TWJM, Goryunova SV, Van der Schoot J, Mitreva M, Salentijn E, Vorst O, Schenk MF, Van Veelen PA, Koning F, Van Soest LJM, Vosman B, Bosch D, Hamer RJ, Gilissen LJWJ, Smulders MJM: Alpha-gliadin genes from the A, B, and D genomes of wheat contain different sets of celiac disease epitopes. BMC Genomics 2006;7:1.

4 Gianibelli MC, Larroque OR, MacRitchie F, Wrigley CW: Biochemical, genetic, and molecular characterization of wheat endosperm proteins. Cereal Chem 2001;78:635–646.

5 Shewry PR, Lookhart GL: Wheat Gluten Protein Analysis. St Paul, American Association of Cereal Chemists, 2003, p 198.

6 Islam N, Tsujimoto H, Hirano H: Proteome analysis of diploid, tetraploid and hexaploid wheat: towards understanding genome interaction in protein expression. Proteomics 2003;3:549–557.

7 Julia EH, Ciclitira PJ: Natural variation in toxicity of wheat. Gastroenterology 2005;129:2129.

8 Koning F, Gilissen LJWJ, Wijmenga C: Gluten: a two-edged sword. Immunopathogenesis of celiac disease. Springer Semin Immun 2005;27:217–232.

9 Ciccocioppo R, Di Sabatino A, Corazza GR: The immune recognition of gluten in coeliac disease. Clin Exp Immunol 2005;140:408–416.

10 Spaenij-Dekking EHA, Kooy-Winkelaar EMC, Nieuwenhuizen WF, Drijfhout JW, Koning F: A novel and sensitive method for detection of T cell stimulatory epitopes of α/β- and γ-gliadin. Gut 2004;53:1267–1273.

11 Spaenij-Dekking L, Kooy-Winkelaar Y, Koning F: The Ethiopian cereal tef in celiac disease. N Engl J Med 2005;353: 1748–1749.

12 Spaenij-Dekking L, Kooy-Winkelaar Y, van Veelen P, Drijfhout JW, Jonker H, van Soest L, Smulders MJM, Bosch D, Gilissen LJWJ, Koning F: Natural variation in toxicity of wheat potential for selection of non-toxic varieties for celiac disease patients. Gastroenterology 2005;129:797–806.

13 Spaenij-Dekking L, Koning F: Natural variation in toxicity of wheat – Reply. Gastroenterology 2005;129:2129–2130.

14 Molberg O, Uhlen AK, Jensen T, Flaete NS, Fleckenstein B, Arentz-Hansen H, Raki M, Lundin KE, Sollid LM: Mapping of gluten T-cell epitopes in the bread wheat ancestors: implications for celiac disease. Gastroenterology 2005;128:393–401.

15 Vader LW, Stepniak DT, Bunnik EM, Kooy YMC, De Haan W, Drijfhout JW, Van Veelen PA, Koning F: Characterization of cereal toxicity for celiac disease patients based on protein homology in grains. Gastroenterology 2003;125:1105–1113.

16 Frewer L, Howard C, Shepherd R: Public concerns in the United Kingdom and specific applications of genetic engineering: risk, benefit, and ethics. Sci Technol Hum Values 1997; 22:98–124.
17 Gilissen LJWJ, Bolhaar STHP, Matos CI, Rouwendal GJA, Boone MJ, Krens FA, Zuidmeer L, van Leeuwen A, Akkerdaas J, Hoffmann-Sommergruber K, Knulst AC, Bosch D, van de Weg WE, van Ree R: Silencing the major apple allergen Mal d 1 by using the RNA interference approach. J Allergy Clin Immunol 2005;115:364–369.
18 Gilissen LJWJ, Bolhaar STHP, Knulst AC, Zuidmeer L, Van Ree R, Gao ZS, Van de Weg WE: Production of hypoallergenic plant foods by selection, breeding and genetic modification; in Gilissen LJWJ, Wichers HJ, Savelkoul HFJ, Bogers RJ (eds): Allergy Matters: New Approaches to Allergy Prevention and Management. Berlin, Springer, 2006, pp 95–105.
19 Wieser H, Koehler P, Folck A, Becker D: Characterization of wheat with strongly reduced α-gliadin content. Proc 9th Int Gluten Workshop, San Francisco, September 14–16, 2006.
20 Bietz JA: Cereal prolamin evolution and homology revealed by sequence analysis. Biochem Genet 1982;20: 1039–1053.
21 Doll H: Nutritional aspects of cereal proteins and approaches to overcome their deficiencies. Phil Trans R Soc Lond B 1984;304:373–380.
22 Thompson T: Oats and the gluten-free diet. J Am Diet Assoc 2003;103: 376–379.
23 Arentz-Hansen H, Fleckenstein B, Molberg Ø, Scott H, Koning F, Jung G, Roepstorff P, Lundin KEA, Sollid LM: The molecular basis for oat intolerance in patients with celiac disease. PLoS Med 2004;1:e1.
24 Salovaara H: 4th European symposium on oats – oats and healthy foods. Cereal Foods World 2006;51:150–151.
25 Janatuinen EK, Kemppainen TA, JulkunenRJK, Kosma V-M, Mäki M, Heikkinen M, Uusitupa MIJ: No harm from five year ingestion of oats in coeliac disease. Gut 2002;50:332–335.
26 Högberg L, Laurin P, Fälth-Magnusson K, Grant C, Grodzinsky E, Jansson G, Ascher H, Browaldh L, Hammersjö J-Å, Lindberg E, Myrdal U, Stenhammar L: Oats to children with newly diagnosed coeliac disease: a randomised double blind study. Gut 2004;53:649–654.
27 Londei M, Maiuri L, Quaratino S: A search for the holy grail: non-toxic gluten for celiac patients. Gastroenterology 2005;129:1111–1113.

Dr. Luud J.W.J. Gilissen
Celiac Disease Consortium, Plant Research International
PO Box 16
NL–6700 AA Wageningen (The Netherlands)
Tel. +31 317 477168, Fax +31 317 418094, E-Mail luud.gilissen@wur.nl

Fasano A, Troncone R, Branski D (eds): Frontiers in Celiac Disease.
Pediatr Adolesc Med. Basel, Karger, 2008, vol 12, pp 148–156

Oral Glutenase Therapy for Celiac Sprue

Jennifer Ehren · Chaitan Khosla

Departments of Chemistry, Chemical Engineering and Biochemistry, Stanford University, Stanford, Calif., USA

Abstract

Early studies determined that proteolytic gluten peptides, not intact gluten protein, were the toxic constituents of wheat, rye and barley for celiac sprue patients. However, only recently have studies correlated gluten sequence to observed toxicity. The discovery of HLA-DQ2 as the primary disease-associated major histocompatibility complex protein, the isolation of DQ2-restricted (and infrequently DQ8-restricted) Th1 cells from mucosal biopsies of celiac patients, and the identification of transglutaminase-2 as the predominant celiac autoantigen led researchers to identify specific T-cell epitopes in gluten proteins. Correlation of proteolytic resistance of gluten peptides and immunotoxicity enabled the identification of oral glutenase supplementation as a possible therapeutic modality. The inability of gastric and pancreatic endoproteases to cleave after proline or glutamine residues and the inability of brush border membrane enzymes to digest long peptides initiated the hypothesis that exogenous proline- and/or glutamine-specific endoproteases would be effective glutenases. This hypothesis has subsequently gained support from in vitro, in vivo animal, and ex vivo human studies. Current and future directions for oral glutenase therapy of celiac sprue are discussed.

In the 1950s and 1960s, several clinical studies explored the origins of gluten toxicity in celiac sprue patients. For example, it was shown that gliadin, the alcohol-soluble fraction of gluten, was sufficient to induce steatorrhea and other disease-associated symptoms in celiac sprue patients [1]. Furthermore, wheat gluten toxicity was not eliminated upon pre-digestion with pancreatin, pepsin, or trypsin [1–4], nor upon exposure to peptic and tryptic dialysates or ultrafiltrates [5]. In contrast, complete acid hydrolysis and complete deamidation of gliadin [6] or extensive treatment of peptic and tryptic gliadin digests with fresh hog intestinal mucosa extracts [7] or crude papain [8] eliminated gluten toxicity. These early studies unambiguously established that proteolytic gluten peptides, not intact gluten protein, were the toxic species in celiac sprue. However, the lack of information correlating the gluten sequence to its observed toxicity limited further insight into celiac sprue pathogenesis.

By the early 1970s, two hypotheses emerged regarding the pathogenesis of celiac sprue. One hypothesis argued that the disease had an immunological basis [5], while the other proposed that celiac patients had an enzyme deficiency, resulting in an accumulation of toxic gluten peptides [9]. Support for the former hypothesis came from the identification of anti-gliadin antibodies in patients and their relatives, but rarely in other populations [5]. Further support was provided by the observation that these anti-gliadin antibodies decreased in patients on a strict gluten-free diet [10]. It was suggested that the immunogenicity of celiac sprue patients resulted from increased permeability of their damaged small intestinal mucosa towards dietary peptides [10]. Although immunofluorescent studies verified that the small bowel epithelium of celiac sprue patients could absorb gluten antigens [11], patients suffering from other diseases that cause intestinal mucosa damage (e.g. ulcerative colitis) did not experience similar high levels of circulating antibodies [5]. Furthermore, the question of how initial damage occurred in order to enable absorption of antigenic gluten peptides was unanswered. Indeed, some studies argued that damage to the intestinal mucosa in celiac sprue patients existed prior to the appearance of anatomically abnormal mucosa [12].

The second hypothesis of the time, the enzyme defect theory, contrasted the immunogenicity theory by postulating that a peptidase deficiency may cause accumulation of partially digested gluten peptides and damage to intestinal mucosa cells [13]. It was known that intestinal disaccharidase and dipeptidase levels decreased in untreated celiac patients compared to normal subjects, although the phenomenon was recognized as secondary to that of the primary mucosal damage [14]. Interestingly, whereas crude papain was believed to detoxify gluten, purified papain did not retain this ability [8]. From these data it was argued that a glutamine cyclotransferase activity in crude papain was likely responsible for gluten detoxification through modification of an N-terminal glutamine in a specific disease-inducing gluten peptide [8]. Independent studies suggested that glutaminase I levels were lower in the small intestinal mucosa of untreated celiac sprue patients compared to that of non-celiac patients, but levels returned to normal in celiac patients adhering to a gluten-free diet [15].

At least two independent experiments disproved the enzyme deficiency theory for celiac sprue pathogenesis. First, it was observed that plasma levels of proline, glutamic acid, and glutamine were similar in celiac sprue patients in remission and control patients [16]. More importantly, the difference between the gluten digestive capacity of biopsies from treated celiac sprue patients and control individuals was insignificant. Therefore, impaired gluten digestion by jejunal mucosa from patients with active disease was viewed as a consequence, not a cause, of the disease [17].

Molecular and cellular insight into gluten pathogenesis in celiac sprue patients received a major boost as a result of the discovery of HLA-DQ2 as the primary disease-associated major histocompatibility complex (MHC) protein [18]. Soon thereafter, gluten-reactive, DQ2-restricted (and in a few instances DQ8-restricted) Th1 cells were isolated from small intestinal biopsies of celiac sprue patients but not from control individuals [19]. Together, these findings clearly established the inflammatory character of the celiac lesion. Further analysis of patient-derived T cells led to the identification of specific epitopes in α- and γ-gliadin polypeptides [20–23]. A critical missing piece in the gluten-induced pathogenic cascade emerged through the identification of transglutaminase 2 (TG2) as the primary disease-associated autoantigen [24]. Treatment of gluten epitopes with TG2 resulted in a dramatic enhancement of their antigenicity as a result of the increased affinity of the deamidated products for HLA-DQ2 [20]. Together, these findings firmly established the immunological basis for celiac sprue pathogenesis (fig. 1).

Notwithstanding considerable progress towards understanding the biology of celiac sprue, the potential relationship between the exceptional proteolytic resistance of dietary gluten and its toxicity to celiac sprue patients had all but been overlooked. Indeed, recombinant α-gliadin was first produced as early as 1987 [25], but was not systematically analyzed for toxic proteolytic fragments until more than a decade later. The availability of heterologous expression systems in *Escherichia coli*, coupled with mass spectrometric methods, had a considerable impact on decoding the structural basis of gluten toxicity.

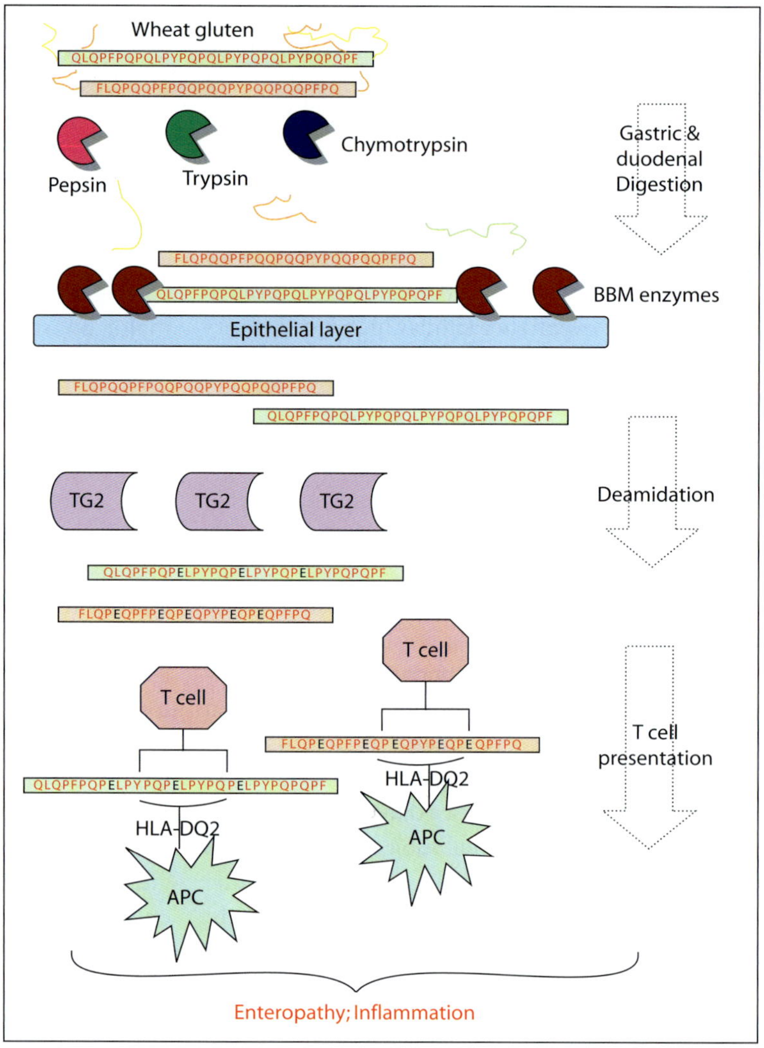

Fig. 1. Celiac sprue pathogenesis. BBM = Brush border membrane; TG2 = tissue transglutaminase 2; APC = antigen-presenting cell; HLA = human leukocyte antigen [36]. Note: The precise mechanism for gluten peptide transport across the epithelium remains unknown.

To our surprise, under simulated gastrointestinal conditions we observed a compelling correlation between the proteolytic resistance of gluten peptides [26] and proteins [27] and their immunotoxicity. Specifically, we recognized that the most immunotoxic gluten peptides were also highly resistant to breakdown by pepsin, the pancreatic proteases, and intestinal brush border membrane (BBM) peptidases [26]. This unusual stability was principally due to two factors: the inability of gastric and pancreatic endoproteases to cleave after proline or glutamine residues and the inability of dipeptidyl peptidase IV and dipeptidyl carboxypeptidase I in the BBM to cleave long peptides. Together, these two features lead to the accumulation of long, metastable intermediates in the small intestinal lumen, which in turn elicited an inflammatory response in celiac sprue patients. These observations led us to hypothesize that addition of exogenous proline- and/or glutamine-specific proteases would provide therapeutic benefit by accelerating gluten detoxification [26]. The hypothesis

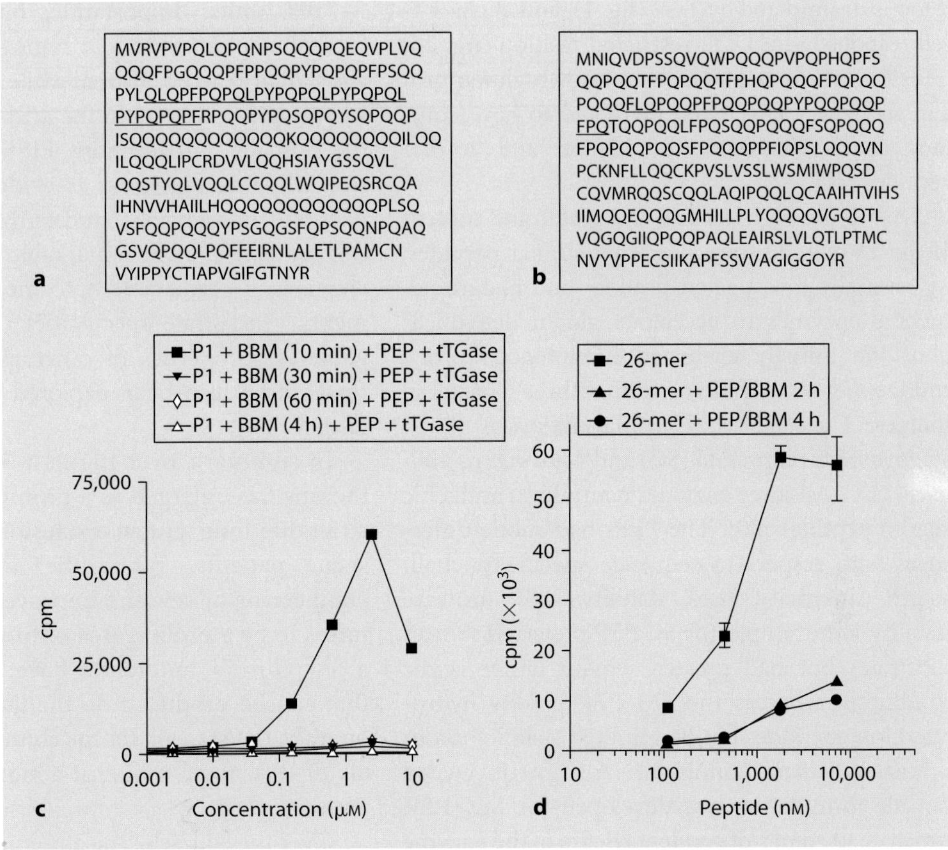

Fig. 2. Origin and immunotoxicity of proteolytically resistant gluten peptides. **a** α_2-Gliadin sequence with the proteolytically resistant immunotoxic peptide sequence (33-mer) underlined. This 33-mer peptide remains intact after α_2-gliadin has been digested with gastric and intestinal proteases [27]. **b** γ_5-Gliadin sequence with analogous 26-mer underlined [36]. **c** Toxicity of 33-mer: stimulation of HLA-DQ2-restricted T-cell clone derived from an intestinal biopsy from a celiac patient by the 33-mer (P1) treated with TG2, prolyl endopeptidase (PEP) derived from *Flavobacterium meningosepticum*, and rat intestinal brush border membrane (BBM) for different time durations [27]. **d** Toxicity of 26-mer: stimulation of HLA-DQ2-restricted T-cell clone derived from an intestinal biopsy from a celiac patient by the 26-mer+TG2 with and without incubation of rat intestinal brush border membrane (BBM) and prolyl endopeptidase (PEP) derived from *Flavobacterium meningosepticum* [36].

has subsequently gained support from a wide range of in vitro, in vivo animal, and ex vivo human studies [28–34].

A vivid example of a proteolytically resistant, pathogenic gluten peptide is the α-gliadin protein-derived 33-mer peptide: LQLQPFPQPQLPYPQ PQLPYPQPQLPYPQPQPF (fig. 2a) [27]. This peptide is not digested by gastric, pancreatic or BBM enzymes; however, it is deamidated by human TG2 at specific residues (fig. 1). The resulting product is recognized with high affinity by HLA-DQ2 on antigen-presenting cells and is presented to disease-specific T cells (fig. 2c) [27]. An analogous proteolytically resistant peptide of 26 residues, FLQPQQPFPQQPQQPYPQQPQQPF PQ, was isolated from a γ-gliadin protein (fig. 2b).

It too is deamidated by TG2 (fig. 1), and elicits a T-cell response in a DQ2-restricted fashion (fig. 2d) [35]. At least 60 peptides from known gluten protein sequences have been predicted to have common characteristics to the 33-mer and 26-mer peptides [36].

Due to the high proline and glutamine content of the 33-mer, 26-mer, and other similar peptides, we naturally investigated proline- and glutamine-specific enzymes to accelerate gluten detoxification. We initially evaluated homologous prolyl endopeptidases (PEPs) from three bacterial sources: *Flavobacterium meningosepticum* (FM), *Sphingomonas capsulata* (SC) and *Myxococcus xanthus* (MX). All three enzymes neutralized antigenic gliadin peptides [30]. The PEPs had subtle differences with respect to sequence specificity, chain length specificity, acid stability, and protease stability. For example, the SC PEP preferred shorter substrates but had greater activity under acidic conditions, whereas the FM PEP readily hydrolyzed long peptides but had limited stability under simulated gastric conditions. An enteric coated capsule formulation was developed for MX PEP, which enabled pH-dependent release of the enzyme in the duodenum [28]. More recently, another promising post-proline cleaving enzyme derived from *Aspergillus niger* (AN PEP) has been identified [37]. In contrast to FM PEP, the AN PEP is active under gastric conditions and can therefore detoxify gluten in the stomach.

The search for a glutenase with therapeutic potential has also led to the study of grain-derived proteases, such as the glutamine-specific cysteine endoprotease B2 (EP-B2) from barley [38]. These proteases play a central role in harnessing the nutritional content in germinating seeds of gluten-producing plants. In addition to their evolutionarily optimized substrate specificity, they have evolved to hydrolyze proteins in an acidic milieu. EP-B2 has a marked specificity for the Q↓XP motif, which also happens to be the preferred recognition site for human TG2. The enzyme is resistant to proteolysis by pepsin and has a broad pH profile range of 3–7 pH units. Importantly, by producing the recombinant enzyme in a zymogen form, its storage stability can be ensured while retaining the ability to rapidly activate in the acidic environment of the stomach. Furthermore, EP-B2 is highly effective at gluten digestion, as evidenced by in vitro [32] and in vivo [33] studies. More significantly, this protease exhibits remarkable synergy with PEP enzymes, a predictable outcome of their complementary substrate specificities (fig. 3) [31]. The glutenase properties of other grain-derived proteases have also been explored in a preliminary fashion [39].

In summary, over the past 5 years, glutenase therapy has emerged as a promising adjunct to a strict life-long gluten exclusion diet for celiac sprue patients. While the identification and engineering of new and improved glutenases promises to be a prolific area of future investigation, a few clinical candidates have already emerged that can be produced on the large scale. Consequently, the stage is set for controlled clinical trials of this novel mode of action in celiac sprue patients.

Over the course of the aforementioned protease studies, several assays have been developed for testing the therapeutic potential of alternative glutenases. They include formal kinetic studies with simple chromogenic substrates [28, 30] as well as antigenic gluten peptides [28], HPLC and mass spectrometric analysis of whole gluten proteolyzed in vitro [28, 31, 34], in vivo measurements of glutenase activity in the stomach [33] and small intestine [29, 33] of rats, quantitative evaluation of residual gluten toxicity using T cells prepared from small intestinal biopsies of celiac sprue patients [31, 33], antibody-based immunoassays [31], and perhaps most significantly, short-term gluten challenge studies in patients (fig. 4) [40, 41].

Clinical investigation into the therapeutic utility of oral glutenases is a subject of particular relevance. A major advantage of this mode of therapy is that it seeks to remedy a fundamental feature of human nutrition (i.e. very slow diges-

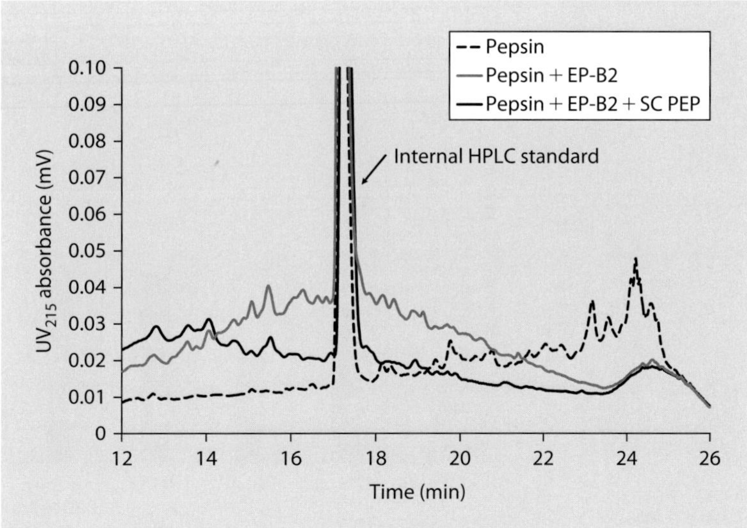

Fig. 3. In vitro digestion of whole wheat bread. Comparison of physiological gastric digestion (pepsin), pepsin + endoprotease B2 (EP-B2) digestion, and pepsin + dual therapy digestion of EP-B2 and *Sphingomonas capsulata* (SC) prolyl endopeptidase (PEP). The efficacy of individual versus combination glutenase therapies was tested by digesting 1 g whole wheat bread in vitro [48]. All enzymes were added prior to the start of the simulated gastric digestion at concentrations of: pepsin = 0.6 mg/ml; EP-B2 = 30 units/mg protein, and SC PEP = 1.67 units/mg protein. All digestions were performed for 60 min at 37°C. The digests were analyzed using HPLC. The internal HPLC standard used was N-α-p-tosyl-L-arginine methyl ester. Under the HPLC conditions used, representative antigenic gluten oligopeptides comprised of 9-, 11-, 12-, 21-, 28-, and 33-residue elutes at 12.5, 18.5, 21.5, 22, 22.5, and 24–25 min, respectively. A lower baseline of the pepsin + EP-B2 + SC PEP sample represents more thorough digestion of oligopeptides in the 14- to 25-min elution times.

tion and assimilation of gluten in the gastrointestinal tract) that occurs in all humans. Thus, the pharmacodynamic efficacy of a glutenase should be assessable in healthy volunteers with considerable accuracy. In contrast to healthy volunteers however, the celiac small intestine reacts adversely to gluten. To test the ability of an oral glutenase to protect against this damage, short-term gluten challenge studies are likely to be very useful [41]. While biopsy read-outs are generally regarded as the gold standard test of diagnosis and monitoring a patient's condition, repeated biopsies in the context of controlled clinical trials are impractical. Therefore, sensitive and specific surrogate markers of gluten-induced small intestinal damage are sorely needed. Some existing markers, such as noninvasive markers of intestinal absorption [42] or mucosal permeability [43], appear to be highly sensitive in the context of short-term challenge studies, although they are not specific for celiac sprue. Other markers, such as anti-TG2 serum autoantibodies [44], are fairly disease-specific but not especially sensitive. Over the next few years, the co-development of new drugs and surrogate markers promises to be an exciting area of research in this disease area.

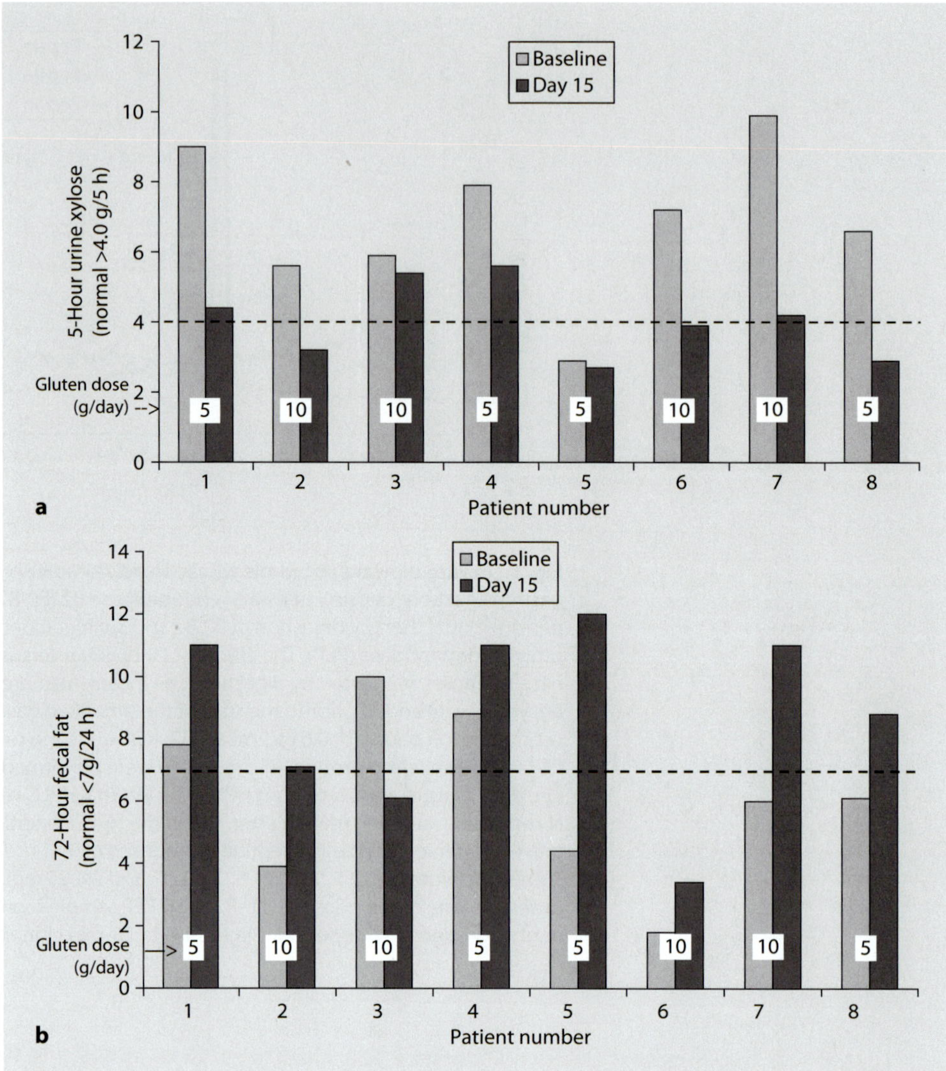

Fig. 4. Patient response to short-term gluten challenge. Eight biopsy-diagnosed celiac sprue patients were given a low-dose gluten challenge (5 or 10 g/day for 2 weeks). The small intestinal absorptive capacity was measured via the 5-hour urinary xylose test (**a**) and the 72-hour quantitative fecal fat test (**b**). The normal range values of these tests are shown as dashed lines [40].

In closing, it is also worth noting the potential for developing other types of non-dietary therapies for celiac sprue [45]. Whereas oral proteases seek to destroy the 'pathogen' (gluten), clinical efficacy could also be achieved by blocking key host proteins, thereby attenuating the gluten-mediated pathogenic response in a celiac patient. For example, as outlined in figure 1, inhibiting TG2 function or blocking HLA-DQ2 binding may also increase their threshold of gluten tolerance. Likewise, cytokine therapies such as interleukin (IL)-10 or anti-IL-15 can be considered to neutralize the inflammatory response to gluten in the celiac small intestine. A key concern that must be addressed early on in the development of such products pertains to drug safety. Antagonists of another putative regulator of intestinal permeability, zonulin, have also been proposed as non-dietary therapeutic candidates. A synthetic peptide based on this strategy increased the transepithelial resistance of intestinal mucosa in a diabetes-prone rat model [46], and is currently undergoing clinical trials in celiac sprue patients [47].

Acknowledgements

Research in the authors' laboratory was supported by a grant from the National Institutes of Health (DK 063158). J.E. is supported by a National Science Foundation fellowship.

References

1 Frazer AC, Fletcher RF, Ross CA, Shaw B, Sammons HG Schneider R: Gluten-induced enteropathy: the effect of partially digested gluten. Lancet 1959;2: 252–255.

2 Alvey C, Anderson CM, Freeman M: Wheat gluten and coeliac disease. Arch Dis Child 1957;32:434–437.

3 Krainick HG, Mohn G: Further investigations on the toxic effect of wheat flour in celiac disease. 2. Effect of enzymatic by-products of gliadin /(in German). Helv Paediatr Acta 1959;14: 124–140.

4 van Roon J, Haex AJ, Seeder WA, de Jong J: Clinical and biochemical analysis of gluten toxicity. I. Experientia 1960;16:209.

5 Reed LS: Pathogenesis of celiac disease in adults. Compatibility of immunologic and enzyme-defect theories. NY State J Med 1970;70:2095–2102.

6 Van De Kamer JH, Weijers HA, Dicke WK: Coeliac disease. IV. An investigation into the injurious constituents of wheat in connection with their action on patients with coeliac disease. Acta Paediatr 1953;42:223–231.

7 Frazer AC: Discussion on some problems of steatorrhea and reduced stature: on the growth defect in coeliac disease. Proc R Soc Med 1956;49:1009–1013.

8 Messer M, Anderson CM, Hubbard L: studies on the mechanism of destruction of the toxic action of wheat gluten in coeliac disease by crude papain. Gut 1964;5:295–303.

9 Beckwith AC, Heiner DC: An immunological study of wheat gluten proteins and derivatives. Arch Biochem Biophys 1966;117:239–247.

10 Alarcon Segovia D, Herskovic T, Wakim KG, Green PA, Scudamore HH: presence of circulating antibodies to gluten and milk fractions in patients with nontropical sprue. Am J Med 1964;36:485–499.

11 Malik GB, Watson WC, Murray D, Cruickshank B: Immunofluorescent antibody studies in idiopathic steatorrhoea. Lancet 1964;13:1127–1129.

12 Dobbins WO 3rd, Rubin CE: studies of the rectal mucosa in celiac sprue. Gastroenterology 1964;47:471–479.

13 Douglas AP, Booth CC: Jejunal mucosal digestion of gluten peptides in adult coeliac disease. Lancet 1968;2:491–492.

14 Berg NO, Dahlqvist A, Lindberg T, Norden A: Intestinal dipeptidases and disaccharidases in celiac disease in adults. Gastroenterology 1970;59: 575–582.

15 Gelfand MD, Spiro HM, Herskovic T: Small intestine glutaminase deficiency in celiac disease. Am J Dig Dis 1968;13: 638–642.

16 Douglas AP, Booth CC: Post-prandial plasma-free amino acids in adult coeliac disease after oral gluten and albumin. Clin Sci 1969;37:643–653.

17 Douglas AP, Booth CC: Digestion of gluten peptides by normal human jejunal mucosa and by mucosa from patients with adult coeliac disease. Clin Sci 1970;38:11–25.

18 Sollid LM, Markussen G, Ek J, Gjerde H, Vartdal F, Thorsby E: Evidence for a primary association of celiac disease to a particular HLA-DQ alpha/beta heterodimer. J Exp Med 1989;169:345–350.

19 Lundin KE, Scott H, Hansen T, Paulsen G, Halstensen TS, Fausa O, Thorsby E, Sollid LM: Gliadin-specific, HLA-DQ(alpha 1*0501,beta 1*0201) restricted T cells isolated from the small intestinal mucosa of celiac disease patients. J Exp Med 1993;178:187–196.

20 Molberg O, McAdam SN, Korner R, Quarsten H, Kristiansen C, Madsen L, Fugger L, Scott H, Noren O, Roepstorff P, Lundin KE, Sjostrom H, Sollid LM: Tissue transglutaminase selectively modifies gliadin peptides that are recognized by gut-derived T cells in celiac disease. Nat Med 1998;4:713–717.

21 van de Wal Y, Kooy YM, van Veelen PA, Pena SA, Mearin LM, Molberg O, Lundin KE, Sollid LM, Mutis T Benckhuijsen WE, Drijfhout JW, Koning F: Small intestinal T cells of celiac disease patients recognize a natural pepsin fragment of gliadin. Proc Natl Acad Sci USA 998;95:10050–10054.

22 Anderson RP, Degano P, Godkin AJ, Jewell DP, Hill AV: In vivo antigen challenge in celiac disease identifies a single transglutaminase-modified peptide as the dominant A-gliadin T-cell epitope. Nat Med 2000;6:337–342.

23 Arentz-Hansen H, Korner R, Molberg O, Quarsten H, Vader W, Kooy YM, Lundin KE, Koning F, Roepstorff P, Sollid LM, McAdam SN: The intestinal T cell response to alpha-gliadin in adult celiac disease is focused on a single deamidated glutamine targeted by tissue transglutaminase. J Exp Med 2000;191:603–612.

24 Dieterich W, Ehnis T, Bauer M, Donner P, Volta U, Riecken EO, Schuppan D: Identification of tissue transglutaminase as the autoantigen of celiac disease. Nat Med 1997;3:797–801.
25 Neill JD, Litts JC, Anderson OD, Greene FC, Stiles JI: Expression of a wheat alpha-gliadin gene in *Saccharomyces cerevisiae*. Gene 1987;55:303–317.
26 Hausch F, Shan L, Santiago NA, Gray GM, Khosla C: Intestinal digestive resistance of immunodominant gliadin peptides. Am J Physiol Gastrointest Liver Physiol 2002;283:G996–G1003.
27 Shan L, Molberg O, Parrot I, Hausch F, Filiz F, Gray GM, Sollid LM, Khosla C: Structural basis for gluten intolerance in celiac sprue. Science 2002;297: 2275–2279.
28 Gass J, Ehren J, Strohmeier G, Isaacs I, Khosla C: Fermentation, purification, formulation, and pharmacological evaluation of a prolyl endopeptidase from *Myxococcus xanthus:* implications for celiac sprue therapy. Biotechnol Bioeng 2005;92:674–684.
29 Piper JL, Gray GM, Khosla C: Effect of prolyl endopeptidase on digestive-resistant gliadin peptides in vivo. J Pharmacol Exp Ther 2004;311:213–219.
30 Shan L, Marti T, Sollid LM, Gray GM, Khosla C: Comparative biochemical analysis of three bacterial prolyl endopeptidases: implications for coeliac sprue. Biochem J 2004;383:311–318.
31 Siegel M, Bethune MT, Gass J, Ehren J, Xia J, Johannsen A, Stuge TB, Gray GM, Lee PP, Khosla C: Rational design of combination enzyme therapy for celiac sprue. Chem Biol 2006;13:649–658.
32 Bethune MT, Strop P, Tang Y, Sollid LM, Khosla C: Heterologous expression, purification, refolding, and structural-functional characterization of EP-B2, a self-activating barley cysteine endoprotease. Chem Biol 2006;13:637–647.
33 Gass J, Vora H, Bethune MT, Gray GM, Khosla C: Effect of barley endoprotease EP-B2 on gluten digestion in the intact rat. J Pharmacol Exp Ther 2006;318: 1178–1186.
34 Marti T, Molberg O, Li Q, Gray GM, Khosla C, Sollid LM: Prolyl endopeptidase-mediated destruction of T cell epitopes in whole gluten: chemical and immunological characterization. J Pharmacol Exp Ther 2005;312:19–26.
35 Piper JL, Gray GM, Khosla C: High selectivity of human tissue transglutaminase for immunoactive gliadin peptides: implications for celiac sprue. Biochemistry 2002;41:386–393.
36 Shan L, Qiao SW, Arentz-Hansen H, Molberg O, Gray GM, Sollid LM, Khosla C: Identification and analysis of multivalent proteolytically resistant peptides from gluten: implications for celiac sprue. J Proteome Res 2005;4: 1732–1741.
37 Stepniak D, Spaenij-Dekking L, Mitea C, Moester M, de Ru A, Baak-Pablo R, van Veelen P, Edens L, Koning F: Highly efficient gluten degradation with a newly identified prolyl endoprotease: implications for celiac disease. Am J Physiol Gastrointest Liver Physiol 2006;291:G621–G629.
38 Davy A, Svendsen I, Sorensen SO, Blom Sorensen M, Rouster J, Meldal M, Simpson DJ, Cameron-Mills V: Substrate specificity of barley cysteine endoproteases EP-A and EP-B. Plant Physiol 1998;117:255–261.
39 Hartmann G, Koehler P, Wieser H: Rapid degradation of gliadin peptides toxic for coeliac disease patients by proteases from germinating cereals. J Cereal Sci 2006;44:368–371.
40 Pyle GG, Paaso B, Anderson BE, Allen D, Marti T, Khosla C, Gray GM: Low-dose gluten challenge in celiac sprue: malabsorptive and antibody responses. Clin Gastroenterol Hepatol 2005;3: 679–686.
41 Pyle GG, Paaso B, Anderson BE, Allen DD, Marti T, Li Q, Siegel M, Khosla C, Gray GM: Effect of pretreatment of food gluten with prolyl endopeptidase on gluten-induced malabsorption in celiac sprue. Clin Gastroenterol Hepatol 2005;3:687–694.
42 Teahon K, Somasundaram S, Smith T, Menzies I, Bjarnason I: Assessing the site of increased intestinal permeability in coeliac and inflammatory bowel disease. Gut 1996;38:864–869.
43 Della Morte MA, Sala MR, Morelli P, Meschi V, Silva A, Valli F: Celiac disease and its diagnostic evolution. Comparisons and experiences in a hospital pediatric department (1975–1992). I (in Italian). Pediatr Med Chir 1992;14:251–271.
44 Korponay-Szabo IR, Laurila K, Szondy Z, Halttunen T, Szalai Z, Dahlbom I, Rantala I, Kovacs JB, Fesus L, Maki M: Missing endomysial and reticulin binding of coeliac antibodies in transglutaminase 2 knockout tissues. Gut 2003;52:199–204.
45 Sollid LM, Khosla C: Future therapeutic options for celiac disease. Nat Rev Clin Gastroenterol Hepatol 2005;2: 140–147.
46 Watts T, Berti I, Sapone A, Gerarduzzi T, Not T, et al: Role of the intestinal tight junction modulator zonulin in the pathogenesis of type I diabetes in BB diabetic-prone rats. Proc Natl Acad Sci USA 2005;102:2916–2921.
47 Paterson BM, Lammers KM, Arrieta MC, Fasano A, Meddings JB: The safety, tolerance, pharmacokinetic and pharmacodynamic effects of single doses of AT-1001 in coeliac disease subjects: a proof of concept study. Aliment Pharmacol Ther 2007;26:757–766.
48 Gass J, Bethune MT, Siegel M, Spencer A, Khosla C: Combination enzyme therapy for gastric digestion of dietary gluten in patients with celiac sprue. Gastroenterology 2007;133:472–480.

Chaitan Khosla
Departments of Chemistry, Chemical Engineering and Biochemistry
Stanford University
Stanford, CA 94305 (USA)
Tel. +1 650 723 6538, Fax +1 650 725 7294, E-Mail khosla@stanford.edu

Fasano A, Troncone R, Branski D (eds): Frontiers in Celiac Disease.
Pediatr Adolesc Med. Basel, Karger, 2008, vol 12, pp 157–171

Inhibitors of Intestinal Barrier Dysfunction

Blake M. Paterson[a] · Jerrold R. Turner[b]

[a]Alba Therapeutics Corporation, Baltimore, Md., and [b]Department of Pathology, University of Chicago, Chicago, Ill., USA

Abstract

In the past decade, literature has increasingly pointed to a proximal intestinal barrier dysfunction and inappropriate paracellular permeability increase that precedes and correlates with inflammatory markers and/or disease expression in inflammatory bowel disease, celiac disease and irritable bowel syndrome. Exogenous and endogenous stimuli are known to induce paracellular permeability and disrupt barrier function. Recent identification of regulatory pathways that induce cytoskeletal reorganization, tight junction disassembly and paracellular permeability provide targets for therapeutic intervention in celiac disease. Here we review the identity, function and regulation of these pathways and propose various approaches to therapeutic intervention in celiac disease with the aim of inhibiting intestinal barrier dysfunction.

Unlike other epithelial barriers in the human body, the gastrointestinal tract must allow for nutrient absorption while maintaining a physical and immunological barrier to massive amounts of potentially harmful agents. This requires an ability to distinguish luminal food antigens and commensal bacteria from pathogens while simultaneously facilitating efficient nutrient digestion and transport. A variety of physiological, anatomic, innate and adaptive immune systems are used to achieve this balance, including peptidase and bile production, mucin barriers, transepithelial cellular transport, dynamic regulation of paracellular diffusion, defensins, recognition of pathogen-associated molecular patterns, elaboration of proinflammatory chemokines and cytokines and the downregulation of these inflammatory signals. When the barrier is violated, a delicate state of controlled inflammation is disrupted and pathology ensues.

Bjarnason et al. [1] have proposed a unified theory that models this complex state of the gut into three compartments: luminal aggressors, barrier function, and mucosal defense. They postulate that whenever an intestinal insult occurs, interaction between luminal factors and mucosal defense results in a permeability and inflammatory cascade whose magnitude eclipses those of the primary insult, regardless of its nature. Three components (fig. 1) are necessary for the development and persistence of intestinal disease: barrier disruption, access of luminal contents to the submucosa, and the consequent immune response [2]. Increases in permeability and inflammation are not simply sequelae of the insult – rather they may be determinant, if not causal, of the pathogenesis

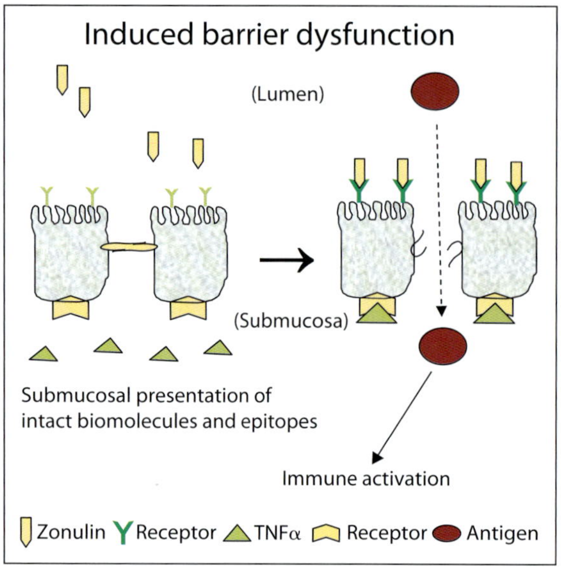

Fig. 1. Intestinal inflammatory disease is the result of 3 converging events: barrier disruption and access of luminal contents to the submucosal gastrointestinal lymphoid tissue, resulting in immune stimulation.

[3]. Many argue that changes in intestinal permeability and inflammation are always correlated and occur hand in hand, leading to the induction of intestinal disease with local and/or systemic expression in susceptible hosts [4], and suggest that defective barrier function is a precondition for any autoimmune disease to occur, regardless of the location of the target tissue [3].

In the absence of epithelial disruption, the functional state of the tight junction (TJ) determines barrier polarity and paracellular permeability [5]. Once considered static structures, TJs are highly dynamic, opening and closing in consonance with a cytoskeletal reorganization that occurs in response to dietary exposure, neurohumoral signaling and inflammatory mediators [6–9]. One example of physiological TJ regulation by an extracellular event is that which occurs following activation of Na^+-nutrient cotransport in the small intestine [10–12]. Although the contribution of Na^+-nutrient cotransport-dependent TJ regulation to mucosal nutrient absorption has remained controversial [13–15], it is clear that this represents both a mechanism by which luminal and apical events regulate cytoskeletal state/TJ structure and paracellular permeability, and a means by which increased paracellular permeability can amplify mucosal absorption in vivo in rodents and human subjects [11, 15–17].

Vibrio cholerae secretes a zonula occludens toxin (ZOT) that binds to a putative receptor on the apical surface of enterocytes, and similarly induces a transient reduction in transepithelial resistance (fig. 2) and increases in paracellular permeability and transepithelial flux along concentration gradients [18–20]. Zonulin, a likely human homolog to ZOT, appears to be a serine protease that functions as an endogenous paracrine signaling protein and whose prokaryotic analogs (e.g., ZOT, ΔG) possess potent immune-stimulating properties when applied, with antigen, to mucosal surfaces in mammals [21–24]. The putative zonulin is secreted in response to various luminal stimuli, including gluten and pathogenic bacteria, and appears to induce intestinal epithelial cell (IEC) rearrangement and TJ disassembly in mammalian tissue [19, 22, 25, 26]. In celiac intestinal tissues and in in vitro, ex vivo, and in vivo animal experiments, gliadin causes rapid zonulin release and consequent increases in paracellular permeability [22, 26–28].

Analyses of isolated rodent mucosa, cultured intestinal epithelial monolayers, and isolated human tissue have demonstrated that contraction of the peri-junctional actomyosin ring is necessary for Na^+-glucose cotransport-dependent TJ regulation [6, 10, 29, 30]; this is also the case for ZOT-dependent TJ disassembly [22, 25–27]. While Na^+-glucose cotransport-dependent TJ regulation is mediated by myosin light chain kinase (MLCK) activation and phosphorylation of the myosin II regulatory light chain [6, 29], ZOT-zonulin-dependent disassembly appears to be associated with protein kinase Cα upregulation and is accompanied by ZO-1 phosphorylation

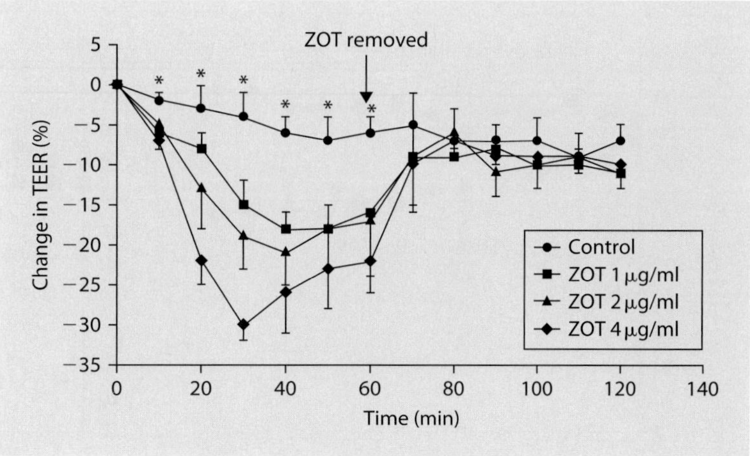

Fig. 2. The induction of paracellular permeability by ZOT is reversible and transient. Percent change in transepithelial electrical resistance (TEER) in blood brain barrier microvascular epithelial cell monolayers (mean ± SD) in the absence and presence of the prokaryotic zonulin analog 'ZOT' (1.0, 2.0, and 4.0 μg/ml). $^*p < 0.05$ versus control. From Karyekar et al. [65], with permission.

and downregulation of peri-junctional claudin and occludin [25–28].

The modulation of epithelial permeability by TJ regulatory pathways such as zonulin and Na^+-glucose cotransport is reversible and transient [2, 20, 22, 29] (fig. 3). If intestinal inflammation and permeability are indeed correlated and causal of intestinal disease, then the ability to reversibly modulate TJs (and thus paracellular permeability) represents an important therapeutic opportunity (fig. 4).

Intestinal Permeability and Celiac Disease

In diseases as diverse as schizophrenia, diabetes type 1, juvenile rheumatoid arthritis, inflammatory bowel disease, irritable bowel syndrome and celiac disease (CD), observations of elevated intestinal permeability and functional enteropathy have been made [31–35]. The greatest correlation between permeability and inflammation has been established in the intestinal diseases [4, 36]. In the past decade, the literature has increasingly pointed to a proximal intestinal permeability that precedes and correlates with inflammatory markers and disease expression in inflammatory bowel disease, irritable bowel syndrome and CD [37–39]. If the hypothesis that intestinal inflammation and permeability are correlated is true, then measures of IP, such as the fractional excretion of unmetabolized sugars, lactulose and mannitol (LA:MA), should provide a fast and sensitive measure of the response to therapeutic intervention, correlating with inflammation markers that have slower response times and are more difficult to measure. In CD, the state of disease activity and histopathology appear to correlate with markers of intestinal inflammation and markers of permeability, as suggested by published data of experimental disease exacerbation induced by gluten challenge and remission induced by dietary gluten withdrawal [40–42].

Like CD, barrier function is compromised in patients with Crohn's disease [43, 44]. The presence of barrier dysfunction is related to Crohn's disease activation, as increased small intestinal permeability predicts clinical relapse in patients with inactive disease [45, 46], and disease suppression with tumor necrosis factor-neutralizing antibodies restores barrier function [47]. Conversely, acute treatment of either cultured monolayers or rodents with tumor necrosis factor causes junctional protein reorganization and intestinal epithelial barrier loss [9, 17, 47]. This

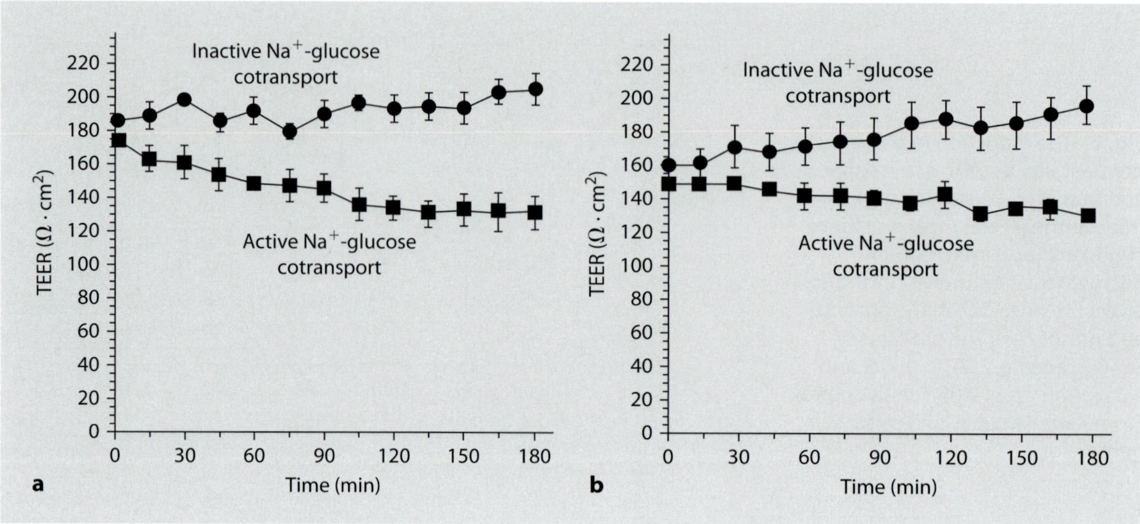

Fig. 3. Na^+-glucose cotransport-dependent tight junction regulation is reversible. **a** Transepithelial electrical resistance (TEER) decreases rapidly following activation of Na^+-glucose cotransport. Caco-2 monolayers were incubated overnight in media with 0.5 mM phloridzin to inhibit SGLT1. Na^+-glucose cotransport was then activated (■) or inhibited (●). Data shown are the mean ± SD (n = 6). **b** TEER rapidly increases following inhibition of Na^+-glucose cotransport. Caco-2 monolayers were incubated overnight in media with 25 mM glucose to activate SGLT1. Na^+-glucose cotransport was then activated (■) or inhibited (●). Data shown are the mean ± SD (n = 6). From Turner et al. [29], with permission.

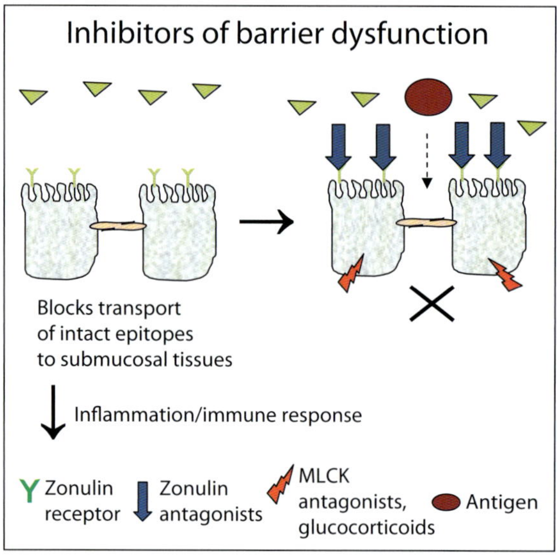

Fig. 4. A new opportunity for the treatment of intestinal inflammatory disease: inhibit the loss of barrier function with permeability inhibitors such as MLCK and zonulin antagonists.

loss of intestinal barrier function is accompanied by both transcriptional and enzymatic activation of MLCK and can be prevented by MLCK inhibition [17, 47–50].

Celiac autoimmunity occurs as a direct result of an inappropriate T-cell-mediated immune response against ingested gluten. After crossing the intestinal epithelium, gliadin fragments are taken up and processed by antigen-presenting cells and presented to CD4 T cells [51]. A leaky gut is sine qua non with the disease and may be one of the primary non-HLA genetic risk factors of the disease [39]; early innate immune responses to gliadin derivatives are also recognized as key to the pathogenesis of the disease [52–54]. Upon exposure to gliadin, IECs undergo immediate cytoskeletal rearrangement, TJs are disassembled (fig. 5) and functional barrier integrity is lost [28]. These changes are directly associated with increases in supernatant zonulin

Fig. 5. Peptic-tryptic digest of gliadin (PTG) induces rapid cytoskeletal rearrangement and disrupts epithelial tight junctions. IEC6 cells were treated with PTG (5 mg/ml) for 60 min at 37°C. Cells were fixed and processed by direct immunofluorescence with anti-ZO-1 antibody and Alexa Fluor 555 phalloidin to detect F-actin. In untreated control cells ZO-1 is seen at cell–cell junctions as a continuous smooth line, whereas in PTG-treated cells the ZO-1 staining is discontinuous indicating a disruption of tight junctions. Untreated cells exhibit robust actin stress fibers. Treatment with PTG results in a loss of stress fibers and is accompanied by the appearance of gaps between cells.

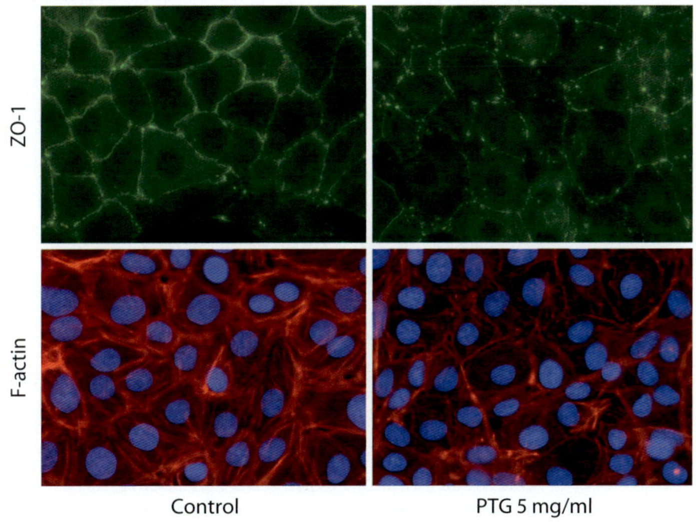

Fig. 6. The ZOT-zonulin analog DeltaG induces rapid cytoskeletal rearrangement and disrupts epithelial tight junctions. IEC6 cells were treated with deltaG (100 μg/ml) for 60 min at 37°C. Cells were fixed and processed by direct immunofluorescence with anti-ZO-1 antibody and Alexa Fluor 555 phalloidin to detect F-actin. In untreated control cells ZO-1 is seen at cell–cell junctions as a continuous smooth line, whereas in deltaG-treated cells the ZO-1 staining is discontinuous or lost from cell–cell junctions. Untreated cells exhibit robust actin stress fibers. Treatment with deltaG results in a loss of stress fibers and is accompanied by the appearance of gaps between cells (arrows).

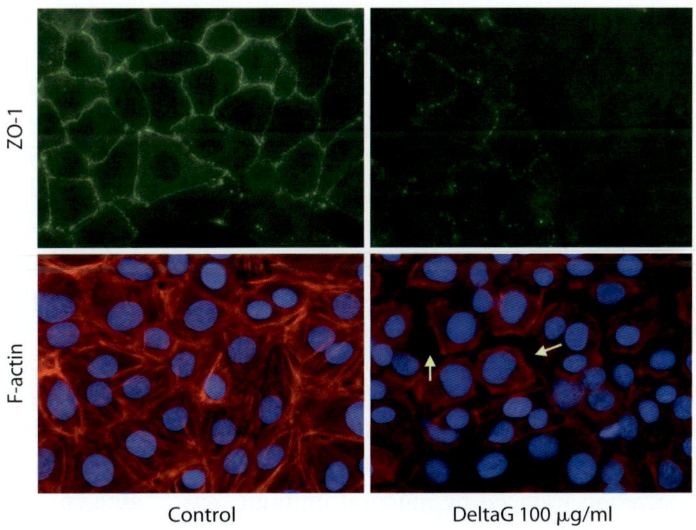

levels [22] as measured by a polyclonal antibody and are reproduced by the local administration of the zonulin analog ΔG (fig. 6). Other studies have demonstrated independent associations between gluten, intestinal permeability, zonulin expression and other autoimmune diseases, including diabetes type 1 and primary biliary cirrhosis [28, 55–62].

Although the mechanisms underlying barrier loss in CD have not been completely elucidated, it

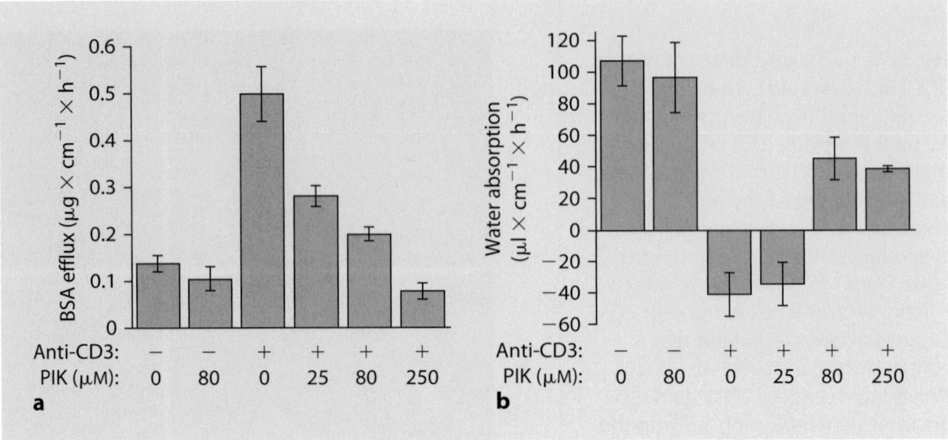

Fig. 7. The specific MLCK inhibitor PIK prevents barrier dysfunction and diarrhea in mice. The specific MLCK inhibitor PIK prevents T-cell activation-induced barrier dysfunction and diarrhea. **a** Increases in paracellular bovine serum albumin efflux induced by anti-CD3 treatment are reduced by PIK perfusion in a dose-dependent manner ($p = 0.015$ between 0 and 80 μM PIK treatment with anti-CD3, $n = 4$). **b** Treatment with 80 μM PIK resulted in the restoration of net water absorption in anti-CD3-treated mice ($p = 0.006$, $n = 4$). From Clayburgh et al. [17], with permission.

seems likely that zonulin or zonulin-like molecules and MLCK may play critical roles. Thus, TJ inhibitors may prove to be effective in CD.

Inhibitors of Barrier Dysfunction

Inhibition of MLCK using a highly specific pseudosubstrate peptide restores barrier function and TJ morphology following tumor necrosis factor treatment [17, 47, 48, 63]. In vivo use of this MLCK inhibitory peptide also restores jejunal mucosal water absorption, thereby preventing the net secretion induced by mucosal immune activation and tumor necrosis factor release (fig. 7) [17, 63]. While only preclinical studies of the MLCK inhibitory peptide in preventing immune-mediated diarrhea have been reported [17, 63], the observation that MLCK expression and activity are increased in Crohn's disease and ulcerative colitis [64] suggests that this may be an effective therapeutic approach for the treatment of various intestinal diseases, including CD.

AT-1001 is an octapeptide that inhibits ZOT- and gliadin-induced IEC cytoskeleton rearrangement, TJ disassembly and peak F-actin increment (fig. 8) [22, 26, 28]. Pretreatment with the peptide fails to inhibit gliadin-induced zonulin release but blocks paracellular permeability in monolayers induced by ZOT analogs (fig. 9) and blocks gliadin-induced leak in diseased (celiac) human duodenal epithelia (fig. 10), suggesting that the effect of the molecule is indirect and may be specific to a putative zonulin receptor [22, 27]. Furthermore, intranasal administration of AT-1001 prevents ZOT-induced immune responses to non-self-antigen challenge (fig. 11) [24], and oral administration mitigates the expression of diabetes type 1 in the BB/wor DP rat (fig. 12) by blocking intestinal permeability and the expression of humoral autoimmunity [61]. Thus AT-1001 appears to block intestinal permeability and the genesis of autoimmune disease, either as a result of a reduction in antigen presentation to immune tissue, or through some unknown inhibitory, direct/indirect effects on immune cells.

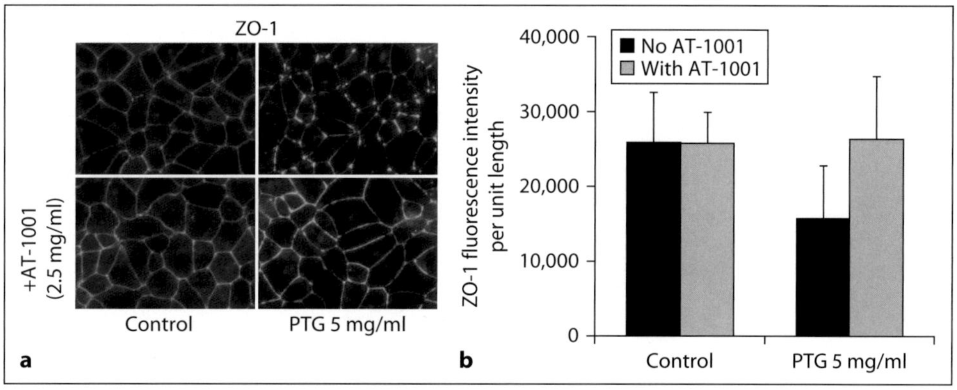

Fig. 8. Permeability inhibitor AT-1001 prevents PT-gliadin (PTG)-mediated tight junction disassembly. **a** IEC6 cells were pretreated with 2.5 mg/ml AT-1001 for 30 min, followed by PTG for 60 min or left untreated in control. Cells were fixed and processed by direct immunofluorescence with anti-ZO-1 antibody. Images were captured on a Nikon TE2000 microscope. PTG-treated cells (in the absence of AT-1001) exhibit punctuate distribution of ZO-1 at cell junctions. In the presence of AT-1001, ZO-1 distribution at cell junctions is smooth and continuous as seen in untreated control cells. **b** Total junctional fluorescence intensity of ZO-1 and length of individual junctions were quantified using NIS-Elements image analysis software. The graph represents ZO-1 fluorescence intensity per unit length of a junction. Approximately 50 cells were analyzed per treatment.

Clinical Implications

Clinical Measures of Intestinal Permeability

Markers of CD progression and remission that are both validated and provide a timely assessment of disease activity are nonexistent. While clinical measurements of intestinal permeability are easily performed in the clinic and provide a means of evaluating immediate changes in disease activity, poor specificity has precluded their use for diagnosis, and they have not been widely adopted for disease monitoring. However, recent improvements in analytical techniques and a standardization of the permeability probe solutions has led to an increase in the precision and accuracies of the LA:MA technique. In our laboratories, these exceed 93% and are performed according to GLP standards.

Different permeability probes provide information about gastrointestinal tract segments; LA:MA ratios quantify functional changes in barrier state versus absorptive surface area of the small bowel (fig. 13). An increased fractional excretion of lactulose suggests that there has been either small intestinal damage or the opening of previously closed TJs. The fractional excretion of mannitol is proportional to villous tip surface area, therefore the LA:MA ratio is often interpreted as damage per unit area. In CD there is a reduction in absorptive surface area (decrease in mannitol fractional excretion) and an increased opening of TJs or epithelial damage (increased lactulose fractional excretion) and both combine to increase the LA:MA ratio [3, 42].

Clinical Studies

The only inhibitor of barrier dysfunction that has been studied in celiac patients is orally administered AT-1001. The oral formulation of AT-1001 is enterically coated and multi-particulate, designed for phasic release in the duodenum and jejunum, and is not systemically bioavailable (fig. 14).

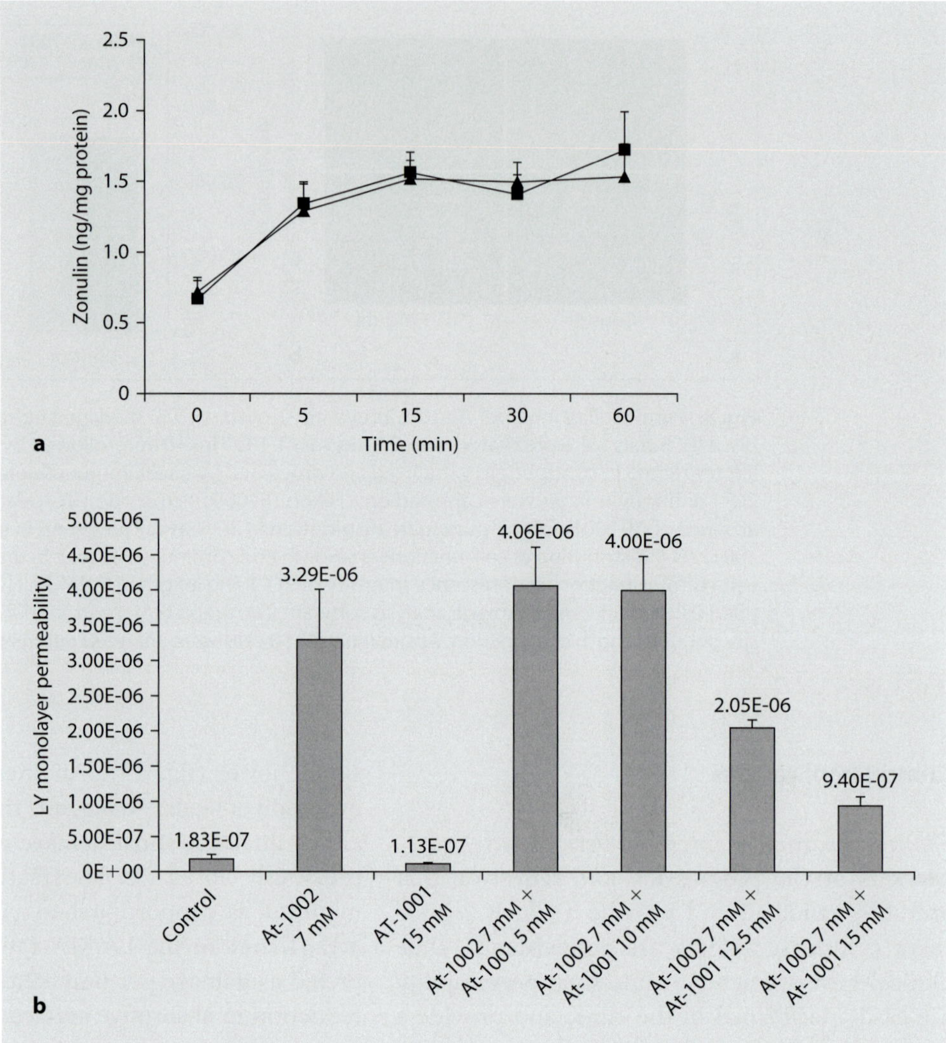

Fig. 9. Effect of AT-1001 on PT-gliadin-induced zonulin release and on ZOT-zonulin analog-induced permeability. **a** Duodenal tissues from CD patients in remission were mounted in the microsnapwell system and exposed to PT-gliadin, either alone or following 15 min preincubation with AT-1001. AT-1001 pretreatment (▲) did not affect the zonulin release by PT-gliadin (■) (n = 17). From Drago et al. [22], with permission. **b** Effect of various concentrations of AT-1001 on increase in Lucifer yellow (LY) Caco-2 monolayer permeability induced by zonulin agonist AT-1002. Results are expressed as mean ± SEM (n = 3). Results indicate a dose-dependent effect of AT-1001 in blocking the AT-1002-induced increase in LY permeability.

As of early 2007, AT-1001 was in phase-II clinical trials in the US and had already completed traditional safety and pharmacokinetic assessment in phase-I studies. One of the phase-I trials was a proof of concept study, designed as an inpatient, double-blind, randomized, placebo-controlled study to determine the safety, tolerability, pharmacokinetic and pharmacodynamic effects of 12 mg doses of

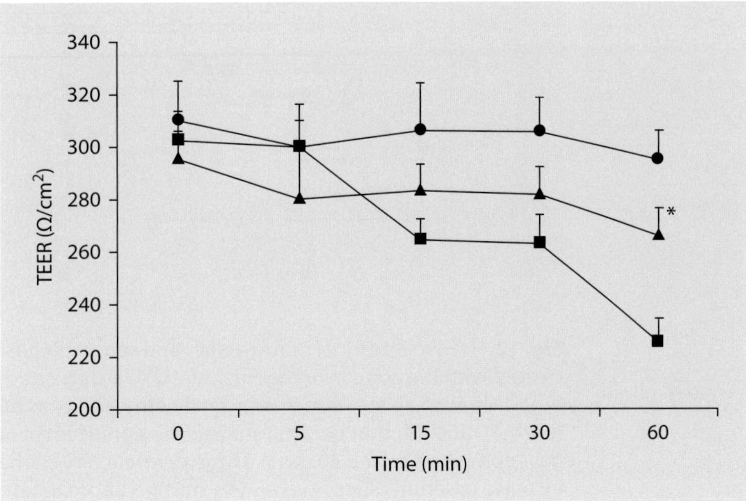

Fig. 10. Effect of the AT-1001 on PT-gliadin-induced zonulin release and transepithelial electrical resistance (TEER) changes in duodenal tissues from CD patients in remission. Duodenal tissues from CD patients in remission were mounted in the microsnapwell system and exposed to PT-gliadin, either alone or following 15 min preincubation with AT-1001. The TEER decrement induced by PT-gliadin (■) was prevented by pretreatment with AT-1001 (▲) (10 mg/ml). PD-casein-treated tissues (●) are shown as negative controls. $^{*}p \leq 0.02$ compared with PT-gliadin alone (n = 17). From Drago et al. [22], with permission.

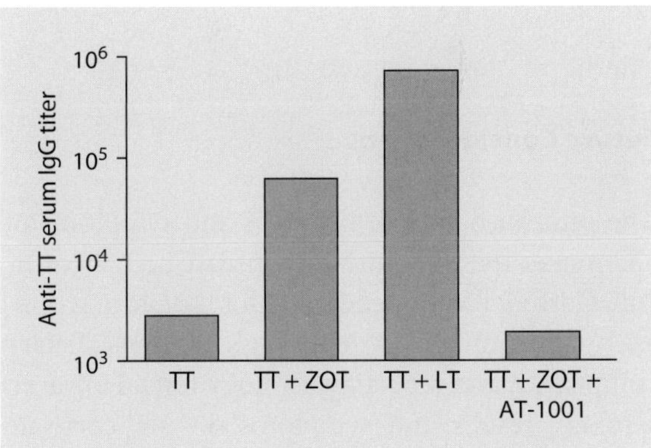

Fig. 11. Inhibition of histidine-tagged ZOT (His-ZOT) adjuvant activity by AT-1001. C57BL/6 mice were intranasally immunized five times with Tetanus toxoid (TT) alone or with TT and His-ZOT in the presence or absence of AT-1001, and with enterotoxin (LT) and TT as positive control. An additional group of mice received TT and AT-1001 to test the potential toxic effect of the inhibitor; however, the octapeptide did not affect the response to the Ag alone (data not shown). Data are expressed as Ab GMTs ± standard errors for 5 mice in each group. From Marinaro et al. [24], with permission.

AT-1001 in CD subjects in remission (fig. 15). Twenty-one subjects previously diagnosed by biopsy and positive antibody screen, on gluten-free diets for at least 6 months prior to enrollment, and presenting with anti-tissue transglutaminase (tTG) titers of ≤10 EU were enrolled. The study involved a 2:1 randomization (drug:placebo) for treatment on days 1, 2 and 3. On day 2, all subjects received a 2.5-gram, blinded oral gluten challenge. Endpoints included changes in urinary LA:MA ratios assessed on study days 1, 2, 3, and 7, self-reported measures of gastrointestinal discomfort, adverse events, global outcomes assessment, urinary nitrites/nitrates and PBMC cell markers and cytokine levels. Urine samples for intestinal permeability measurement were collected for 8 h after dietary challenge on days 1, 2, 3, and 7; subjects remained on a strict gluten-free diet throughout the study.

Following acute gluten exposure, a 70% increase in intestinal permeability was detected in the placebo group (table 1), while no changes were seen in the AT-1001 treatment group. After

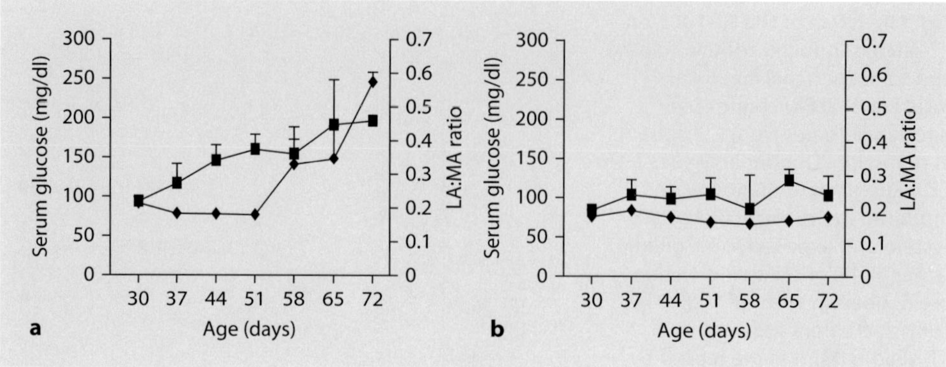

Fig. 12. In vivo intestinal permeability and serum glucose levels in diabetic prone BBDP rats treated with the zonulin antagonist AT-1001. **a** Untreated BBDP animals that evolved to diabetes type 1 showed an increase in intestinal permeability as measure by the lactulose/mannitol (LA/MA) ratio (■) that became statistically significant at age 44 days ($p < 0.05$–0.002 age 44–72 days compared to age 30 days). These permeability changes were followed by a significant increase in serum glucose levels (◆) starting approximately 2 weeks after the increase in intestinal permeability ($p < 0.05$–0.0001 age 65–72 days compared to age 30 days). **b** Conversely, BBDP rats treated with AT-1001 and that did not develop diabetes type 1 had no changes in either intestinal permeability or serum glucose levels. The AT-1001-treated animals that developed diabetes ($n = 4$) and the untreated animals that did not develop diabetes ($n = 3$) were eliminated from the final analysis. Therefore, the treated group had 11 animals, and the untreated group had 12. From Watts et al. [61], with permission.

gluten exposure, IFN-γ levels increased in 4 of 7 patients (57.1%) of the placebo group, but only in 4 of 14 patients (28.6%) of the AT-1001-group. Gastrointestinal symptoms were more frequently detected among patients of the placebo group as compared to the AT-1001 group (table 2).

Inhibition of intestinal barrier dysfunction has the potential to provide suppression of mucosal inflammation and modification of disease in a manner that is safe, effective and well tolerated. Oral AT-1001 reduces gluten-induced intestinal barrier dysfunction, cytokine production, and gastrointestinal symptoms in celiac patients, and has great potential for the treatment and induction of remission in celiac patients. Further studies are required to better elucidate the potential risks and benefits of this innovative therapeutic approach.

Future Considerations

The protean nature of the signs and symptoms of CD makes the monitoring of disease activity difficult. Current recommendations for monitoring disease progression include assessing symptoms, dietary compliance and repeating serology tests. However, serology results and symptoms do not correlate well with symptomatology or the histopathology of the mucosal lining of the small intestine. Indeed, markers of CD progression and remission that are both validated and provide a timely assessment of disease activity are nonexistent. In conjunction with various clinical and epidemiological experts in the field, we are presently undertaking the creation of a disease index that can account for the differences in periodicity (timing) of change in symptoms, histopathology, intestinal permeability and serology that occur with change in disease state,

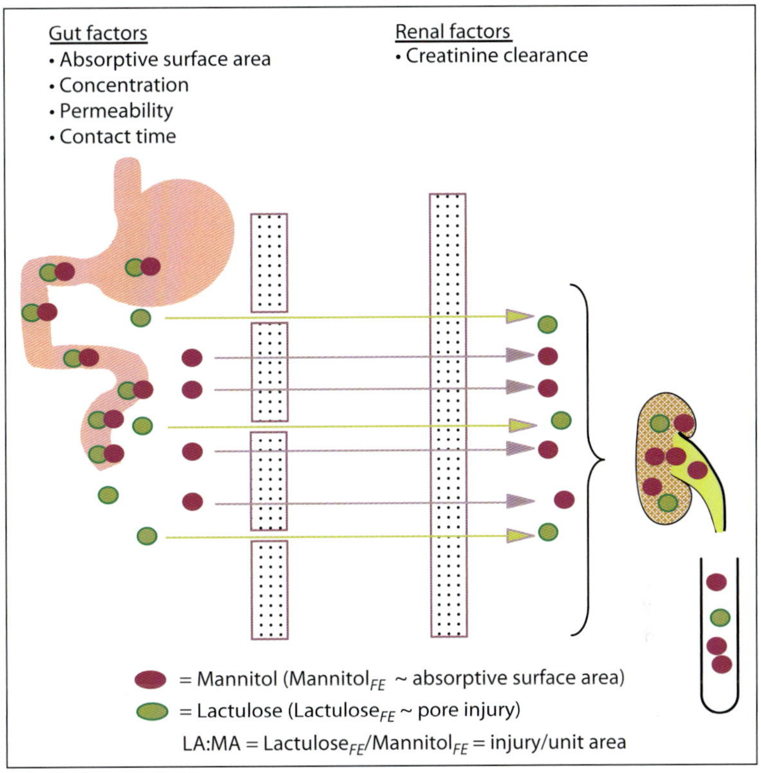

Fig. 13. The use of lactulose and mannitol as oral permeability probes to noninvasively determine small bowel paracellular permeability. Lactulose is absorbed only upon disruption of the tight junction. Factors such as gut transit time, intestinal length, surface area and renal function alter the absolute absorption and fractional excretion of lactulose (lactulose$_{FE}$), so mannitol is required as a control. Mannitol is passively absorbed through both transcellular and paracellular routes, correlating with the area of absorptive tissue.

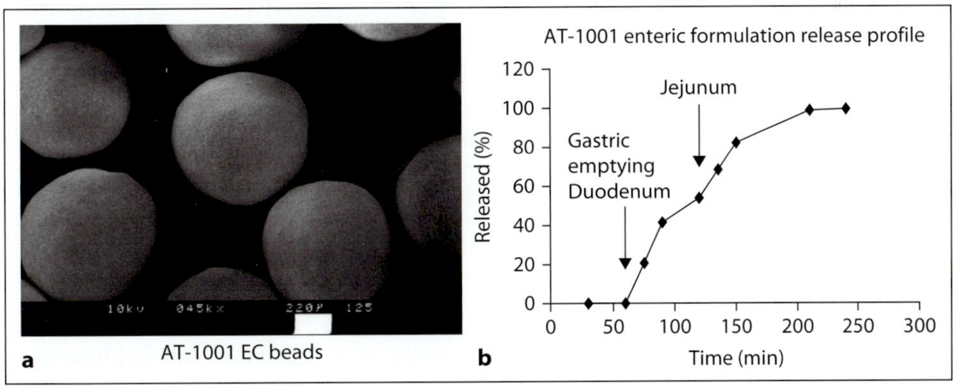

Fig. 14. AT-1001 EC oral formulation. **a** Scanning electron micrograph of enterically coated AT-1001 beads. **b** In vitro release profile of multi-particulate AT-1001 enterically coated beads filled into hard gelatin capsules. Results are expressed as mean ± SEM (n = 3). Results indicate no AT-1001 release in simulated gastric fluid within the first 60 min. Results also indicate a delayed release of AT-1001 in simulated intestinal fluid over the next 120 min.

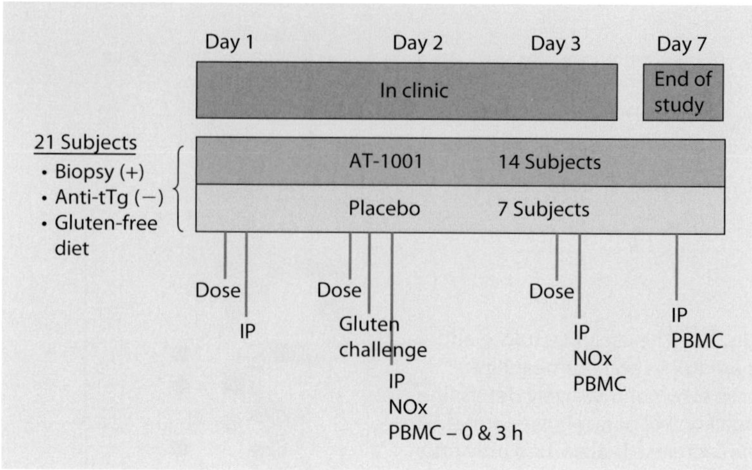

Fig. 15. A randomized, double-blind, placebo-controlled study to determine the safety, tolerance, pharmacokinetic and pharmacodynamic effects of single doses of AT-1001 in celiac disease subjects. IP = Intestinal permeability.

Table 1. Summary of lactulose to mannitol ratio findings

	Geometric mean (95% CI)				
	day 1	day 2	day 3	day 7	
Observed values	Placebo (n = 7)	0.012 (0.009–0.016)	0.020 (0.012–0.031)	0.015 (0.008–0.029)	0.015 (0.009–0.023)
	AT-1001 (n = 14)	0.015 (0.011–0.022)	0.016 (0.011–0.022)	0.014 (0.010–0.021)	0.015 (0.011–0.02)[1]
Ratios compared to day 1 by group[1]	Placebo (n = 7)		1.70 (1.03–2.77) p = 0.041	1.33 (0.76–2.35) p = 0.26	1.27 (0.87–1.86) p = 0.17
	AT-1001 (n = 14)		1.02 (0.73–1.44) p = 0.88	0.92 (0.58–1.46) p = 0.71	0.98 (0.62–1.54) p = 0.92
Placebo to AT-1001 summary[2]			1.65 (0.95–2.87) p = 0.074	1.45 (0.71–2.97) p = 0.30	1.30 (0.67–2.54) p = 0.42

[1]p value for a paired t test, based on $\log_{10}$ (lactulose/mannitol ratio) of no within-group change.
[2]p value for a t test of no between-group difference in the hour 0 to later hour ratio.

while weighing the different correlations of each of these with fundamental assessments such as body mass, clinical impression of change and each other. The literature suggests that changes in intestinal permeability will precede symptomatology, which precedes serology and histopathology. It is expected that this index will facilitate bedside assessment of changes in disease state within hours, days, weeks or months after intervention. Prospective validation of the index is currently underway, which should enable the development and registration of therapies for the treatment of CD.

Table 2. Summary of gastrointestinal adverse events

	Subject count (%) by treatment		p value (Fisher's exact test)
	placebo (n = 7)	AT-1001 (n = 14)	
Gastrointestinal disorders*	7 (100%)	6 (43%)	0.018
Celiac disease-related			
Abdominal discomfort	2 (29%)	0 (0%)	0.10
Constipation	1 (14%)	0 (0%)	0.33
Diarrhea*	5 (71%)	2 (14%)	0.017
Flatulence	2 (29%)	2 (14%)	0.57
Vomiting	1 (14%)	3 (21%)	1
Not celiac disease-related			
Eructation	0 (0%)	1 (7%)	1
Gastroesophageal reflux	1 (14%)	1 (7%)	1
Nausea	2 (29%)	4 (29%)	1
Stomach discomfort	0 (0%)	2 (14%)	0.53
Dyspepsia	0 (0%)	3 (21%)	0.52

*$p < 0.05$.

References

1 Bjarnason I, Takeuchi K, Bjarnason A, Adler SN, Teahon K: The G.U.T. of gut. Scand J Gastroenterol 2004;39:807–815.

2 Clayburgh DR, Shen L, Turner JR: A porous defense: the leaky epithelial barrier in intestinal disease. Lab Invest 2004;84:282–291.

3 Arrieta MC, Bistritz L, Meddings JB: Alterations in intestinal permeability. Gut 2006;55:1512–1520.

4 Suenaert P, Bulteel V, Vermeire S, Noman M, Van Assche G, Rutgeerts P: Hyperresponsiveness of the mucosal barrier in Crohn's disease is not tumor necrosis factor-dependent. Inflamm Bowel Dis 2005;11:667–673.

5 Stevenson BR: Understanding tight junction clinical physiology at the molecular level. J Clin Invest 1999;104:3–4.

6 Berglund JJ, Riegler M, Zolotarevsky Y, Wenzl E, Turner JR: Regulation of human jejunal transmucosal resistance and MLC phosphorylation by Na(+)-glucose cotransport. Am J Physiol Gastrointest Liver Physiol 2001;281: G1487–G1493.

7 Sander GR, Cummins AG, Henshall T, Powell BC: Rapid disruption of intestinal barrier function by gliadin involves altered expression of apical junctional proteins. FEBS Lett 2005;579: 4851–4855.

8 Fukudo S: Role of corticotropin-releasing hormone in irritable bowel syndrome and intestinal inflammation. J Gastroenterol 2007;42(suppl 17):48–51.

9 Bruewer M, Luegering A, Kucharzik T, Parkos CA, Madara JL, Hopkins AM, Nusrat A: Proinflammatory cytokines disrupt epithelial barrier function by apoptosis-independent mechanisms. J Immunol 2003;171:6164–6172.

10 Madara JL, Pappenheimer JR: Structural basis for physiological regulation of paracellular pathways in intestinal epithelia. J Membr Biol 1987;100:149–164.

11 Pappenheimer JR, Reiss KZ: Contribution of solvent drag through intercellular junctions to absorption of nutrients by the small intestine of the rat. J Membr Biol 1987;100:123–136.

12 Turner JR: Show me the pathway! Regulation of paracellular permeability by Na(+)-glucose cotransport. Adv Drug Deliv Rev 2000;41:265–281.

13 Turner JR: 'Putting the squeeze' on the tight junction: understanding cytoskeletal regulation. Semin Cell Dev Biol 2000;11:301–308.

14 Sadowski DC, Meddings JB: Luminal nutrients alter tight-junction permeability in the rat jejunum: an in vivo perfusion model. Can J Physiol Pharmacol 1993;71:835–839.

15 Meddings JB, Westergaard H: Intestinal glucose transport using perfused rat jejunum in vivo: model analysis and derivation of corrected kinetic constants. Clin Sci (Lond) 1989;76:403–413.

16 Turner JR, Cohen DE, Mrsny RJ, Madara JL: Noninvasive in vivo analysis of human small intestinal paracellular absorption: regulation by Na+-glucose cotransport. Dig Dis Sci 2000;45:2122–2126.

17 Clayburgh DR, Musch MW, Leitges M, Fu YX, Turner JR: Coordinated epithelial NHE3 inhibition and barrier dysfunction are required for TNF-mediated diarrhea in vivo. J Clin Invest 2006;116: 2682–2694.

18 Lee A, White N, van der Walle CF: The intestinal zonula occludens toxin (ZOT) receptor recognises non-native ZOT conformers and localises to the intercellular contacts. FEBS Lett 2003; 555:638–642.
19 Fasano A: Regulation of intercellular tight junctions by zonula occludens toxin and its eukaryotic analogue zonulin. Ann NY Acad Sci 2000;915: 214–222.
20 Salama NN, Eddington ND, Fasano A: Tight junction modulation and its relationship to drug delivery. Adv Drug Deliv Rev 2006;58:15–28.
21 Antalis TM, Shea-Donohue T, Vogel SN, Sears C, Fasano A: Mechanisms of disease: protease functions in intestinal mucosal pathobiology. Nat Clin Pract Gastroenterol Hepatol 2007;4:393–402.
22 Drago S, El Asmar R, Di Pierro M, Grazia Clemente M, Tripathi A, Sapone A, Thakar M, Iacono G, Carroccio A, D'Agate C, Not T, Zampini L, Catassi C, Fasano A: Gliadin, zonulin and gut permeability: effects on celiac and non-celiac intestinal mucosa and intestinal cell lines. Scand J Gastroenterol 2006;41:408–419.
23 Marinaro M, Di Tommaso A, Uzzau S, Fasano A, De Magistris MT: Zonula occludens toxin is a powerful mucosal adjuvant for intranasally delivered antigens. Infect Immun 1999;67: 1287–1291.
24 Marinaro M, Fasano A, DeMagistis M: Zonula occludens toxin acts as an adjuvant through different mucosal routes and induces protective immune responses. Infect Immun 2003;71: 1897–1902.
25 Fasano A, Not T, Wang W, Uzzau S, Berti I, Tommasini A, Goldblum SE: Zonulin, a newly discovered modulator of intestinal permeability, and its expression in coeliac disease. Lancet 2000; 355:1518–1519.
26 Wang W, Uzzau S, Goldblum SE, Fasano A: Human zonulin, a potential modulator of intestinal tight junctions. J Cell Sci 2000;113:4435–4440.
27 Fasano A, Uzzau S, Fiore C, Margaretten K: The enterotoxic effect on zonula occludens toxin on rabbit small intestine involves the paracellular pathway. Gastroenterology 1997;112:839–846.
28 Clemente M, De Virgiliis S, Kang JS, Macatagney R, Musu MP, Di Pierro MR, Drago S, Congia M, Fasano A: Early effect of gliadin on enterocyte intracellular signaling in intestinal barrier function. Gut 2003;52:218–223.
29 Turner JR, Rill BK, Carlson SL, Carnes D, Kerner R, Mrsny RJ, Madara JL: Physiological regulation of epithelial tight junctions is associated with myosin light-chain phosphorylation. Am J Physiol 1997;273:C1378–C1385.
30 Atisook K, Carlson S, Madara JL: Effects of phlorizin and sodium on glucose-elicited alterations of cell junctions in intestinal epithelia. Am J Physiol 1990;258:C77–C85.
31 Wei J, Hemmings GP: Gene, gut and schizophrenia: the meeting point for the gene-environment interaction in developing schizophrenia. Med Hypotheses 2005;64:547–552.
32 Bosi E, Molteni L, Radaelli MG, Folini L, Fermo I, Bazzigaluppi E, Piemonti L, Pastore MR, Paroni R: Increased intestinal permeability precedes clinical onset of type 1 diabetes. Diabetologia 2006;49:2824–2827.
33 Cordain L, Toohey L, Smith MJ, Hickey MS: Modulation of immune function by dietary lectins in rheumatoid arthritis. Br J Nutr 2000;83:207–217.
34 Bruewer M, Samarin S, Nusrat A: Inflammatory bowel disease and the apical junctional complex. Ann NY Acad Sci 2006;1072:242–252.
35 Dunlop SP, Hebden J, Campbell E, Naesdal J, Olbe L, Perkins AC, Spiller RC: Abnormal intestinal permeability in subgroups of diarrhea-predominant irritable bowel syndromes. Am J Gastroenterol 2006;101:1288–1294.
36 Porras M, Martín MT, Yang PC, Jury J, Perdue MH, Vergara P: Correlation between cyclical epithelial barrier dysfunction and bacterial translocation in the relapses of intestinal inflammation. Inflamm Bowel Dis 2006;12:843–852.
37 D'Inca R, Annese V, di Leo V, Latiano A, Quaino V, Abazia C, Vettorato MG, Sturniolo GC: Increased intestinal permeability and NOD2 variants in familial and sporadic Crohn's disease. Aliment Pharmacol Ther 2006;23: 1455–1461.
38 Barbara G: Mucosal barrier defects in irritable bowel syndrome. Who left the door open? Am J Gastroenterol 2006; 101:1295–1298.
39 Monsuur AJ, de Bakker PI, Alizadeh BZ, Zhernakova A, Bevova MR, Strengman E, Franke L, van't Slot R, van Belzen MJ, Lavrijsen IC, Diosdado B, Daly MJ, Mulder CJ, Mearin ML, Meijer JW, Meijer GA, van Oort E, Wapenaar MC, Koeleman BP, Wijmenga C: Myosin IXB variant increases the risk of celiac disease and points toward a primary intestinal barrier defect. Nat Genet 2005;37: 1341–1344.
40 Pizzuti D, Bortolami M, Mazzon E, Buda A, Guariso G, D'Odorico A, Chiarelli S, D'Incà R, De Lazzari F, Martines D: Transcriptional downregulation of tight junction protein ZO-1 in active coeliac disease is reversed after a gluten-free diet. Dig Liver Dis 2004;36:337–341.
41 Di Cagno R, De Angelis M, Auricchio S, Greco L, Clarke C, De Vincenzi M, Giovannini C, D'Archivio M, Landolfo F, Parrilli G, Minervini F, Arendt E, Gobbetti M: Sourdough bread made from wheat and non-toxic flours and started with selected lactobacilli is tolerated in celiac sprue patients. Appl Environ Microbiol 2004;70:1088–1096.
42 Smecuol E, Bai JC, Vazquez H, Kogan Z, Cabanne A, Niveloni S, Pedreira S, Boerr L, Mauriño E, Meddings JB: Gastrointestinal permeability in celiac disease. Gastroenterology 1997;112:1129–1136.
43 Hollander D: Crohn's disease – a permeability disorder of the tight junction? Gut 1988;29:1621–1624.
44 Ukabam SO, Clamp JR, Cooper BT: Abnormal small intestinal permeability to sugars in patients with Crohn's disease of the terminal ileum and colon. Digestion 1983;27:70–74.
45 Wyatt J, Vogelsang H, Hübl W, Waldhöer T, Lochs H: Intestinal permeability and the prediction of relapse in Crohn's disease. Lancet 1993;341:1437–1439.
46 D'Inca R, Di Leo V, Corrao G, Martines D, D'Odorico A, Mestriner C, Venturi C, Longo G, Sturniolo GC: Intestinal permeability test as a predictor of clinical course in Crohn's disease. Am J Gastroenterol 1999;94:2956–2960.
47 Wang F, Graham WV, Wang Y, Witkowski ED, Schwarz BT, Turner JR: Interferon-gamma and tumor necrosis factor-alpha synergize to induce intestinal epithelial barrier dysfunction by up-regulating myosin light chain kinase expression. Am J Pathol 2005;166:409–419.

48 Zolotarevsky Y, Hecht G, Koutsouris A, Gonzalez DE, Quan C, Tom J, Mrsny RJ, Turner JR: A membrane-permeant peptide that inhibits MLC kinase restores barrier function in in vitro models of intestinal disease. Gastroenterology 2002;123:163–172.
49 Ma TY, Boivin MA, Ye D, Pedram A, Said HM: Mechanism of TNF-{alpha} modulation of Caco-2 intestinal epithelial tight junction barrier: role of myosin light-chain kinase protein expression. Am J Physiol Gastrointest Liver Physiol 2005;288:G422–G430.
50 Graham WV, Wang F, Clayburgh DR, Cheng JX, Yoon B, Wang Y, Lin A, Turner JR: Tumor necrosis factor-induced long myosin light chain kinase transcription is regulated by differentiation-dependent signaling events. Characterization of the human long myosin light chain kinase promoter. J Biol Chem 2006;281:26205–26215.
51 Ciclitira PJ, Johnson MW, Dewar DH, Ellis HJ: The pathogenesis of coeliac disease. Mol Aspects Med 2005;26: 421–458.
52 Maiuri L, Ciacci C, Ricciardelli I, Vacca L, Raia V, Auricchio S, Picard J, Osman M, Quaratino S, Londei M: Association between innate response to gliadin and activation of pathogenic T cells in coeliac disease. Lancet 2003;362:30–37.
53 Gianfrani C, Auricchio S, Troncone R: Adaptive and innate immune responses in celiac disease. Immunol Lett 2005; 99:141–145.
54 Thomas KE, Sapone A, Fasano A, Vogel SN: Gliadin stimulation of murine macrophage inflammatory gene expression and intestinal permeability are MyD88-dependent: role of the innate immune response in celiac disease. J Immunol 2006;176:2512–2521.
55 Ventura A, Magazzu G, Greco L: Duration of exposure to gluten and risk for autoimmune disorders in patients with celiac disease. SIGEP Study Group for auto immune disorders in celiac disease. Gastroenterology 1999;117:297–303.
56 Schuppan D: Current concepts of celiac disease pathogenesis. Gastroenterology 2000;119:234–242.
57 National Institutes of Health Consensus Development on Celiac Disease. Consensus Development Conference, Bethesda, 2004.
58 Feld JJ, Meddings J, Heathcote EJ: Abnormal intestinal permeability in primary biliary cirrhosis. Dig Dis Sci 2006;51:1607–1613.
59 Funda DP, Kaas A, Bock T, Tlaskalová-Hogenová H, Buschard K: Gluten-free diet prevents diabetes in NOD mice. Diabetes Metab Res Rev 1999;15:323–327.
60 Meddings JB, Jarand J, Urbanski SJ, Hardin J, Gall DG: Increased gastrointestinal permeability is an early lesion in the spontaneously diabetic BB rat. Am J Physiol 1999;276:G951–G957.
61 Watts T, Berti I, Sapone A, Gerarduzzi T, Not T, Zielke R, Fasano A: Role of the intestinal tight junction modulator zonulin in the pathogenesis of type I diabetes in BB diabetic-prone rats. Proc Natl Acad Sci USA 2005;102:2916–2921.
62 Norris JM, Barriga K, Klingensmith G, Hoffman M, Eisenbarth GS, Erlich HA, Rewers M: Timing of initial cereal exposure in infancy and risk of islet autoimmunity. JAMA 2003;290:1713–1720.
63 Clayburgh DR, Barrett TA, Tang Y, Meddings JB, Van Eldik LJ, Watterson DM, Clarke LL, Mrsny RJ, Turner JR: Epithelial myosin light chain kinase-dependent barrier dysfunction mediates T cell activation-induced diarrhea in vivo. J Clin Invest 2005;115:2702–2715.
64 Blair SA, Kane SV, Clayburgh DR, Turner JR: Epithelial myosin light chain kinase expression and activity are upregulated in inflammatory bowel disease. Lab Invest 2006;86:191–201.
65 Karyekar CS, Fasano A, Raje S, Lu R, Dowling TC, Eddington ND: Zonula occludens toxin increases the permeability of molecular weight markers and chemotherapeutic agents across the bovine brain microvessel endothelial cells. J Pharm Sci 2003;92:414–423.

Blake M. Paterson, MD
Alba Therapeutics Corporation
800 W. Baltimore St., Baltimore, MD 21201 (USA)
Tel. +1 410 319 0780, Fax +1 410 319 0782, E-Mail bpaterson@albatherapeutics.com

Fasano A, Troncone R, Branski D (eds): Frontiers in Celiac Disease.
Pediatr Adolesc Med. Basel, Karger, 2008, vol 12, pp 172–180

Development of a Vaccine for Celiac Disease

R.P. Anderson

Autoimmunity and Transplantation Division, Walter and Eliza Hall Institute of Medical Research, Parkville, Victoria, Australia

Abstract

Celiac disease is the result of an immune response to gluten. Gluten exclusion removes the antigen that stimulates CD4 T-cell-mediated tissue damage in the gut, but does not remove the immune response. In fact, gluten exclusion may heighten the immune response stimulated by gluten since regulatory T cells are typically not maintained unless antigen exposure continues. This may explain why gluten exposure triggers more dramatic symptoms following adoption of a gluten-free diet than during chronic gluten exposure associated with untreated celiac disease. Peptide-based therapeutic vaccines aim to strengthen the antigen-specific regulatory T-cell response to suppress proinflammatory adaptive and innate immunity in an antigen-specific and nonspecific fashion. Peptide-based therapeutic vaccines require detailed understanding of the peptides derived from pathogenic antigens that stimulate pathogenic CD4 T cells. The present knowledge of gluten peptides recognized by CD4 T cells largely derives from T-cell clones and lines isolated from celiac-disease-affected intestinal tissue. In this chapter, it is argued that T cells mobilized into blood by acute gluten exposure facilitate a more reliable mapping of gluten peptides recognized by relevant CD4 T cells. Understanding not only the specificity, but also the hierarchy (immunodominance) of peptides is critical to the practical design of a peptide-based therapeutic vaccine. The effort is worthwhile and the debate important since peptide-based therapeutic vaccines offer the possibility of a qualitative change in the pathogenic immune response to gluten and for patients to return to a virtually normal lifestyle.

In principle, any human allergic or autoimmune disease for which there is a known causative antigen could be amenable to peptide-based or antigen-specific immunotherapy. Whole-antigen immunotherapy provides long-term remission in allergic diseases such as hay fever [1], while a prototype vaccine using allergen-derived (Fel d 1) peptides recognized by CD4 T cells in cat-sensitive asthma shows efficacy in phase II clinical trials [2]. Provided that suitable immunodominant gluten peptides can be selected, peptide-based therapeutic vaccines may be ideally suited to the treatment of celiac disease. In contrast to other proposed nondietary therapies [3], peptide-based therapeutic vaccines would specifically modify the pathogenic T-cell response rather than reduce the amount of gluten peptide presented to the T cell or compromising other aspects of the immune system. This overview addresses the development of a peptide-based therapeutic vaccine for HLA-DQ2 (*HLA-DQA1*05* and *-DQB1*02)*-associated celiac disease. HLA-DQ8-associated celiac disease will not be discussed.

Peptide-based therapeutic vaccines utilize immunodominant peptides derived from defined environmental or self-antigens that trigger disease by activating pathogenic T cells, a small fraction of the body's total T-cell population [4]. In common with traditional whole-antigen immunotherapy, peptide-based therapeutic vaccines delivered in multiple small doses over a course of injections or mucosal applications can induce immune tolerance not only to the selected immunodominant epitopes or protein, but also potentially spreading to involve other subdominant pathogenic epitopes [5].

Whole-antigen immunotherapy for allergic diseases carries a small risk of triggering clinically significant anaphylaxis. Anaphylaxis occurs because the administered antigen/allergen is sufficiently large to allow cross-linking of membrane-bound IgE on mast cells [6]. Peptides less than 20 amino acids in length are sufficiently small to avoid IgE cross-linking and promise to be safer than protein-based strategies [6].

In celiac disease, a T-cell- rather than IgE-mediated disease, it is the insolubility of gluten proteins and their requirement of selective deamidation by tissue transglutaminase (tTG) to facilitate T-cell recognition [7] that makes whole-protein immunotherapy unattractive. In celiac disease, peptide-based therapeutic vaccines would be anticipated to minimize the risk of anaphylaxis and allow selection of soluble peptides with immunological properties suitable for a pharmaceutical agent with predictable efficacy and safety.

Peptide-Based Therapeutic Vaccine – Proof of Principle

In contrast to celiac disease, there are no strong HLA associations in allergic diseases such as asthma, and the epitopes recognized by allergen-specific T cells are rather inconsistent between individuals [4]. In cat-sensitive asthma caused by skin dander protein (Fel d 1), rather than use defined CD4 T-cell epitopes, a successful peptide-based therapeutic vaccine has been designed according to the binding affinity of Fel d 1 16-mers for various common HLA-DR molecules [2]. Intradermal escalating doses (0.1, 1, 5, 10, 25, 50 and 100 μg) of peptide cocktail administered every 3–7 days leads to clinical nonresponsiveness and abolishes cutaneous CD4 T-cell-mediated late-phase reactions to Fel d 1 [2, 5]. This protocol using Fel d 1 16-mers does not cause acute anaphylaxis.

Three to six hours after administration, the Fel d 1 peptide-based therapeutic vaccine is occasionally followed by bronchospasm. The delayed reaction is readily controlled and typically occurs after the first administration of peptide or with dose escalation. This delayed reaction is due to activation of effector T cells in the lungs [2, 6, 8]. Such T cells are likely to be 'effector memory' T cells. Upon activation by cognate antigen, effector memory T cells are characterized by cytokine secretion rather than proliferation [9].

In contrast, activation and proliferation of central memory T cells residing in secondary lymphoid organs are dependent upon antigen carried and presented by tissue-derived dendritic cells [9]. Amplification of T-cell responses by antigen-driven proliferation is due to central memory T cells. Following proliferation, relevant T cells exit secondary lymphoid tissue and travel via lymphatics to eventually appear in peripheral blood in the days after antigen encounter. Both effector and central memory T cells are present in blood.

Indeed, peripheral blood T cells are qualitatively altered by Fel d 1 peptide immunotherapy. Regulatory CD4+CD25+ T cells in blood 1 week after Fel d 1 peptide therapy effectively suppress Fel d 1-stimulated proliferation of peripheral blood T cells drawn before therapy, and in vitro Fel d 1-stimulated γ-interferon (IFN-γ) is reduced but interleukin (IL) 10 secretion is increased [5, 10]. Interestingly, regulatory T cells are capable of suppressing established asthma in rats and require ongoing allergen exposure both to suppress disease and for their own maintenance [11]. Consistent with this observation, tolerance induced by peptide and allergen-based immunotherapy is durable for weeks or months, but is not indefinite

[1, 4]. Hence, without some form of maintenance, immune tolerance induced by peptide-based therapeutic vaccines is likely to be reversible and to require ongoing monitoring utilizing a marker of disease remission and/or immune tolerance.

Relevant T-Cell Epitopes in Human HLA-Associated Disease

Celiac disease and many autoimmune diseases are strongly associated with MHC class II molecules, HLA-DR3-DQ2 and/or HLA-DR4-DQ8 [12]. These consistent associations suggest that specific CD4 T-cell epitopes presented by HLA-DR3 and/or -DR4, or HLA-DQ2 and/or -DQ8 are critical to initiation or maintenance of these diseases. However, the identity and hierarchy of epitopes for pathogenic autoreactive CD4 T cells in human autoimmune diseases are poorly defined, handicapping the rational design of peptide-based therapy.

Celiac disease does have a known causative antigen, gluten, and characterization of T-cell epitopes is well advanced. Could a peptide-based therapeutic vaccine be designed for celiac disease?

T Cells and the Immunopathogenesis of Celiac Disease

Celiac disease is unequivocally an immune disease caused by dietary gluten. Almost all individuals with celiac disease possess genes encoding either HLA-DQ2 or HLA-DQ8. Gluten-specific T-cell clones and lines have been successfully isolated from intestinal biopsies and expanded in vitro using gluten combined with various mitogens. Almost all such T-cell clones are HLA-DQ2 or -DQ8 restricted and secrete Th1-associated cytokines dominated by IFN-γ [13, 14]. Their presence supports the contention that gluten-specific CD4+ T cells play a central role in celiac disease.

T-Cell Expansion in vitro: Gold Standard or Contrivance?

Despite gluten-specific CD4+ T cells isolated from disaggregated intestinal tissue proliferating when incubated with growth factors and gluten in vitro, 24-hour incubation of celiac intestinal tissue with gluten stimulates expression of the nuclear proliferation-associated marker Ki-67 in intraepithelial CD8+ γ/δ T cells but not lamina propria CD4+ T cells [15]. Although gluten does not stimulate proliferation, it increases expression of the activation marker CD25 in celiac lamina propria CD4+ T cells [16]. In vivo, ingestion of gluten is followed by crypt hyperplasia, villous atrophy and intraepithelial lymphocytosis in the small intestine within 4–6 h [17], yet ex vivo incubation of celiac intestinal biopsies with gluten does not cause crypt hyperplasia but increases the density of intraepithelial lymphocytes [16]. In other words, there is no compelling evidence that lamina propria gluten-specific CD4 T cells proliferate in intestinal tissue. But in vitro, various protocols utilizing gluten and nonspecific lymphocyte growth factors do drive CD4 T-cell proliferation and allow expansion of polyclonal gluten-specific T-cell lines from which monoclonal T cells can be isolated, further expanded and characterized.

Polyclonal intestinal T-cell lines and clones from celiac donors raised against gliadin or gluten commonly recognize certain epitopes such as DQ2-αI (PFPQPELPY) [18]. Cognizant of the artifacts that may result from in vitro expansion, biological relevance of epitopes characterized using T-cell lines and clones is established by demonstrating that the same epitope is also recognized by T cells from tissue or blood that have not been expanded in vitro. MHC peptide tetramers directly identify epitope-specific T cells. However, the frequency of DQ2-αI-specific CD4 T cells in freshly disaggregated celiac intestinal biopsies is below the level of detection for MHC tetramers, yet the same DQ2-αI MHC tetramer detects T cells from polyclonal lines expanded from the same tissue [19]. The scarcity of gluten-specific T cells in celiac intestinal tissue and their failure to proliferate in situ upon gluten stimulation emphasizes the nonphysiological measures that are required to expand these cells. In the absence of information regarding fresh unmanipulated T cells, immunodominance of epitopes inferred using T-cell lines and clones should be interpreted with caution. Unless efforts are made to select antigen-experienced cells, the relevance of T-cell clones is further compromised by the possibility that naïve gluten-responsive T cells may be activated, expanded and cloned.

Gluten Epitopes of Intestinal T-Cell Lines and Clones

Notwithstanding these reservations, intestinal T-cell clones or lines specific for either of the overlapping α-gliadin epitopes DQ2-αI (PFPQPELPY) or DQ2-αII (PQPELPYPQ) are isolated from half of Dutch children and adults [20] and all Norwegian adults with HLA DQ2-associated celiac disease [18]. The observed inconsistencies between the Dutch and Norwegian studies may be due to differences in methodology. Although immunodominance is less clear-cut in Dutch studies, intestinal T-cell lines raised against gliadin from Norwegian celiac donors respond equally well to deamidated gluten as to the α-gliadin 33-mer [21, 22] that encompasses serial overlapping versions of DQ2-αI, DQ2-αII and a variant of DQ2-αI (PYPQPELPY, referred to as DQ2-αIII) [23]. In addition, the majority of intestinal T-cell lines raised against deamidated wheat gluten also recognize deamidated secalin and hordein peptides homologous to DQ2-αI or DQ2-αII (PFPQPEQPF and PQPEQPFPQ) and T-cell clones specific for DQ2-αI or DQ2-αII also respond to deamidated secalin, hordein and γ-gliadin sequences (e.g. PFPQPQQTF) [23, 24].

Although DQ2-αI and DQ2-αII are the epitopes most commonly recognized by celiac intestinal T-cell lines raised against gluten, the first gluten peptide to be identified as an HLA-DQ2-restricted epitope was α-gliadin p31–47, albeit for a single peripheral blood T-cell clone [25]. At that time, this peptide had recently been shown to cause intestinal damage in vivo [26] but is now implicated as an innate immunostimulatory peptide [27].

The second HLA-DQ2-restricted gluten epitope reported, recognized by intestinal T cells from 3 celiac donors, and the first to be widely replicated was the γ-gliadin peptide PQQSFPQQQ (DQ2-γI) with glutamines at positions 7 and 9 deamidated to glutamate by the action of tTG [28]. Indeed, the majority of T-cell epitopes relevant to celiac disease are deamidated rather than wild-type gluten sequences, deamidation most likely to be due to intestinal mucosal tTG activity [29]. However, proliferative responses to DQ2-γI by gluten-specific intestinal T-cell lines are less frequent and substantially weaker than to DQ2-αI or DQ2-αII [22].

After discovery of DQ2-αI and DQ2-αII published in 2000 by Arentz-Hansen et al. [18], other HLA-DQ2-restricted mostly deamidated wheat gluten epitopes have been reported. DQ2-γII (IQPQQPAQL), DQ2-γIII (QQPQQPYPQ) and DQ2-γVI (QQPFPQQPQ) are generally recognized by fewer than half of celiac intestinal T-cell lines, and rarely do responses match those to the α-gliadin 33-mer encompassing DQ2-αI, DQ2-αII and DQ2-αIII [20, 22, 23]. Intestinal T-cell lines infrequently recognize other γ-gliadin epitopes, DQ2-γIV (SQPQQQFPQ) and DQ2-γVII (PQPQQQFPQ) [22, 23]. HLA-DQ2-restricted T-cell clones and lines also occasionally recognize the low-molecular-weight glutenin epitopes Glt-17 (QQPPFSQQQQQPLPQ) and Glt-156 (PFSQQQQSPF), the α-gliadin Glia-α20 (PFRPQQPYPQPQPQ), and the gluten sequences Glu-21 (QSEQSQQPFQPQ) and Glu-5 [Q(I/L)PQQPQQF] [20].

On the Origins of Intestinal T Cells in Celiac Disease

Crypt hyperplasia occurs within 4 h of gluten challenge in vivo, yet gluten-specific CD4 T cells do not proliferate and crypt hyperplasia does not occur in celiac intestinal tissue when exposed to gluten ex vivo. So how do T cells arrive in the intestinal lamina propria? An attractive explanation supported by recent experimental data could be that IL-21 secreted by activated lamina propria CD4+ T cells is responsible for release of the chemokine macrophage inflammatory protein 3α (MIP-3α) from intestinal epithelium [30]. MIP-3α is a highly selective chemoattractant for peripheral blood memory T cells expressing CCR-6, the receptor for MIP-3α [31]. Interestingly, IL-21 also blocks the antiproliferative effects of regulatory T cells [32]. So is there evidence for gluten-specific T cells in peripheral blood?

Based upon data derived from T-cell clones and lines, it has been accepted wisdom that peripheral blood T cells are not reflective of the intestinal (disease-relevant) gluten-specific T-cell response in celiac disease [7]. Gluten-reactive T-cell clones expanded from intestinal tissue are almost exclusively HLA-DQ2- or -DQ8-restricted and preferentially recognize deamidated gliadin [7, 13]. In contrast, the majority of blood-derived T-cell clones raised against gluten are HLA-DR restricted and show no preference for deamidated gliadin [7, 25, 33].

Beginning in 2000, the assertion that peripheral blood T cells are irrelevant to the intestinal immune response to gluten in celiac disease has been challenged [34]. Six days after HLA-DQ2+ celiac volunteers commence in vivo gluten challenge, HLA-DQ2-restricted CD4+ T cells specific for deamidated gliadin and various gliadin epitopes appear in blood [34]. The frequency of gliadin-specific T cells, expressed as 'spot-forming units per million peripheral blood mononuclear cells' (PBMCs, i.e. SFU/million), is measurable by overnight incubation of PBMCs with gliadin or peptides in single-cell IFN-γ secretion (ELISpot) assays (the overnight ELISpot assay does not involve T-cell proliferation). More recently, blood drawn from American HLA-DQ2+ celiac donors on a gluten-free diet but not challenged with gluten has been used to assess T-cell proliferation stimulated by deamidated gliadin [35]. The highly sensitive carboxyfluorescein succinimidyl ester dye dilution method utilizing fluorescence-activated cell sorting analysis indicates that deamidated gliadin does indeed stimulate proliferation of HLA-DQ2-restricted peripheral blood CD4+ T cells. These gliadin-specific T cells also express the β_7-integrin that is associated with homing to the intestinal lamina propria.

In general, the findings based upon peripheral blood T cells drawn from English and Australian adults with celiac disease after in vivo wheat gluten challenge are consistent with findings based upon intestinal T-cell lines raised against wheat gluten obtained from Norwegian adult donors. The finding of peripheral blood T cells specific for DQ2-αI and DQ2-αII following gluten challenge has now been replicated in adult Norwegian volunteers (see below) using MHC tetramers and by IFN-γ ELISpot assay [36].

In vivo Gluten Challenge and Peripheral Blood T Cells

'Gluten challenge' for T-cell studies involves adult celiac volunteers on a strict gluten-free diet to consume 2 slices of wheat bread for breakfast and lunch (approx. 20 g/day gluten) in addition to their normal gluten-free diet [34]. Various other sources of gluten can be used in the challenge, for example purified oats, rye, barley or any 'safe' edible test compound. Typically, 1 in 5 volunteers experiences nausea and vomiting 2–4 h after the first gluten meal, but these symptoms do not persist even in those that persevere with gluten challenge. Often the highest frequencies of gluten-specific T cells found on day 6 are in those volunteers who experience the most noticeable symptoms during the 3-day challenge. Conversely, celiac volunteers who report no symptoms with gluten challenge often have low-frequency or undetectable gluten-specific T cells in the blood on day 6. On further questioning, at least some of the celiac volunteers asymptomatic on gluten challenge are not strictly compliant with the gluten-free diet, while those with symptoms tend to be scrupulously compliant. Indeed, recruitment for gluten challenge studies may attract volunteers who know they are asymptomatic with gluten exposure. Our practice is to screen volunteers for suboptimal compliance and exclude those with elevated tTG IgA levels.

Time course studies consistently indicate that T cells specific for gliadin peptides and deamidated gliadin are maximal 6 days after commencing gluten challenge whether the challenge is for 3 or 10 days [34, 37]. Hence, blood drawn on day 6 has been exploited to map the consistency and hierarchy of gluten epitopes induced by in vivo gluten exposure. Unlike intestinal T-cell clones and lines, over 1,000 peptides can be screened using a single donor's blood, and epitopes can be characterized within 1 week of a volunteer commencing gluten challenge.

When screened by overnight IFN-γ ELISpot using overlapping 15-mers spanning α-gliadin with or without pretreatment with tTG, T cells present in the blood of HLA-DQ2+ celiac volunteers 6 days after commencing gluten challenge are specific for only one region centerd upon the deamidated 11-mer PFPQPELPYPQ encompassing DQ2-αI and DQ2-αII [34]. For optimal activity in the IFN-γ ELISpot assay using PBMCs, the 11-mer PFPQPELPYPQ is flanked at either end by 3 additional amino acids (p57–73 QE65: QLQPFPQPELPYPQPQS). PBMCs preincubated with anti-HLA-DQ antibody or depleted of T cells expressing CD4 or β_7-integrin but not α^E-integrin abolishes IFN-γ ELISpot responses to deamidated gliadin as well as p57–73 QE65 [37].

Peripheral blood T cells specific for p57–73 QE65 are not detectable by IFN-γ ELISpot before gluten challenge in HLA-DQ2+ celiac donors on a long-term gluten-free diet, or in healthy HLA-DQ2+ donors 6 days after commencing gluten challenge having been gluten free for the previous 4 weeks [34]. In untreated celiac donors before adopting the gluten-free diet, the frequency of spot-forming units stimulated by p57–73 QE65 is typically only twice that to medium alone (13 vs. 7 SFU/million) [37].

The frequency of T cells specific for deamidated gliadin or p57–73 QE65 measured by IFN-γ ELISpot varies widely between celiac donors and is dependent upon adoption of a strict gluten-free diet for at least 2 weeks prior to 3-day gluten challenge. In 50/59 (85%) HLA-DQ2+ celiac donors reportedly on a strict gluten-free diet, IFN-γ ELISpot responses to p57–73 QE65 were between 10 and 1,500 SFU/million. At optimal concentrations, IFN-γ ELISpot responses stimulated by deamidated gliadin and p57–73 QE65 are closely correlated. Typically, p57–73 QE65 spot-forming units per million are half those of deamidated gliadin [37]. Clearly, T cells specific for p57–73 QE65 (DQ2-αI and DQ2-αII) represent a substantial proportion of the IFN-γ-secreting T cells specific for deamidated gliadin induced by in vivo exposure to wheat gluten. Interestingly, deamidated gliadin does stimulate strong IL-10 secretion measurable by ELISpot but p57–73 QE65 does not [37].

In vitro Culture May Alter the Composition and Function of the T-Cell Population of Interest and May Favor the Growth of Certain Subpopulations

The first independent replication study of in vivo gluten challenge appeared in 2007 [36]. Raki et al. [36] demonstrated that a 3-day gluten challenge mobilizes peripheral blood T cells specific for either DQ2-αI or DQ2-αII in all (9/9) HLA-DQ2+ celiac volunteers but not in healthy HLA-

DQ2+ controls on a gluten-free diet. In this study, T cells were detected by MHC tetramers and by IFN-γ ELISpot assay. The frequency of T cells specific for DQ2-αI or DQ2-αII was approximately 3 times higher using MHC tetramers than by IFN-γ ELISpot. The median frequency of peripheral blood CD4 T cells specific for either epitope detected by MHC tetramers is approximately 1:1,000 to 1:5,000 of CD4 T cells (or 1:5,000 to 1:25,000 PBMCs); the minimal detection limit is approximately 1:6,700 CD4 T cells (or 1:33,000 PBMCs), similar to IFN-γ ELISpot (1:50,000 PBMCs). All T cells specific for DQ2-αI or DQ2-αII detected by MHC tetramer express β_7-integrin, and many express markers of memory T-cell function. After sorting by FACS, fewer than 1:100 MHC tetramer-positive T cells proliferated in vitro and seldom do they retain specificity for the gliadin peptide.

These findings contrast with the reported scarcity of DQ2-αI-specific T cells detected by MHC tetramers in lamina propria mononuclear cells [19]. The authors, who have pioneered the cultivation of gluten-specific intestinal T-cell clones and reported that T-cell clones from blood and intestinal tissue do not share key characteristics such as preference for deamidated gliadin or exclusivity of HLA-DQ2 restriction [7, 13, 33], reflected that 'in vitro culture may alter the composition and function of the T cell population of interest and may favor the growth of certain subpopulations'. Hence, it would seem that the mainstay for mapping T-cell epitopes in celiac disease – isolating and expanding T-cell lines and clones based upon proliferation in vitro – is susceptible to substantial experimental artifact.

Peripheral Blood T-Cell Epitope Hierarchy

Peripheral blood T cells induced by in vivo gluten challenge have been used to screen 20-mer peptide libraries that encompass all unique 12-amino-acid sequences in gluten proteins of bread-making wheat *(Triticum aestivum)*, barley, rye and oats found in Genbank [38]. The key findings of this extensive mapping study are: (1) hundreds of structurally related gluten sequences stimulate T cells induced by gluten challenge; (2) amongst these stimulatory sequences, there is substantial redundancy; (3) certain gluten epitopes are consistently immunodominant; (4) the hierarchy of epitopes differs according to the toxic grain ingested; (5) certain epitopes are immunodominant whether wheat, rye or barley is consumed; the immunodominance of other peptides is grain specific, for example p57–73 QE65 is only immunodominant after wheat challenge [39–41].

Utilizing this comprehensive epitope map, cocktails of immunodominant and apparently nonredundant epitopes have been screened to maximize T-cell-stimulatory activity, minimize the number of peptides and optimize peptide stability and solubility. A prototype therapeutic peptide-based vaccine for HLA-DQ2+ celiac disease is under investigation.

Conclusion

Celiac disease is well suited to the possibility of a therapeutic peptide-based vaccine. Proof of principle for peptide immunotherapy has been established in animal as well as human immune diseases. In allergic disease, desensitization immunotherapy is administered as an induction course with dose escalation followed by maintenance injections. In celiac disease the primary obstacle to the development of a therapeutic peptide-based vaccine has been the definition of immunodominant gluten epitopes that are consistently recognized by a large proportion of the T-cell population specific for gluten peptides in vivo. Immunodominance and consistency of T-cell epitopes is readily demonstrable using peripheral blood after in vivo gluten challenge. A therapeutic peptide-based vaccine for celiac disease is in preclinical development and will be assessed in clinical trials.

References

1 Durham SR, Walker SM, Varga EM, Jacobson MR, O'Brien F, Noble W, Till SJ, Hamid QA, Nouri-Aria KT: Long-term clinical efficacy of grass-pollen immunotherapy. N Engl J Med 1999; 341:468–475.

2 Oldfield WL, Larche M, Kay AB: Effect of T-cell peptides derived from Fel d 1 on allergic reactions and cytokine production in patients sensitive to cats: a randomized controlled trial. Lancet 2002; 360:47–53.

3 Sollid LM, Khosla C: Future therapeutic options for celiac disease. Nat Clin Pract Gastroenterol Hepatol 2005;2: 140–147.

4 Larche M, Wraith DC: Peptide-based therapeutic vaccines for allergic and autoimmune diseases. Nat Med 2005; 11:S69–S76.

5 Verhoef A, Alexander C, Kay AB, Larche M: T cell epitope immunotherapy induces a CD4+ T cell population with regulatory activity. PLoS Med 2005;2:e78.

6 Haselden BM, Kay AB, Larche M: Immunoglobulin E-independent major histocompatibility complex-restricted T cell peptide epitope-induced late asthmatic reactions. J Exp Med 1999;189: 1885–1894.

7 Molberg O, McAdam SN, Korner R, Quarsten H, Kristiansen C, Madsen L, Fugger L, Scott H, Noren O, Roepstorff P, Lundin KE, Sjostrom H, Sollid LM: Tissue transglutaminase selectively modifies gliadin peptides that are recognized by gut-derived T cells in celiac disease. Nature Medicine 1998;4: 713–717 (erratum appears in Nat Med 1998;4:974).

8 Ali FR, Oldfield WL, Higashi N, Larche M, Kay AB: Late asthmatic reactions induced by inhalation of allergen-derived T cell peptides. Am J Respir Crit Care Med 2004;169:20–26.

9 Lanzavecchia A, Sallusto F: Understanding the generation and function of memory T cell subsets. Curr Opin Immunol 2005;17:326–332.

10 Alexander C, Ying S, Kay AB, Larche M: Fel d 1-derived T cell peptide therapy induces recruitment of CD4+CD25+; CD4+interferon-gamma+ T helper type 1 cells to sites of allergen-induced late-phase skin reactions in cat-allergic subjects. Clin Exp Allergy 2005;35:52–58.

11 Strickland DH, Stumbles PA, Zosky GR, Subrata LS, Thomas JA, Turner DJ, Sly PD, Holt PG: Reversal of airway hyperresponsiveness by induction of airway mucosal CD4+CD25+ regulatory T cells. J Exp Med 2006;203:2649–2660.

12 Jones EY, Fugger L, Strominger JL, Siebold C: MHC class II proteins and disease: a structural perspective. Nat Rev Immunol 2006;6:271–282.

13 Lundin KE, Scott H, Hansen T, Paulsen G, Halstensen TS, Fausa O, Thorsby E, Sollid LM: Gliadin-specific, HLA-DQ(alpha 1*0501,beta 1*0201) restricted T cells isolated from the small intestinal mucosa of celiac disease patients. J Exp Med 1993;178:187–196.

14 Lundin KE, Scott H, Fausa O, Thorsby E, Sollid LM: T cells from the small intestinal mucosa of a DR4, DQ7/DR4, DQ8 celiac disease patient preferentially recognize gliadin when presented by DQ8. Hum Immunol 1994;41:285–291.

15 Halstensen TS, Brandtzaeg P: Activated T lymphocytes in the celiac lesion: non-proliferative activation (CD25) of CD4+ alpha/beta cells in the lamina propria but proliferation (Ki-67) of alpha/beta and gamma/delta cells in the epithelium. Eur J Immunol 1993;23:505–510.

16 Halstensen TS, Scott H, Fausa O, Brandtzaeg P: Gluten stimulation of celiac mucosa in vitro induces activation (CD25) of lamina propria CD4+ T cells and macrophages but no crypt-cell hyperplasia. Scand J Immunol 1993; 38:581–590.

17 Freedman AR, Macartney JC, Nelufer JM, Ciclitira PJ: Timing of infiltration of T lymphocytes induced by gluten into the small intestine in celiac disease. J Clin Pathol 1987;40:741–745.

18 Arentz-Hansen H, Korner R, Molberg O, Quarsten H, Vader W, Kooy YM, Lundin KE, Koning F, Roepstorff P, Sollid LM, McAdam SN: The intestinal T cell response to alpha-gliadin in adult celiac disease is focused on a single deamidated glutamine targeted by tissue transglutaminase. J Exp Med 2000; 191:603–612.

19 Quarsten H, McAdam SN, Jensen T, Arentz-Hansen H, Molberg O, Lundin KE, Sollid LM: Staining of celiac disease-relevant T cells by peptide-DQ2 multimers. J Immunol 2001;167:4861–4868.

20 Vader W, Kooy Y, Van Veelen P, De Ru A, Harris D, Benckhuijsen W, Pena S, Mearin L, Drijfhout JW, Koning F: The gluten response in children with celiac disease is directed toward multiple gliadin and glutenin peptides. Gastroenterology 2002;122:1729–1737.

21 Shan L, Molberg O, Parrot I, Hausch F, Filiz F, Gray GM, Sollid LM, Khosla C: Structural basis for gluten intolerance in celiac sprue. Science 2002;297: 2275–2279.

22 Qiao SW, Bergseng E, Molberg O, Jung G, Fleckenstein B, Sollid LM: Refining the rules of gliadin T cell epitope binding to the disease-associated DQ2 molecule in celiac disease: importance of proline spacing and glutamine deamidation. J Immunol 2005;175:254–261.

23 Arentz-Hansen H, McAdam SN, Molberg O, Fleckenstein B, Lundin KE, Jorgensen TJ, Jung G, Roepstorff P, Sollid LM: Celiac lesion T cells recognize epitopes that cluster in regions of gliadins rich in proline residues. Gastroenterology 2002;123:803–809.

24 Vader LW, Stepniak DT, Bunnik EM, Kooy YM, de Haan W, Drijfhout JW, Van Veelen PA, Koning F: Characterization of cereal toxicity for celiac disease patients based on protein homology in grains. Gastroenterology 2003;125:1105–1113.

25 Gjertsen HA, Lundin KE, Sollid LM, Eriksen JA, Thorsby E: T cells recognize a peptide derived from alpha-gliadin presented by the celiac disease-associated HLA-DQ (alpha 1*0501, beta 1*0201) heterodimer. Hum Immunol 1994;39:243–252.

26 Sturgess R, Day P, Ellis HJ, Lundin KE, Gjertsen HA, Kontakou M, Ciclitira PJ: Wheat peptide challenge in celiac disease. Lancet 1994;343:758–761.

27 Maiuri L, Ciacci C, Ricciardelli I, Vacca L, Raia V, Auricchio S, Picard J, Osman M, Quaratino S, Londei M: Association between innate response to gliadin and activation of pathogenic T cells in celiac disease. Lancet 2003;362:30–37.

28 Sjostrom H, Lundin KE, Molberg O, Korner R, McAdam SN, Anthonsen D, Quarsten H, Noren O, Roepstorff P, Thorsby E, Sollid LM: Identification of a gliadin T-cell epitope in celiac disease: general importance of gliadin deamidation for intestinal T-cell recognition. Scand J Immunol 1998;48:111–115.

29 Molberg O, McAdam S, Lundin KE, Kristiansen C, Arentz-Hansen H, Kett K, Sollid LM: T cells from celiac disease lesions recognize gliadin epitopes deamidated in situ by endogenous tissue transglutaminase. Eur J Immunol 2001;31:1317–1323.

30 Caruso R, Fina D, Peluso I, Stolfi C, Fantini MC, Gioia V, Caprioli F, Del Vecchio Blanco G, Paoluzi OA, Macdonald TT, Pallone F, Monteleone G: A functional role for interleukin-21 in promoting the synthesis of the T-cell chemoattractant, MIP-3alpha, by gut epithelial cells. Gastroenterology 2007;132:166–175.

31 Liao F, Rabin RL, Smith CS, Sharma G, Nutman TB, Farber JM: CC-chemokine receptor 6 is expressed on diverse memory subsets of T cells and determines responsiveness to macrophage inflammatory protein 3 alpha. J Immunol 1999;162:186–194.

32 Peluso I, Fantini MC, Fina D, Caruso R, Boirivant M, MacDonald TT, Pallone F, Monteleone G: IL-21 counteracts the regulatory T cell-mediated suppression of human CD4+ T lymphocytes. J Immunol 2007;178:732–739.

33 Gjertsen HA, Sollid LM, Ek J, Thorsby E, Lundin KE: T cells from the peripheral blood of celiac disease patients recognize gluten antigens when presented by HLA-DR, -DQ, or -DP molecules. Scand J Immunol 1994;39: 567–574.

34 Anderson RP, Degano P, Godkin AJ, Jewell DP, Hill AV: In vivo antigen challenge in celiac disease identifies a single transglutaminase-modified peptide as the dominant A-gliadin T-cell epitope. Nat Med 2000;6:337–342.

35 Ben-Horin S, Green PH, Bank I, Chess L, Goldstein I: Characterizing the circulating, gliadin-specific CD4+ memory T cells in patients with celiac disease: linkage between memory function, gut homing and Th1 polarization. J Leukoc Biol 2006;79:676–685.

36 Raki M, Fallang LE, Brottveit M, Bergseng E, Quarsten H, Lundin KE, Sollid LM: Tetramer visualization of gut-homing gluten-specific T cells in the peripheral blood of celiac disease patients. Proc Natl Acad Sci USA 2007;104:2831–2836.

37 Anderson RP, van Heel DA, Tye-Din JA, Barnardo M, Salio M, Jewell DP, Hill AV: T cells in peripheral blood after gluten challenge in celiac disease. Gut 2005;54:1217–1223.

38 Beissbarth T, Tye-Din JA, Smyth GK, Speed TP, Anderson RP: A systematic approach for comprehensive T-cell epitope discovery using peptide libraries. Bioinformatics 2005;21(suppl 1): i29–37.

39 Tye-Din JA, Beissbarth T, Anderson RP: A comprehensive bioinformatic and functional screen of wheat gluten T-cell epitopes in HLA-DQ2 celiac disease in vivo. Gastroenterology 2005;128:A-2.

40 Tye-Din JA, Beissbarth T, Anderson RP: T-cell epitope hierarchy after rye and barley ingestion in celiac disease. Gastroenterology 2005;128:A-259.

41 Tye-Din JA, Beissbarth T, Anderson RP: A 35mer peptide with T cell stimulatory activity comparable to whole gliadin: a lead compound for peptide immunotherapy in celiac disease? Gastroenterology 2006;130:A-95.

R.P. Anderson, PhD, FRACP
Autoimmunity and Transplantation Division
Walter and Eliza Hall Institute of Medical Research
1G Royal Parade, Parkville, Vic. 3050 (Australia)
Tel. +61 3 9345 2458, Fax +61 3 9347 0852, E-Mail banderson@wehi.edu.au

Fasano A, Troncone R, Branski D (eds): Frontiers in Celiac Disease.
Pediatr Adolesc Med. Basel, Karger, 2008, vol 12, pp 181–187

Regulatory T Cells in the Coeliac Intestinal Mucosa

A New Perspective for Treatment?

Carmen Gianfrani[a,b] · Alessandra Camarca[a,b] · Virginia Salvati[b] · Giuseppe Mazzarella[a,b] · Maria Grazia Roncarolo[c] · Riccardo Troncone[b]

[a]Institute of Food Sciences, CNR Avellino, Avellino, [b]Department of Paediatrics and European Laboratory for the Investigation of Food-Induced Diseases, University Federico II, Naples, and [c]San Raffaele Telethon Institute of Gene Therapy, San Raffaele Scientific Institute Milan, Milan, Italy

Abstract

In the physiological condition, the immune system tolerizes the huge amount of proteins that are daily introduced into the gastro-intestinal tract with the diet, a phenomenon known as oral tolerance. Many and complex immunological mechanisms are involved in the induction of oral tolerance including suppression by regulatory T cells (T_{reg}). In addition, a key role in the gut homoeostasis is sustained by immuno-suppressive cytokines, such as interleukin (IL)-10 and transforming growth factor (TGF) β, released by T_{reg}. Coeliac disease is a common, and almost worldwide spread, intolerance to wheat gluten and related proteins from barley and rye. Coeliac disease is caused by abnormal pro-inflammatory responses to ingested gluten in which gliadin-reactive T cells are one of the main actors in orchestrating the complex adverse immune reactions following gluten ingestion. Our recent studies have revealed that the treatment with IL-10 of small-intestinal mucosa from coeliac disease patients in remission prevents the massive immune activation induced by gluten challenge. Furthermore, we have observed that coeliac intestinal mucosa harbours a subset of T_{reg}, the Tr1, that through the release of both IL-10 and TGF-β inhibit the pathogenic response to in vitro gluten challenge. Herein we discuss these recent studies on T_{reg} in coeliac disease mucosa and envision an IL-10-based therapeutic approach for coeliac disease.

In coeliac disease patients, a diet containing gluten leads to severe lesions of the small intestine that result in severe malabsorption [1]. Several studies have shown that T lymphocytes resident in intestinal mucosa upon encountering gluten peptides release high levels of the pro-inflammatory cytokines γ-interferon (IFN-γ), tumour necrosis factor α and interleukin (IL)-2 [for a review, see 2]. Nevertheless, concomitantly with this pro-inflammatory response, high amounts of the anti-inflammatory cytokines IL-10 and IL-4 are also produced in the untreated intestinal mucosa [3, 4]. This apparent paradoxical milieu of both pro-inflammatory and suppressive cytokines strongly suggests that regulatory mechanisms might operate to counterbalance the gluten-triggered, abnormal immune activation in untreated mucosa [5].

It is well known that IL-10 is required for the establishment and maintenance of intestinal immune homoeostasis [6–10] and that IL-10-deficient mice develop chronic inflammatory colitis [6]. It has been demonstrated that this cytokine suppresses

T-cell-mediated immune responses by inhibiting the expression of costimulatory molecules on antigen-presenting cells, and by inducing long-term unresponsiveness of antigen-specific T cells [11]. Importantly, IL-10 is a key mediator for the in vitro and in vivo differentiation of type 1 regulatory (Tr1) T cells that have a crucial role in controlling intestinal immune responses to dietary proteins and micro-organisms [9, 12]. Collectively, IL-10 and Tr1 cells down-regulate the pro-inflammatory immune responses by decreasing the cytokine release and proliferation of antigen-specific T cells.

This review discusses the potential role of regulatory T cells (T_{reg}) and suppressive cytokines in controlling the gluten-dependent inflammation in coeliac intestinal mucosa.

Regulatory T Cells: Key Players in Modulating Intestinal Inflammatory Responses

Immunological tolerance, a lack of responsiveness towards self- and non-self-antigens, is acquired in both central and peripheral tissues. To date, several T-cell subsets have been described that mediate immune tolerance. CD8+ suppressor cells, Th3, Tr1 and, most recently, the naturally occurring CD4+CD25+ cells have been largely described to suppress activation of effector T cells both in humans and in mice [13]. These T_{reg} share a number of inhibitory mechanisms that involve production of the anti-inflammatory cytokines IL-10 and transforming growth factor (TGF)-β, and cell-cell contact via the ligation of inhibitory receptors such as CTLA4, GITR and Fas [13].

The gut-associated immune system has the capability to discriminate, among the plenty of antigens daily introduced, between harmful agents, against which a vigorous immune response is mandatory, and innocuous antigens, which are tolerized as 'self-antigens' [9]. Several cellular and molecular mechanisms operate to maintain the gut homoeostasis. Among them, integrity of the intestinal epithelial layer, innate immunity and humoral responses contrast the adhesion and colonization of pathogens [14], while T_{reg} control the undesired immune responses towards food antigens and commensal micro-organisms [15]. Several T_{reg} subsets have been described to play a central role in controlling intestinal inflammation. In the eighties, suppressor CD8+ T cells were described to be involved in the induction and maintenance of oral tolerance in mice [16]. Studies in knockout mice have shown that intestinal TCRγδ+ T cells, which preferentially infiltrate the epithelium compartment and have an important role in maintaining its integrity, can transfer tolerance to specific dietary antigens from fed mice into naïve mice [17]. By contrast, very little is known about the immunoregulatory function of TCRγδ+ T cells in the human gut. Among the CD4+ T_{reg}, TGF-β-secreting Th3 cells have been extensively shown to mediate, by bystander suppression, the tolerance to dietary antigens when these are ingested at low doses [18]. CD4+CD45RB^{low} cells were shown to prevent colitis in SCID mice adoptively transferred with inflammatory CD4CD45RB^{high} cells, via the production of IL-10 and TGF-β [19]. Later studies have shown that Tr1, antigen-specific cells producing high levels of IL-10 and TGF-β, are pivotal in controlling intestinal immune responses to dietary proteins [20] and to the enteric flora [21]. Further studies are required to determine whether the Th3, Tr1 and CD4+CD45RB^{low} cells, which control gut inflammation by secreting the IL-10 and/or TGF-β, are 3 different regulatory lineage cells or belong to the same CD4+ T-cell subset.

In recent years, the naturally occurring CD4+CD25+ T_{reg} have been extensively shown to have an important role in controlling the immune response to both self- and non-self-antigens [22]. These cells constitutively express high levels of CD25, the IL-2 receptor and of the forkhead (winged helix) transcription factor P3 (Foxp3) [23], this latter representing their phenotypic hallmark. It was demonstrated that CD4+CD25+ T_{reg}

have a role also in maintaining gut homoeostasis. In mice, proliferation of CD4+CD25– cells in response to entero-antigens was markedly suppressed by CD4+CD25+ cells [24]. Similarly, in human lamina propria CD4+CD25+ cells were found significantly increased in patients with inflammatory bowel disease and suppressed proliferation of peripheral CD4+CD25– effector cells [25]. Interestingly, an increased percentage of circulating CD4+CD25+ cells was reported in children which outgrew milk allergy compared to those with a clinically active allergy [26].

Regulatory T Cells and Regulatory Cytokines in Coeliac Mucosa

It is well documented that coeliac disease represents a wide spectrum due to the several clinical presentations (ranging from overt to silent or potential disease). For many years coeliac disease has been considered prevalently as a childhood disease, since most diagnoses were made immediately after gluten introduction. Nevertheless, diagnoses of coeliac disease in adults, in some cases older than 60 and with apparent absence of previous symptoms, are indeed increasing in the last decade. This suggests 2 possible scenarios: (1) the immune system ignores this important dietary protein, or (2) an immune tolerance to gluten occurs in the gut to some extent. If this latter is the case, it may be of crucial importance to define the mechanisms underlying the gluten tolerance firstly in healthy individuals and in those developing coeliac disease later in life. Why and when these regulatory mechanisms are lost in coeliac disease patients are two important and unsolved questions.

Foxp3+CD4+CD25+ Regulatory T Cells

A recent study investigated the presence of Foxp3+ CD4+CD25+ cells in the coeliac small-intestinal mucosa and their correlation with disease state and gluten stimulation [27]. The expression of Foxp3, CD4 and CD25 was analysed by immunohistochemistry in duodenal biopsies taken from patients with treated coeliac disease, with untreated coeliac disease and from healthy controls. The presence of Foxp3+ T_{reg} was also investigated in treated coeliac disease biopsies upon challenge with gliadin, which represents the in vitro model of coeliac disease [4]. The number of Foxp3+CD4+ cells per square millimetre of lamina propria was found to be significantly higher in untreated coeliac disease mucosa compared to treated coeliac disease and control mucosa. Lamina propria Foxp3+ cells were significantly more frequent in treated coeliac disease biopsies cultured with gliadin than in those cultured with medium alone. Taken together, these results show that in coeliac disease mucosa there is no basic defect of Foxp3+ T_{reg}. Furthermore, the finding that these T_{reg} are more frequent in untreated intestinal mucosa compared to non-inflamed mucosa (either treated or control subjects) strongly supports the hypothesis that an expansion or recruitment of this cell subset in coeliac disease mucosa could act as a self-regulatory mechanism of the immune system to counteract the pro-inflammatory immune response induced by gluten ingestion.

Interleukin-10

Both IL-10 and IFN-γ are found significantly up-regulated, either as mRNA transcripts or proteins, in duodenal explants from untreated patients compared to treated ones and controls [3–5]. Therefore, the ratio of IL-10/IFN-γ transcripts was found consistently reduced in untreated mucosa compared to treated or control mucosa [4]. Ex vivo ELISPOT assay [4, 5] and intracytoplasmic cytokine staining [Salvati et al., unpubl.] revealed that IL-10 is mainly produced by intestinal CD3+ T cells as a consequence, presumably, of a compensatory feedback mechanism. In order to investigate whether the exogenous addition of IL-10 to coeliac

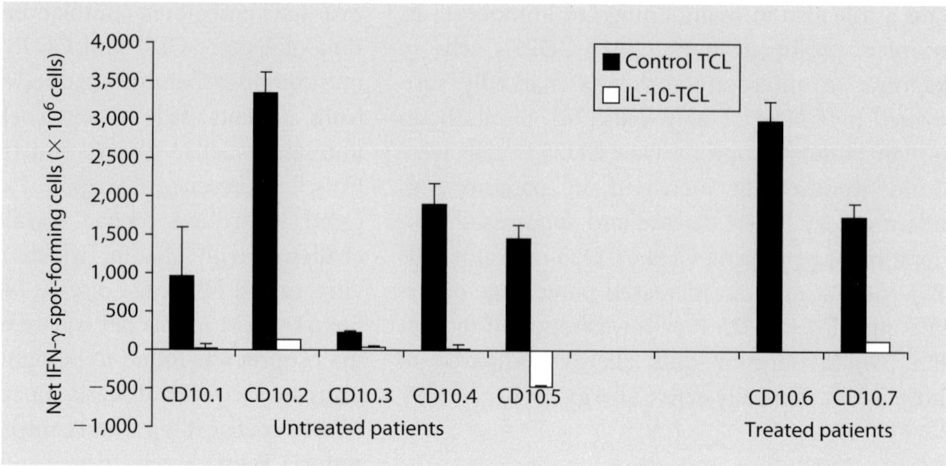

Fig. 1. IL-10 treatment down-regulates the IFN-γ production to gliadin stimulation in short-term T-cell lines from coeliac disease intestinal mucosa. T-cell lines were obtained from jejunal biopsies from treated or untreated coeliac disease patients by stimulating mucosal cells twice with gliadin in the presence or absence of IL-10 (100 U/ml). Gliadin-specific T-cell responses were detected following culture with irradiated autologous peripheral blood mononuclear cells which had been pulsed with medium or gliadin (100 μg/ml), as antigen-presenting cells. All experiments were performed in duplicate. Results are shown as net IFN-γ spot-forming cells per total cells plated (means ± SD). One representative experiment out of 2 performed for each iTCL is illustrated.

disease mucosa could suppress gliadin-induced intestinal T-cell activation and cytokine production, we cultured treated coeliac disease explants with a peptic tryptic digest of gliadin in the presence or absence of recombinant human (rh) IL-10 [4]. Immune activation was evaluated by IFN-γ mRNA and the expression of activation and costimulatory markers by immunohistochemistry. The addition of rhIL-10 markedly reduced the gliadin-induced IFN-γ mRNA expression and the number of CD25+ and B7-1+ cells. A reduced intra-epithelial infiltration of CD3+ cells following gliadin challenge was also observed in biopsies cultured with rhIL-10 [4].

Importantly, IL-10 induced a long-term hyporesponsiveness in gliadin-specific T-cell lines, since T-cell lines generated from treated coeliac disease biopsies (iTCLs) cultured for 24 h in the presence of rhIL-10 and peptic-tryptic-digest-gliadin failed to produce IFN-γ upon subsequent rechallenge with gliadin until 3 weeks later [4].

Long-Term in vitro IL-10-Treatment-Induced Anergy of Gliadin-Specific T Cells

To further investigate the suppressive effect of IL-10 on gliadin-specific T-cells, we generated short-term iTCL from untreated and treated coeliac disease patients by stimulating mucosal cells with gliadin in the absence or presence of IL-10 for 2 weeks. Gliadin-specific IFN-γ-secreting cells were detected in all cell cultures generated in the absence of IL-10 (control TCL; fig. 1). In contrast, iTCLs generated in the presence of IL-10 (IL-10-TCLs) showed a drastic reduction of the number of cells releasing IFN-γ upon gliadin stimulation.

To exclude that the down-regulation of gliadin-specific T-cell activation was due to an overall toxic effect of IL-10, we analysed the capacity of the iTCLs to proliferate in response to polyclonal stimuli. In parallel to the antigen specificity assays, control and IL-10-TCLs were stimulated with immobilized anti-CD3 and anti-CD28 mono-

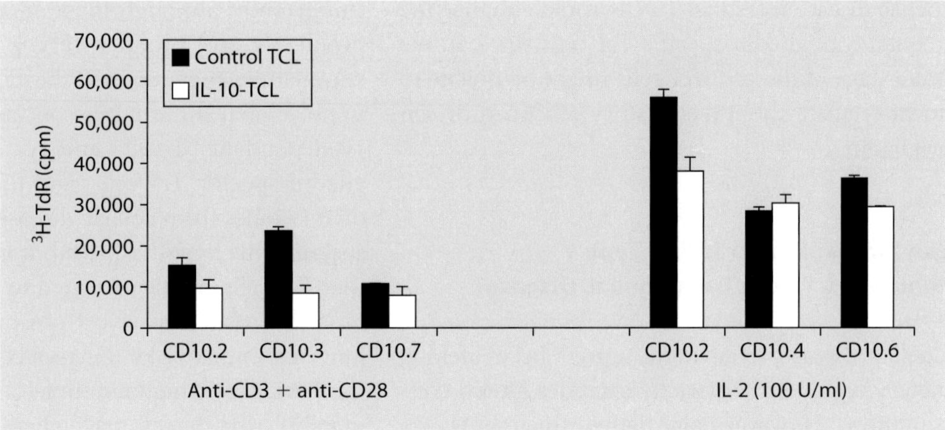

Fig. 2. IL-10 treatment does not affect the proliferative capacity to polyclonal stimuli of short-term T-cell lines from coeliac disease intestinal mucosa. iTCLs were analysed for the capacity to proliferate in response to immobilized anti-CD3 and soluble anti-CD28 monoclonal antibodies or to IL-2 (100 U/ml). All experiments were performed in duplicate. Results are shown as means ± SD of counts per minute. The spontaneous proliferation was less than 500 cpm. Representative experiments out of 2 performed for each iTCL are illustrated.

clonal antibody. As clearly shown in figure 2, IL-10-TCLs proliferated following a TCR polyclonal activation although to a lesser extent than control TCLs. A sustained proliferation to IL-2 was also observed (fig. 2). Collectively, these data indicated that IL-10 treatment is able to induce an anergic state of mucosa-derived, gliadin-reactive T cells.

Gliadin-Specific, Interleukin-10-Secreting Type 1 Regulatory T Cells Are Present in Coeliac Mucosa

Since IL-10 is the differentiation factor of Tr1 cells [12], in the next series of experiments we looked at the presence of these cells in our iTCLs. When the function of IL-10 and TGF-β (the two main Tr1 cytokines) are blocked with specific neutralizing antibodies, an increased immune activation to gliadin stimulation was observed in the great majority of iTCLs generated. Interestingly, this increment of immune response to gliadin was observed in iTCLs from both treated and untreated mucosa, thus suggesting that cellularly mediated, immune regulation might occur in coeliac disease mucosa, aimed to silence or counteract the activation of pathogenic T cells. Subsequently, the cell cloning of gliadin-specific iTCLs revealed that coeliac intestinal mucosa harbour gliadin-reactive Tr1 cells that show a low proliferative rate to gliadin stimuli, but are able to suppress pathogenic T cells through the release of both IL-10 and TGF-β [28]. Collectively, these ex vivo and in vitro results suggested that gliadin-specific Tr1 cells can differentiate in vivo as, most likely, a consequence of the marked IL-10 production in inflamed coeliac disease mucosa. It could also be hypothesized that gliadin-reactive Tr1 cells may have a role in keeping under control the inflammatory reaction in the case of latent coeliac disease or in subjects with a high genetic risk to develop coeliac disease. To dissect this aspect, experiments on the presence of T-cell-mediated regulatory mechanisms in these cohorts of patients are ongoing in our laboratories. Furthermore, it would be of great importance to investigate whether IL-10 in vitro treatment of coeliac disease intestinal T cells could enhance the frequency of gliadin-specific Tr1 cells since, in the acute stage of disease, Tr1 cells might be unable to down-regulate the inflammatory reactions driven by gliadin.

Can Interleukin-10 and/or Type 1 Regulatory T Cells Treat Coeliac Disease?

Coeliac disease is currently cured by a lifelong dietary regimen that strictly excludes gluten consumption. However, alternative treatments are required, as compliance is quite poor especially in young patients [29]. Given the key role of adaptive, gliadin-reactive T cells in coeliac disease lesions, we have investigated the feasibility of using IL-10 to specifically target the ex vivo and in vitro activation and propagation of mucosa-derived, pathogenic T cells. The rationale of this approach resides in several pieces of evidence. Firstly, IL-10 is highly up-regulated in untreated coeliac disease mucosa compared to treated and normal mucosa, as demonstrated in several studies [9, 10]. Then, the finding that the magnitude of IFN-γ released by iTCLs upon gliadin stimulation is enhanced in the presence of antibodies neutralizing IL-10 and/or TGF-β [28] suggests the existence in coeliac disease mucosa of endogenous anti-inflammatory mechanisms aimed to control locally the gliadin-induced inflammation. Furthermore, effector T lymphocytes infiltrating intestinal coeliac disease mucosa and reactive to dietary gliadin can be rendered anergic by in vitro stimulation with IL-10. Importantly, although these anergic cells failed to proliferate and produce IFN-γ following gliadin stimulation, they retained the capacity to respond to polyclonal stimuli. It is conceivable that this IL-10-dependent T-cell anergy is mediated by gliadin-specific Tr1 cells, and the recent isolation of Tr1 clones from coeliac disease mucosa strongly sustains this hypothesis [28]. It is also conceivable that Tr1 cells can be recruited to inflamed mucosa or differentiated in vivo from naïve cells by prolonged stimulation of mucosal cells with gliadin in the presence of high amounts of IL-10. So far, the inability to detect any gliadin-specific T-cell responses (of either inflammatory or regulatory phenotype) in control mucosa could be explained by the fact that these T cells are only generated in coeliac disease patients. Further studies are required to address this important question.

Several ways of IL-10 administration are currently under investigation. The engineering of IL-10-producing cells either of eukaryotic (CD4+ T cells with homing for the gut) [30] or of prokaryotic phenotype [10] is currently being investigated for the treatment of inflammatory bowel disease. Alternatively, lipopolysaccharide capsules with a pronounced resistance to gastric degradation could represent a valid way to deliver IL-10 directly to the inflamed intestine.

In conclusion, the findings that IL-10 could specifically inhibit the intestinal pro-inflammatory T-cell responses to the dietary gliadin indeed encourage the investigation of the possible therapeutic use for coeliac disease of this potent immune-regulatory cytokine.

References

1 Gianfrani C, Troncone R, La Cava A: Autoimmunity and celiac disease. Mini Rev Med Chem, in press.

2 Gianfrani C, Auricchio S, Troncone R: Adaptive and innate immune responses in celiac disease. Immunol Lett 2005;99:141–145.

3 Lahat N, Shapiro S, Karban R, Gerstein R, Kinarty A, Lerner A: Cytokine profile in coeliac disease. Scand J Immunol 1999;49:441–446.

4 Salvati V, Mazzarella G, Gianfrani C, Levings M, Stefanile R, De Giulio B, Iaquinto G, Giardullo N, Auricchio S, Roncarolo MG, Troncone R: Recombinant human IL-10 suppresses gliadin-dependent T-cell activation in ex vivo cultured celiac intestinal mucosa. Gut 2005;54:46–53.

5 Forsberg G, Hernell O, Melgar S, Israelsoon A, Hammarstrom S, Hammarstrom ML: Paradoxical coexpression of proinflammatory and down-regulatory cytokines in intestinal T-cells in childhood celiac disease. Gastroenterology 2002;123:667–678.
6 Khun R, Lohler J, Rennick D, Rajewsky K, Muller W: Interleukin-10 deficient mice develop chronic enterocolitis. Cell 1993;75:263–274.
7 De Winter H, Elewaut D, Turovskaya O, Huflejt M, Shimeld, Hagenbaugh A, Binder S, Takahashi I, Kronenberg M, Cheroutre H: Regulation of mucosal immune responses by recombinant interleukin 10 produced by intestinal epithelial cells in mice. Gastroenterology 2002;122:1829–1841.
8 Braunstein J, Qiao L, Autschbach F, Schurmann G, Meuer S: T-cells of the human intestinal lamina propria are high producers of interleukin-10. Gut 1997;41:215–220.
9 Battaglia M, Gianfrani C, Gregori, S, Roncarolo MG: IL-10-producing T regulatory type 1 cells and oral tolerance. Ann NY Acad Sci 2004;1029:142–153.
10 Steidler L, Hans R, Schotte L, Neirynck S, Obermeier F, Falk W, Fiers W, Remaut E: Treatment of murine colitis by *Lactococcus lactis* secreting interleukin-10. Science 2000;289:1352–1355.
11 Groux H, Bigler M, de Vries J, Roncarolo MG: Interleukin-10 induces a long-term antigen specific anergic state in human CD4+ T-cells. J Exp Med 1996;184:19–29.
12 Roncarolo MG, Bacchetta R, Bordignon C, Narula S, Levings MK: Type 1 T regulatory cells. Immunol Rev 2001;181: 1–12.
13 Roncarolo MG, Levings MK: The role of different subsets of T regulatory cells in controlling autoimmunity. Curr Opin Immunol 2000;12:676–683.
14 Rumbo M, Anderle P, Didierlaurent A, Sierro F, Debard N, Sirard JC, Finke D, Kraehenbuhl JP: How the gut links innate and adaptive immunity. Ann NY Acad Sci 2004;1029:17–21.
15 Izcue A, Coombes JL, Powrie F: Regulatory T-cells suppress systemic and mucosal immune activation to control intestinal inflammation. Immunol Rev 2006;212:256–271.
16 Ke Y, Kapp JA: Oral antigen inhibits priming of CD8+ CTL, CD4+ T-cells, and antibody responses while activating CD8+ suppressor T-cells. J Immunol 1996;156:916–921.
17 Ke Y, Pearce K, Lake JP, Ziegler HK, Kapp JA: Gamma delta T lymphocytes regulate the induction and maintenance of oral tolerance. J Immunol 1997;158:3610–3618.
18 Miller A, Lider O, Roberts AB, Sporn MB, Weiner HL: Suppressor T-cells generated by oral tolerization to myelin basic protein suppress both in vitro and in vivo immune responses by the release of transforming growth factor beta after antigen-specific triggering. Proc Natl Acad Sci USA 1992;89:421–425.
19 Powrie F, Leach MW, Mauze S, Menon S, Caddle LB, Coffman RL: Inhibition of Th1 responses prevents inflammatory bowel disease in SCID mice reconstituted with CD45RBhiCD4+ T-cells. Immunity 1994;1:553–562.
20 Groux H, O'Garra A, Bigler M, de Vries J, Roncarolo MG: A CD4+ T-cell subset inhibits antigen-specific T-cell responses and prevents colitis. Nature 1997;389:737–742.
21 Cong Y, Weaver C, Lazenby A, Elson CO: Bacterial-reactive T regulatory cells inhibit pathogenic immune responses to the enteric flora. J Immunol 2002;169:6112–6119.
22 Levings MK, Allan S, d'Hennezel E, Piccirillo CA: Functional dynamics of naturally occurring regulatory T-cells in health and autoimmunity. Adv Immunol 2006;92:119–155.
23 Hori S, Nomura T, Sakaguchi S: Control of regulatory T-cell development by the transcription factor Foxp3. Science 2003;299:1057–1061.
24 Gad M, Pedersen A, Kristensen N, Claesson H: Demonstration of strong enterobacterial reactivity of CD4+CD25– T-cells from conventional and germ-free mice which is counter-regulated by CD4+CD25+ T-cells. Eur J Immunol 2004;34:695–704.
25 Makita S, Kanai T, Oshima S, Uraushihara K, Totsuka T, Sawada T, Nakamura T, Koganei K, Fukushima T, Watanabe M: CD4+CD25bright T-cells in human intestinal lamina propria as regulatory cells. J Immunol 2004;173: 3119–3130.
26 Karlsson MR, Rugtveit J, Brandtzaeg P: Allergen-responsive CD4+CD25+ regulatory T-cells in children who have outgrown cow's milk allergy. J Exp Med 2004;199:1679–1688.
27 Mazzarella G, Stefanile R, Gianfrani C, Zanzi D, Salvati VM, Iaquinto G, Giardullo N, Auricchio S, Troncone R: Foxp3+ regulatory T cells are increased in the untreated coeliac mucosa and are expanded by gliadin in the in vitro cultured treated mucosa. 12th Int Celiac Dis Symp, New York, November 2006.
28 Gianfrani C, Leving M, Sartirana C, Mazzarella G, Iaquinto G, Giardullo N, Zanzi D, Camarca A, Auricchio S, Troncone R, Roncarolo MG: Gliadin-specific type-1 regulatory T-cells from intestinal mucosa of treated celiac patients inhibit pathogenic T-cells. J Immunol 2006;177:4178–4186.
29 Gianfrani C, Auricchio S, Troncone R: Possibile drug targets for celiac disease. Expert Opin Ther Targets 2006;10:601–611.
30 Van Montfrans C, Hooijberg E, Rodriguez Pena M, De Jong E, Spits H, Velde A, Van Deventer S: Generation of regulatory gut-homing human T lymphocytes using ex vivo interleukin 10 gene transfer. Gastroenterology 2002;123:1877–1888.

Carmen Gianfrani, Dr Biol. Sc.
Institute of Food Sciences, CNR Avellino
Via Roma 52A/C
IT–83100 Avellino (Italy)
Tel. +39 0825 299 411, Fax +39 0825 781 585, E-Mail cgianfrani@isa.cnr.it

Fasano A, Troncone R, Branski D (eds): Frontiers in Celiac Disease.
Pediatr Adolesc Med. Basel, Karger, 2008, vol 12, pp 188–197

Strategies for Prevention of Celiac Disease

C.E. Hogen Esch[a] · J.C. Kiefte-de Jong[b] · E.G.D. Hopman[b] · F. Koning[c] · M.L. Mearin[a, d]

Departments of [a]Pediatric Gastroenterology, [b]Dietetics and Nutrition and [c]Immunohematology and Blood Bank, Leiden University Medical Center, Leiden, and [d]Free University Medical Center Amsterdam, Amsterdam, The Netherlands

Abstract

Approximately 1% of the population is intolerant to the immunogenic food antigen gluten, which results in the chronic illness celiac disease (CD). In genetically predisposed individuals, gluten evokes a T-cell response resulting in disease development. The only treatment of CD is a gluten-free diet (GFD), which is demanding for CD patients, and prevention of the disease would be desirable. Prevention is usually defined as any activity which reduces the burden of mortality or morbidity from disease, and which takes place at the primary, secondary or tertiary level. Adherence to the GFD reduces the complications of CD, and may be considered as a tertiary preventive measurement. Early diagnosis and treatment of CD represents secondary prevention. Primary prevention is based on avoiding disease development. The possibilities for primary prevention of CD are based on the modulation of environmental factors involved in the disease and in the development of tolerance to gluten.

Celiac disease (CD) is a chronic disorder caused by an inflammatory T-cell response to wheat proteins called gluten. CD has a multifactorial etiology, and both genetic and environmental factors contribute to disease development. It is an HLA-associated disorder, and the majority of CD patients express HLA-DQ2 and to a lesser extent HLA-DQ8 [1]. Disease development is a consequence of ingestion of immunogenic fragments in gluten by genetically predisposed subjects [2]. The prevalence of CD is high in the western countries; approximately 1% of the western population is intolerant to gluten [2–4], which means that around 2.5 million Europeans have CD. CD is considered to be an important health problem because it is associated with specific and nonspecific morbidity and long-term complications like chronic anemia, infertility, autoimmune disorders, malignancy and osteoporosis [2, 5]. The standard treatment of CD, the gluten-free diet (GFD), was discovered by the Dutch pediatrician Willem-Karel Dicke (1905–1962) and introduced after the Second World War [6]. The treatment of CD consists of a lifelong diet which may bring difficulties along since avoiding gluten completely is almost impossible, because gluten is widely used in many food products. For many patients, adherence to the diet is difficult to achieve and may decrease their quality of life [7–10]. While adherence to a GFD may have negative nutritional consequences [11, 12], nonadherence may lead to complications such as diarrhea, abdominal pain, anemia, osteoporosis, infertility and cancer [2]. Another difficulty of the GFD is that gluten-free products are in general more expensive than normal food: according to an estimation by the Dutch Celiac Disease Society (www.glutenvrij.nl) the necessary GFD gives extra costs of EUR 1,200–1,300 per patient a year (www.CDEUSSA.com). Hereby, a GFD is a treatment and no cure.

Moreover, CD is frequently unrecognized by physicians, because of its variable clinical presentation and symptoms [13, 14]. Both in Europe and in America, approximately 85% of the CD cases are unrecognized and thus also untreated. Findings from mass screening studies in the USA show that CD is a much greater problem in the USA and South America than previously assumed [15]. This possibly means that CD has worldwide substantial negative economical consequences due to lost working-time and misspent healthcare cost. However, during the last few years new studies have suggested that prevention of CD may be possible [16, 17].

Prevention

The statement 'prevention is better than cure' is desirable for every disease, that is also for the chronic illness CD. Prevention is usually defined as any activity which reduces the burden of mortality or morbidity from disease, and can take place at the primary, secondary or tertiary level [18].

The aim of tertiary prevention is to reduce the negative impact of an already established disease by restoring function and reducing disease-related complications [18]. Since adherence to a GFD might reduce complications, this may be considered as a tertiary preventive measurement [5, 19].

Secondary prevention activities are aimed at early disease detection, thereby increasing opportunities for interventions to prevent progression of the disease and emergence of symptoms [18]. That may only be achieved on a large scale by mass screening in the general population [4]. However, it is not clear if mass screening for CD should be performed, since CD does not comply with all 10 principles for early disease detection elaborated by Wilson and Jungner (table 1) [4, 15, 21, 22]. One important aspect in this respect is that the natural history of CD is not well understood; for example, it is not clear if patients with none or subtle symptoms of CD identified by mass screening have the same health risk and long-term complications as those with clinically diagnosed CD.

Primary prevention avoids the development of a disease. In CD primary prevention would aim to avoid this chronic disease by intervening before the disease processes have been initiated. In the next section we will outline the rationale for primary prevention in CD, which is based on: (1) factors contributing to CD; (2) the possibility to improve tolerance to (food) allergens.

Factors Contributing to Celiac Disease

Gluten

The development of agriculture has led to the widespread use of wheat products in the normal daily diet as well as to an increase in the amount of gluten intake in the general population. As a matter of fact this is a remarkable development, because gluten has been proven to be highly immunogenic. Gluten is derived from wheat, barley and rye, and it consists of a heterogenic set of proteins that contain multiple sequences that can elicit immune responses in the intestine of genetically predisposed individuals [6, 23, 24]. It is unclear, why only a minority of predisposed individuals actually develops CD and that the majority of the population (approx. 99%) is tolerant to these highly immunogenic food antigens. Theoretically, CD could be prevented by no introduction of gluten into the diet of infants genetically predisposed to CD, but this is not an option.

Infections

A seasonal variation in the risk of developing CD has been suggested by Ivarsson et al. [25]. Children who were born during the summer had a higher risk to develop CD than children born in

Table 1. The principles of Wilson and Jungner [20] for early disease detection in CD

	Principles	CD	Comment
(1)	The condition should be an important health problem	Yes	Morbidity and mortality complications
(2)	There should be an accepted treatment for the disease	Yes	GFD
(3)	Facilities for diagnosis and treatment of the disease	Yes	In hospital and at home
(4)	There should be a recognizable latent or early symptomatic stage	Yes	Diarrhea, distension of abdomen, failure to thrive, lassitude etc.
(5)	There should be a suitable test for disease detection	Yes	Serological antibodies
(6)	The test should be acceptable for the population	Yes	Noninvasive; venous puncture
(7)	The natural history of the condition, including development from latent to declared disease should be understood	No	Not clear whether cases found by screening have the same risk for long-term complications as clinically diagnosed cases
(8)	There should be an agreed policy of whom to treat as patient	No	Not clear whether asymptomatic cases should be treated
(9)	The costs of case finding should be economically balanced in relation to possible expenditure on medical care as a whole	Yes	More studies need to be done in different countries
(10)	Case finding should be a continuous process	Yes	Implementation studies needed

the winter (relative risk = 1.4, 95% confidence interval = 1.2–1.7), which may reflect causal environmental exposure(s) with a seasonal pattern. One possible explanation for this observation is that children born in the summer may have been more exposed to intrauterine infections during the winter, and intrauterine rubella virus and enterovirus infections have been reported to increase the risk of type 1 diabetes in the offspring [26]. On the other hand, maternal enterovirus infection during pregnancy is not associated with an increased risk for CD in the offspring [27]. Another reason to implicate seasonality and infection in the etiology of CD is that most children born in the summer are introduced to dietary gluten, and also frequently weaned off the breast, during the winter when there is the highest likelihood of becoming infected.

The finding of rod-shaped bacteria attached to the small-intestinal epithelium of some untreated and treated celiac patients, but not to the epithelium of healthy controls, suggests the notion that bacteria may be involved in the pathogenesis of CD and may trigger the aberrant innate immunity [28, 29]. On the other hand, few studies have demonstrated the role of infections and specifically of gastrointestinal infections in the development of CD. Intestinal infection and inflammation may increase intestinal permeability, a phenomenon which is frequently observed in CD which may increase the absorption of antigenic gluten peptides [30]. More than 20 years ago Kagnoff et al. [31] suggested the possible role of human adenovirus type 12 in the development of CD, but there is no evidence of persistent adenovirus 12 infection in CD patients [32]. Recently, frequent rotavirus infections have been suggested as a plausible risk factor for developing CD, since it has been shown prospectively that there is a correlation between repeated infection with rotavirus and the expression of tissue transglutaminase autoantibodies and the development of CD [33]. Rotavirus is the most common cause of acute gastroenteritis in children worldwide, and most children have already been infected by 3 years of age. Rotavirus infection has also been implicated in the development of another autoimmune disorder strongly associated with CD, diabetes type 1, by triggering islet autoimmunity by molecular mimicry with T-cell epitopes in the islet autoantigens glutamic acid decarboxylase and tyrosine phosphatase IA-2 [34]. The implication of rotavirus infection in the development of CD may have important consequences for the primary prevention of CD, for example by rotavirus vaccination in genetically predisposed children [33, 35]. Therefore, the role of infections in CD and the possible preventive potential of immunization should be explored.

Breastfeeding

Breastfeeding provides the immunological integration between mother and neonate. Breastfeeding has immunological advantages as it protects against infections. Moreover, there is evidence that it protects against cardiovascular disorders, obesity, Crohn's disease, colitis ulcerosa, allergies, diabetes mellitus type I and other (autoimmune) disorders such as CD [36–38]. The risk of these disorders could increase if the duration of breastfeeding is less than 3–6 months [37].

During the lactation period, breast milk has 3 different phases with different milk composition: colostrum, first milk and mature milk [39]. Colostrum, the milk produced during the first 5 days postpartum, contains high amounts of β-carotene, antioxidants, cholesterol, immunoglobulins, lysozymes and lactoferrin. First milk, produced during the 5th to 10th days of lactation, has reduced amounts of immunoglobulins compared to colostrum, but still in high proportions, and it also contains high levels of lactoferrin and lysozymes. The mature breast milk, produced after 10 days of lactation, has a high amount of lipids and smaller amounts of immunoglobulins, lactoferrin, lysozymes and mucins, and it also contains enzymes which stimulate the physiological changes of the mammary glands and the digestive functions and further development of the newborn. Breast milk provides a large amount of granulocytes, macrophages and lymphocytes to the newborn during early lactation and thereby transfers immunological information from the mother to the infant [40]. Breast milk contains all immunoglobulins (IgA, IgE, IgG, IgD and IgM) [41], but for the newborns, the most important ones are IgA and IgG. IgA, mainly secretory IgA, provides mucosal defense, and IgG antibodies support tissue defense. Several studies describe the detection of wheat gliadins and other gluten peptides in breast milk, as well as specific IgA antibodies against gliadin [42]. The low levels of gluten in breast milk could potentially be involved in the induction of oral tolerance to gluten in breastfed infants. The concentration of IgA antigliadin is the highest in colostrum and becomes reduced after a month [43].

Many studies have been published regarding the preventive effect of breastfeeding in CD. An important systematic review and meta-analysis of observational studies on breastfeeding and CD by Akobeng et al. [44] concludes that breastfeeding offers protection against the development of CD. However, it is unclear if breastfeeding protects permanently against the development of CD or whether it only delays the onset of symptoms [44].

The mechanism of protection against CD by breast milk is not well understood. Hanson et al.

cells. The function of innate immunity is to identify and eliminate pathogens that might cause infections by the production of cytokines such as IFN-γ, TGF-β, TNF-α, IL-10 and IL-15 [24]. The dendritic cells have a central role in the process of antigen presentation and serve as a link between the innate and adaptive immune systems [24, 65].

The intestinal immune system has several arms of adaptive defense to avoid systemic and peripheral inflammatory immune responses by activation of regulatory T cells to tolerate innocuous antigens bombarding the mucosal surfaces, such as food proteins and commensal bacteria. This hyporesponsiveness to dietary protein antigens in the intestine is a phenomenon termed 'oral tolerance' [66–68].

Oral tolerance involves several immunoregulatory mechanisms, and experiments in rodents based on feeding of soluble proteins have revealed an overwhelming complexity. Identifiable variables are genetics, age, feeding dose and timing, antigenic structure, epithelial barrier integrity and the degree of concurrent local immune activation, as reflected in the maturation state of mucosal antigen-presenting cells and the microenvironmental cytokine profiles [66–68]. Many studies have investigated the interface mechanisms of innate and adaptive immunity that determine how the body responds to orally administered proteins and how local bacteria modify these [68]. It has been shown that dendritic cells in the intestinal mucosa are the critical antigen-presenting cells that take up dietary proteins and migrate to the draining mesenteric lymph node, where they induce regulatory CD4+ T-cell differentiation [69]. After 'being primed' in these lymph nodes, the regulatory T cells migrate back to the gut mucosa to maintain local homeostasis and in this manner create 'oral tolerance' [68, 70].

Early exposure to antigen by breastfeeding, the frequency and amount of antigen exposure, the genetic profile and the immunological status of the child could also play an important role in the induction of tolerance [65, 71].

The immunopathological origin of CD can be explained by poorly developed intestinal tolerance against gluten and similar dietary proteins in infancy – or tolerance abrogation – leading to disrupted proximal gut homeostasis in genetically susceptible individuals [65]. However, it seems possible to regulate this hypersensitive reaction since in animal models immunomodulatory strategies could tolerize the gliadin-specific T-cell response. Rossi et al. [71] showed in mice that intravenous or intranasal administration of multiple doses of gliadin was able to downregulate the specific immune response. Experiments in the CD model in young AVN rats show that breastfeeding has a protective effect on the development of CD-like lesions in these animals, possibly mediated by epidermal growth factor, one of the components of breastfeeding [72]. Finally, probiotics may prove an alternative means to promote tolerance to gluten in genetically predisposed individuals.

Use of Probiotics

Probiotics, defined as live bacterial preparations with clinically documented health effects in humans, are suggested to play an important role in inducing oral tolerance [63, 73]. Nowadays probiotic products are extremely popular. In Europe more than 1,000 million kg of daily-dose probiotic drinks are sold annually, that is said to account for over 1.2 billion euros [73]. Only a handful of representative microbial strains have been used in clinial trials, namely *Lactobacillus casei* (commercial brand names are Actimel® and Yakult®), *Lactobacillus johnsonii* (brand name LC1®), *Lactobacillus rhamnosus* (e.g Actifit plus®, LGG® or Vifit®), *Lactobacillus plantarum* (ProViva®) and *Bifidobacterium lactis* (various brand names), and, to our knowledge, none has been reported in CD [73]. The mechanisms of probiotics are based on the regulation of microflora composition, which offers the possibility to influence the development of mucosal and systemic immunity as well as the treatment and prevention of disease [73]. Probiotic bacteria may influence the immune system by modulating the innate immune response both to anti-inflammatory (IL-10) and pro-inflammatory (TNF-α, IL-6 and IL-12) directions [73, 74]. In vitro, *L. rhamnosus* seems to modulate dendritic cell functions by inducing hyporesponsiveness of CD4+ T cells by reducing the production of IL-2 and IFN-γ [75] which suggests an anti-inflammatory effect of probiotics. Future research will determine the possible role of probiotics in the treatment and prevention of CD.

Future Prospects

- Prospective nutritional intervention studies in representative populations are necessary to clarify the role of early feeding, gluten introduction and (ongoing) breastfeeding in the prevention of the development of CD.
- At the beginning of 2007, a European multicenter project funded by the EU has been launched to investigate these aspects (PREVENTCD, FP6-Food-036383; www.preventcd.com). The study will involve 1,000 European infants who have an increased risk of 10% to develop CD because they have a first-degree family member with CD. Theoretically 100 of these 1,000 infants would develop CD. The study is a double-blind prospective randomized food intervention study whereby the newborns will be divided into 2 groups; 'a tolerance induction group for gluten' and a 'control' group. At the age of 4 months gluten will be introduced during the period of breastfeeding in order to promote tolerance to gluten. The infants will be followed up to the age of 3 years. If among the intervention group 50% of CD cases are reduced, the intervening strategy will be considered as effective prevention.
- Long-term prospective cohort studies in large representative populations of young children, which are performed in Sweden (ETICS study, www.umu.se/phmed/epidemi/celiaki/etics; PREVENTCD, www.preventcd.com), are needed to elucidate the environmental factors implicated in the disease whose modification may represent primary prevention.

References

1 Mearin ML, Biemond I, Pena AS, Polanco I, Vazquez C, Schreuder GT, de Vries RR, van Rood JJ: HLA-DR phenotypes in Spanish coeliac children: their contribution to the understanding of the genetics of the disease. Gut 1983;24:532–537.

2 Green PHR, Jabri B: Coeliac disease. Lancet 2003;362:383–391.

3 Catassi C, Ratsch IM, Fabiani E, Rossini M, Bordicchia F, Candela F, Coppa GV, Giorgi PL: Coeliac disease in the year 2000: exploring the iceberg. Lancet 1994;343:200–203.

4 Mearin ML, Ivarsson A, Dickey W: Coeliac disease: is it time for mass screening? Best Pract Res Clin Gastroenterol 2005;19:441–452.

5 Holmes GK, Prior P, Lane MR, Pope D, Allan RN: Malignancy in coeliac disease – effect of a gluten free diet. Gut 1989;30: 333–338.

6 Dicke WK: Coeliac Disease: Investigation of the Harmful Effects of Certain Types of Cereal on Patients with Celiac Disease (in Dutch); thesis, University of Utrecht, 1950.

7 Lamontagne P, West GE, Galibois I: Quebecers with celiac disease: analysis of dietary problems. Can J Diet Pract Res 2001;62:175–181.

8 Ciacci C, D'Agate C, De Rosa A, Franzese C, Errichiello S, Gasperi V, Pardi A, Quagliata D, Visentini S, Greco L: Self-rated quality of life in celiac disease. Dig Dis Sci 2003;48: 2216–2220.

9 Lee A, Newman J: Celiac diet: its impact on quality of life. J Am Diet Assoc 2003;103:1533–1535.

10 Hallert C, Sandlund O, Broqvist M: Perceptions of health-related quality of life of men and women living with coeliac disease. Scand J Caring Sci 2003;17:301–307.

11 Kemppainen T, Uusitupa M, Janatuinen E, Jarvinen R, Julkunen R, Pikkarainen P: Intakes of nutrients and nutritional status in coeliac patients. Scand J Gastroenterol 1995;30: 575–579.

12 Hopman EGD, le Cessie S, von Blomberg BME, Mearin ML: Nutritional management of the gluten-free diet in young people with celiac disease in the Netherlands. J Pediatr Gastroenterol Nutr 2006;43:102–108.

13 Steens RFR, Csizmadia CGDS, George EK, Ninaber MK, Hira Sing RA, Mearin ML: Better recognition of childhood celiac disease in the Netherlands and its changing clinical picture: a national prospective study 1993–2000. J Pediatr 2005;147:239–242.

14 Mearin ML, Catassi C, Brousse N, Brand R, Collin P, Fabiani E, Schweizer JJ, Abuzakouk M, Szajewska H, Hallert C, Farre Masip C, Holmes GK: Biomed Study Group on Coeliac Disease and Non-Hodgkin Lymphoma: European multicenter study on coeliac disease and non-Hodgkin lymphoma. Eur J Gastroenterol Hepatol 2006;18:187–194.

15 Fasano A: European and North-American populations should be screened for celiac disease. Gut 2003; 52:168–169.

16 Ivarsson A, Hernell O, Stenlund H, Persson LÅ: Breast-feeding protects against celiac disease. Am J Clin Nutr 2002;75:914–921.

17 Ivarsson A: The Swedish epidemic of coeliac disease explored using an epidemiological approach – some lessons to be learnt. Best Pract Res Clin Gastroenterol 2005;19:425–440.

18 van der Maars PJ, Mackenbach JP: Volksgezondheid en gezondheidszorg. Maarsen, Elsevier/Bunge, 1999.

19 Mora S, Weber G, Barera G, Bellini A, Pasolini D, Prinster C, Bianchi C, Chiumello G: Effect of gluten-free diet on bone mineral content in growing patients with coeliac disease. Am J Clin Nutr 1993;57:224–230.

20 Wilson JM, Jungner G: Principles and Practice of Screening for Disease. Geneva, World Health Organisation, 1968.

21 Tommasini A, Not T, Kiren V, Baldas V, Santon D, Trevisiol C, Berti I, Neri E, Gerarduzzi T, Bruno I, Lenhardt A, Zamuner E, Spano A, Crovella S, Martellossi S, Torre G, Sblattero D, Marzari R, Bradbury A, Tamburlini G, Ventura A: Mass screening for coeliac disease using antihuman transglutaminase antibody assay. Arch Dis Child 2004;89:512–515.

22 Shamir R, Hernell O, Leshno M: Cost-effectiveness analysis of screening for celiac disease in the adult population. Med Decis Making 2006;26:282–293.

23 Spaenij-Dekking L, Kooy-Winkelaar Y, van Veelen P, Drijfhout JW, Jonker H, van Soest L, Smulders MJ, Bosch D, Gilissen LJ, Koning F: Natural variation in toxicity of wheat: potential for selection of nontoxic varieties for celiac disease patients. Gastroenterology 2005;129: 797–806.

24 Stepniak D, Koning F: Celiac disease – sandwiched between innate and adaptive immunity. Hum Immunol 2006;67: 460–468.

25 Ivarsson A, Hernell O, Nystrom L, Persson LA: Children born in the summer have increased risk for coeliac disease. J Epidemiol Community Health 2003;57:36–39.

26 Hyoty H, Hiltunen M, Knip M, Laakkonen M, Vahasalo P, Karjalainen J, Koskela P, Roivainen M, Leinikki P, Hovi T, et al: A prospective study of the role of coxsackie B and other enterovirus infections in the pathogenesis of IDDM. Childhood Diabetes in Finland (DiMe) Study Group. Diabetes 1995;44:652–657.

27 Carlsson AK, Lindberg BA, Bredberg AC, Hyoty H, Ivarsson SA: Enterovirus infection during pregnancy is not a risk factor for celiac disease in the offspring. J Pediatr Gastroenterol Nutr 2002;35:649–652.

28 Sollid LM, Gray GM: A role for bacteria in celiac disease? Am J Gastroenterol 2004;99:905–906.

29 Forsberg G, Fahlgren A, Horstedt P, Hammarstrom S, Hernell O, Hammarstrom ML: Presence of bacteria and innate immunity of intestinal epithelium in childhood celiac disease. Am J Gastroenterol 2004;99:894–904.

30 Fasano A: Regulation of intercellular tight junctions by zonula occludens toxin and its eukaryotic analogue zonulin. Ann NY Acad Sci 2000;915: 214–222.

31 Kagnoff MF, Austin RK, Hubert JJ, Bernardin JE, Kasarda DD: Possible role for a human adenovirus in the pathogenesis of celiac disease. J Exp Med 1984;160:1544–1557.

32 Lawler M, Humphries P, O'Farrelly C, Hoey H, Sheils O, Jeffers M, O'Brian DS, Kelleher D: Adenovirus 12 E1A gene detection by polymerase chain reaction in both the normal and coeliac duodenum. Gut 1994;35: 1226–1232.

33 Stene LC, Honeyman MC, Hoffenberg EJ, Haas JE, Sokol RJ, Emery L, Taki I, Norris JM, Erlich HA, Eisenbarth GS, Rewers M: Rotavirus infection frequency and risk of celiac disease autoimmunity in early childhood: a longitudinal study. Am J Gastroenterol 2006;101:2333–2340.

34 Honeyman MC, Coulson BS, Stone NL, Gellert SA, Goldwater PN, Steele CE, Couper JJ, Tait BD, Colman PG, Harrison LC: Association between rotavirus infection and pancreatic islet autoimmunity in children at risk of developing type 1 diabetes. Diabetes 2000;49:1319–1324.

35 Offit PA: The future of rotavirus vaccines. Semin Pediatr Infect Dis 2002; 13:190–195.

36 Hanson LA: Human milk and host defense: immediate and long-term effects. Acta Paediatr 1999;88(suppl): 42–46.

37 Oddy WH: The impact of breast milk on infant and child health. Breastfeed Rev 2002;10:5–18.

38 Brandtzaeg PE: Mucosal immunity: integration between mother and the breast-fed infant. Vaccine 2003;21: 3382–3388.

39 McLaren DS, Burmad D, Belton NR, Williams NF: Textbook of Paediatric Nutrition, ed 3. Edinburgh, Churchill Livingstone, 1991, pp 31–32, 47–53.

40 Hanson LA, Korotkova M, Haversen L, Mattsby-Baltzer I, Hahn-Zoric M, Silfverdal SA, Strandvik B, Telemo E: Breast-feeding, a complex support system for the offspring. Pediatr Int 2002; 44:347–352.

41 Hanson LA, Korotkova M: The role of breastfeeding in prevention of neonatal infection. Semin Neonatol 2002;7: 275–281.

42 Troncone R, Scarcella A, Donatiello A, Cannataro P, Tarabuso A, Auricchio S: Passage of gliadin into human breast milk. Acta Paediatr Scand 1987;76: 453–456.

43 Ozkan T, Ozeke T, Meral A: Gliadin-specific IgA antibodies in breast milk. J Int Med Res 2000;28:234–240.

44 Akobeng AK, Ramanan AV, Buchan I, Heller RF: Effect of breast feeding on risk of coeliac disease: a systematic review and meta-analysis of observational studies. Arch Dis Child 2006;91:39–43.

45 Sollid LM: Breast milk against coeliac disease. Gut 2002;51:767–768.
46 Juto P, Meeuwisse G, Mincheva-Nilsson L: Why has coeliac disease increased in Swedish children? Lancet 1994;343: 1372.
47 Complementary feeding; in WHO (ed): Feeding and Nutrition of Infants and Young Children. WHO Regional Publications, European Series, No 87. Geneva, WHO, 2000.
48 WHO: The Optimal Duration of Exclusive Breastfeeding. Systematic Review. Geneva, WHO, 2001, pp 28–30.
49 Wharton B: Patterns of complementary feeding (weaning) in countries of European Union: topics for research. Pediatrics 2000;106:1273.
50 Weile B, Cavell B, Nivenius K, Krasilnikoff PA: Striking differences in the incidence of childhood celiac disease between Denmark and Sweden: a plausible explanation. J Pediatr Gastroenterol Nutr 1995;21:64–68.
51 Mitt K, Uibo O: Low cereal intake in Estonian infants: the possible explanation for the low frequency of coeliac disease in Estonia. Eur J Clin Nutr 1998;52:85–88.
52 Briefel RR, Reidy K, Karwe V, Devaney B: Feeding infants and toddlers study: improvements needed in meeting infant feeding recommendations. J Am Diet Assoc 2004;104(suppl 1):s31–s37.
53 Hopman EGD, Kiefte-de Jong JC, le Cessie S, Moll HA, Witteman JC, Bleeker SE, Mearin ML: Food questionnaire for assessment of infant gluten consumption. Clin Nutr 2007;26:264–271.
54 Auricchio S, Follo D, de Ritis G, Giunta A, Marzorati D, Prampolini L, Ansaldi N, Levi P, Dall'Olio D, Bossi A, et al: Does breast feeding protect against the development of clinical symptoms of celiac disease in children? J Pediatr Gastroenterol Nutr 1983;2:428–433.
55 Greco L, Auricchio S, Mayer M, Grimaldi M: Case control study on nutritional risk factors in celiac disease. J Pediatr Gastroenterol Nutr 1988;7:395–399.
56 van den Boom SAM, Kimber AC, Morgan JB: Weaning practices in children up to 19 months of age in Madrid. Acta Paediatr 1995;84:854–858.
57 Falth-Magnusson K, Franzen L, Jansson G, Laurin P, Stemhammer L: Infant feeding history shows distinct differences between Swedish celiac and reference children. Pediatr Allergy Immunol 1996;7:1–5.
58 Ascher H, Holm K, Kristiansson B, Mäki M: Influence of infant feeding and gluten intake on coeliac disease. Arch Dis Child 1997;76:113–117.
59 Challacombe DN, Mecrow IK, Elliott K, Clarke FJ, Wheeler EE: Changing infant feeding practices and declining incidence of celiac disease in West Somerset. Arch Dis Child 1997;77:206–209.
60 Peters U, Schneeweiss S, Trautwein EA, Erbersdobler HF: A case-control study of the effect of infant feeding on celiac disease. Ann Nutr Metab 2001;45: 135–142.
61 Norris JM, Barriga K, Hoffenberg EJ: Risk of celiac disease autoimmunity and timing of gluten introduction in the diet of infants at increased risk of disease. JAMA 2005;293:2343–2351.
62 Ziegler AG, Schmid S, Huber D, Hummel M, Bonifacio E: Early infant feeding and risk of developing type 1 diabetes-associated autoantibodies. JAMA 2003;290:1721–1728.
63 Ivarsson A, Persson LA, Nystrom L, Ascher H, Cavell B, Danielsson L, Dannaeus A, Lindberg T, Lindquist B, Stenhammar L, Hernell O: Epidemic of celiac disease in Swedish children. Acta Paediatr 2000;89:65–71.
64 Brandtzaeg PE: Current understanding of gastrointestinal immunoregulation and its relation to food allergy. Ann NY Acad Sci 2002;964:13–45.
65 Brandtzaeg PE: The changing immunological paradigm in coeliac disease. Immunol Lett 2006;105:127–139.
66 Brandtzaeg PE: History of oral tolerance and mucosal immunity. Ann NY Acad Sci 1996;778:1–27.
67 Mowat AM: Anatomical basis of tolerance and immunity to intestinal antigens. Nat Rev immunol 2003;3:331–341.
68 Strobel S, Mowat AM: Oral tolerance and allergic response to food proteins. Curr Opin Allergy Clin Immunol 2006; 6:207–213.
69 Viney JL, Mowat AM, O'Malley JM, Williamson E, Fanger NA: Expanding dendritic cells in vivo enhances the induction of oral tolerance. J Immunol 1998;160:5815–5825.
70 Strobel S: Oral tolerance, systemic immunoregulation and autoimmunity. Ann NY Acad Sci 2002;968:47–58.
71 Rossi M, Maurano F, Caputo N, Auricchio S, Sette A, Capparelli R, Troncone R: Intravenous or intranasal administration of gliadin is able to down-regulate the specific immune response in mice. Scand J Immunol 1999;50:177–182.
72 Stepankova R, Kofronova O, Tuckova L, Kozakova H, Cebra JJ, Tlaskalova-Hogenova H: Experimentally induced gluten enteropathy and protective effect of epidermal growth factor in artificially fed neonatal rats. J Pediatr Gastroenterol Nutr 2003;36:96–104.
73 Saxelin M, Tynkkynen S, Mattila-Sandholm T, de Vos WM: Probiotic and other functional microbes: from markets to mechanisms. Curr Opin Biotechnol 2005;16:204–211.
74 Veckman V, Miettinen M, Pirhonen J, Siren J, Matikainen S: Lactobacilli and streptococci activate NF-kappa and STAT signaling pathways in human macrophages. J Immunol 2000;164: 3733–3740.
75 Braat H, van den Brande J, van Tol E, Hommes D, Peppelenbosch M, van Deventer S: *Lactobacillus rhamnosus* induces peripheral hyporesponsiveness in stimulated CD4+ T cells via modulation of dendritic cell function. Am J Clin Nutr 2004;80:1618–1625.

C.E. Hogen Esch, MD
Department of Pediatric Gastroenterology, Leiden University Medical Center
Postbus 9600
NL–2300 RC Leiden (The Netherlands)
Tel. +31 71 526 2806, Fax +31 71 524 8198, E-Mail c.e.hogen_esch@lumc.nl

Fasano A, Troncone R, Branski D (eds): Frontiers in Celiac Disease.
Pediatr Adolesc Med. Basel, Karger, 2008, vol 12, pp 198–209

Towards Preventing Celiac Disease – An Epidemiological Approach

A. Ivarsson · A. Myléus · S. Wall

Epidemiology and Public Health Sciences, Department of Public Health and Clinical Medicine, Umeå University, Umeå, Sweden

Abstract

Celiac disease has emerged as a world wide public health problem. Based on lessons learnt from epidemiological studies – both descriptive and analytical – it is likely that the disease has a multifactorial etiology. Genetic susceptibility and dietary gluten are necessary but not sufficient for the disease to develop. Thus, environmental and lifestyle factors, also other than gluten exposure, contribute to disease onset. Exposures during the whole lifespan may contribute, including the fetal period, childhood, adolescence and adulthood. Importantly, when identified, some environmental and lifestyle factors might be suitable for primary prevention initiatives. Increasing evidence suggests that fetal exposures contribute to disease risk. Notably, infant feeding practices influence the risk, and a gradual introduction of gluten-containing foods seems most favorable, preferably in parallel with breastfeeding. Reducing infectious episodes might also be favorable. It is urgent to explore any relation between the increased world consumption of wheat and fast foods and the increase in celiac disease frequency, as such a relation would have large implications for both food production and dietary advice. An epidemiological approach to identify further potential risk factors and protective factors in relation to celiac disease is warranted. When such contributing causal factors have been identified, an evaluation with respect to their public health impact is warranted. In this chapter an epidemiological approach built on lessons learnt so far is outlined, and a way towards preventive initiatives is suggested. If future primary preventive initiatives are widely spread, a large public health effect can be expected.

Celiac disease, or permanent gluten-sensitive enteropathy, has emerged as a worldwide public health problem; being fairly common, mostly undiagnosed and thereby also untreated with negative short- and long-term health consequences [1, 2]. Once diagnosed, the recommended gluten-free diet excluding all food containing wheat, rye and barley, improves wellbeing and health in almost all. In daily life, compliance with the treatment is a challenge as gluten-containing foods are widespread.

Previously, celiac disease was considered genetically determined. Once a person with a genetic susceptibility was exposed to dietary gluten, the disease inevitably developed. Thus, it was surprising when, in the mid 1980s, an epidemic of symptomatic celiac disease was reported among Swedish children. Also, it was unexpected that the epidemic was partly explained by changes over time in infant feeding practices [3]. This suggests a multifactorial etiology where genetic susceptibility and exposure to dietary gluten are not sufficient, although necessary, for celiac disease onset. It is likely that throughout life, possibly even during fetal life, an individual's genetic disposition interacts with environmental and lifestyle exposures jointly shaping the immunological responses to

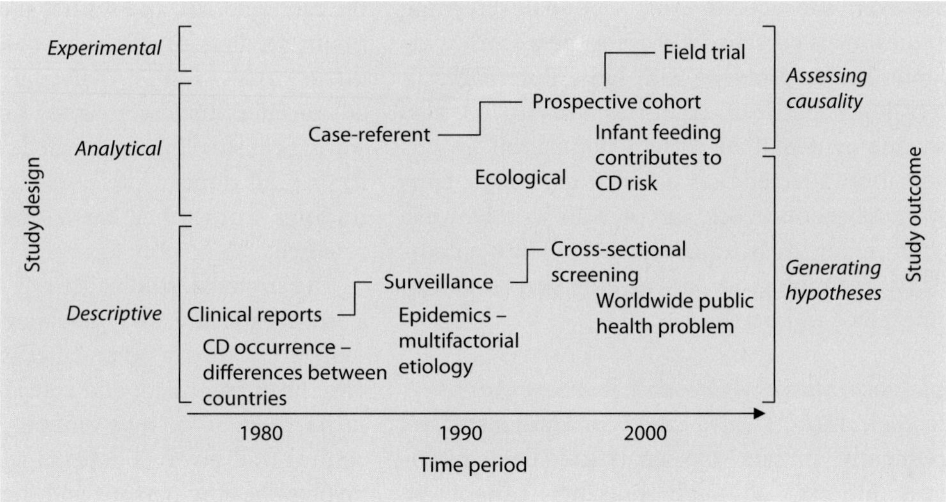

Fig. 1. An epidemiological approach to celiac disease (CD) research.

dietary gluten. The search for such exposures has so far been limited.

When environmental and lifestyle causal factors have been identified, primary prevention interventions will be possible. Such interventions may reduce the likelihood of celiac disease onset also without completely excluding gluten-containing foods. The search for a large variety of contributing environmental and lifestyle exposures, which exhibit their effect during different periods of the lifespan, should therefore be intensified. When contributing causal exposures have been identified, an evaluation with respect to their public health impact is warranted. In this chapter an epidemiological approach built on lessons learnt so far is outlined, and a way towards preventive initiatives is suggested.

Epidemiology Applied to Public Health

Epidemiology has evolved rapidly during recent years, and now encompasses all phenomena related to health in populations [4]. It is commonly defined as, 'The study of the distribution and determinants of health-related states or events in specified populations, and the application of this study to control of health problems' [5]. In the case of celiac disease it would thus imply exploring the role of environmental and lifestyle exposures as potential risk factors beyond genetic susceptibility and gluten exposure, and assessing their suitability for intervention. Both descriptive and analytical study designs and, when feasible, field studies with an experimental design are contributive (fig. 1).

Descriptive Studies – Surveillance and Hypotheses Generation

In the 1980s surveillance studies from England, Scotland and Ireland demonstrated a decreasing incidence rate of celiac disease [6–8]. Later a European child study revealed large differences in celiac disease prevalence between countries from highest in Sweden to lowest in neighboring Denmark [9]. It was debated whether these findings reflected true differences in disease frequency or merely variation in case ascertainment.

However, subsequent cross-sectional screening studies revealed celiac disease to be a worldwide public health problem with large differences in prevalence between countries [10–13]. It also became evident that certain population groups were more affected than others, e.g. females, family members of celiacs, and persons with Downs's syndrome or diabetes mellitus [1]. Thus, a complex epidemiological pattern emerged related to time, place and person.

Analytical Studies – Causality Assessment

Ecological studies, also called correlation studies, frequently initiate the analytical epidemiological process, although causality cannot be proven. In the 1980s such an approach demonstrated that the decline in incidence of celiac disease on the British Isles had been accompanied by changes in infant feeding [6, 8]. In the 1990s celiac disease was more frequently reported for children in Sweden and Italy as compared to Finland, Denmark and Estonia, and infants in the former countries had a larger consumption of wheat gluten [14–16]. Also, a Swedish surveillance revealed an epidemic of celiac disease in children where changes in incidence had a temporal correlation with changes in infant feeding [17].

Epidemiological studies to explore the etiology of celiac disease, however, require exposure information for the individual. This is needed to control for confounders, i.e. exposures that can bias the interpretation of an association between an exposure under study and the disease by being related to both. In cross-sectional studies both exposures and outcome are measured at the same time, and thus the study itself cannot reveal whether the exposure precedes or follows the outcome. A prospective cohort study is preferable as exposure information is collected before the outcome; however, with respect to celiac disease it has only been used for selected high-risk groups [18, 19], which reduces generalizability of the results. Another longitudinal design used is the case-referent, and several such studies suggest infant feeding practices to contribute to celiac disease risk [20]. Analytical studies require advanced statistical analyses and scientific reasoning considering established criteria for causality [4], all done while also taking into account findings from other basic sciences and clinical research.

Experimental studies actively attempt to change a causal exposure, and thereafter evaluate the consequences. Thus, a potential causal exposure must have been identified, and considered safe enough to be used in an intervention. The randomized control trial involves patients while the field trial involves healthy persons and the community trial whole groups of people. A field trial for celiac disease primary prevention is presently being launched with recruitment of pregnant mothers from families with already known celiac disease, and where the infants are randomly allocated to different regimens for exposure to gluten proteins (www.preventcd. com).

A Multifactorial Etiology

Nowadays celiac disease is considered to have a multifactorial etiology, while previously genetic susceptibility and dietary gluten were considered sufficient for the disease to develop. Thus, interactions between genes and lifestyle exposures, also other than dietary gluten, are likely to influence immunological responses, and confer either increased or reduced risk for the disease (fig. 2). The gut immunological system must distinguish between potentially hazardous foreign antigens and food constituents, a process known as oral tolerance [21], and in celiac disease gluten proteins are regarded by the immune system as unsafe. Celiac disease may therefore be viewed as a failure of oral tolerance when it develops close to the introduction of gluten into the diet of infants, or a later loss of oral tolerance to gluten when the disease develops later in life.

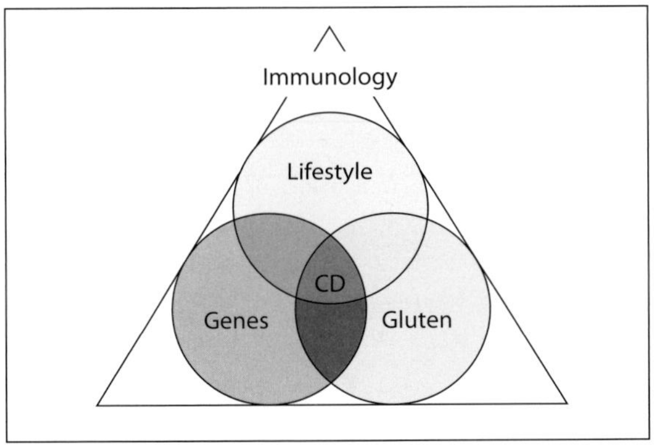

Fig. 2. The multifactorial etiology of celiac disease (CD) in interplay with immunology.

A Life Course Approach

Celiac disease was previously thought to promptly and inevitably develop when a genetically susceptible infant was introduced to dietary gluten, while it was later clearly demonstrated that the disease can develop at any age, including adulthood [22]. Many celiac disease cases are still diagnosed in early childhood, but reports from several countries reveal an increasing median age for diagnosis over time [2]. Adults diagnosed may have symptoms compatible with celiac disease dating back into childhood, and have thus gone unrecognized, while others have developed the disease later in life. Knowledge on which environmental and lifestyle exposures contribute to celiac disease onset during different parts of the lifespan is limited. Also the age distribution for developing the disease is not well described, although variations between countries are expected due to differences in both genetic susceptibility and lifestyle.

It has been increasingly recognized that adult health is largely influenced by events earlier in life, during childhood or sometimes already during fetal life [23]. Such events, which refer both to the physical and psychosocial environment, have been suggested to have a more pronounced effect during certain age periods, so-called 'critical periods'. Norris et al. [18] suggest, for example, that the age at which gluten is introduced affects celiac disease risk. Theoretically such critical periods in life could be the result of a natural development of the immune system over time.

In addition, a cumulative model has been suggested, i.e. that unfavorable exposures accumulate from fetal life through childhood to adulthood and eventually result in health problems [23]. Thus, with respect to celiac disease it can be hypothesized that tolerance to gluten develops during infancy, but that it is later broken down due to one or several exposures, such as an infectious episode, a stressful life situation, a daily high consumption of gluten-containing foods or other environmental and lifestyle factors. So far most of the lifespan after infancy is largely unexplored with respect to exposures contributing to celiac disease risk.

A Model of Causation

A life course approach to modeling the multifactorial etiology of celiac disease is suggested in figure 3. In this model factors are defined according to their level of action, i.e. structural and associated factors, or directly causal exposures which are defined depending on their role in disease development as either necessary or component (i.e. contributing) causes [24]. For celiac disease development both genetic susceptibility and the presence of dietary gluten are necessary causes, i.e. without these disease will not develop. Other environmental and lifestyle exposures are suggested as component causes. The necessary causes when combined with one or several component causes produce a sufficient cause, i.e. development of disease is unavoidable. This implies that celiac disease onset can be avoided by lifelong exclusion of a necessary cause, e.g. dietary gluten. More importantly, the disease might also be avoided, at least in some subjects, through a change of one or several component causes. Focus has mainly been on breastfeeding and the timing and dose when gluten is

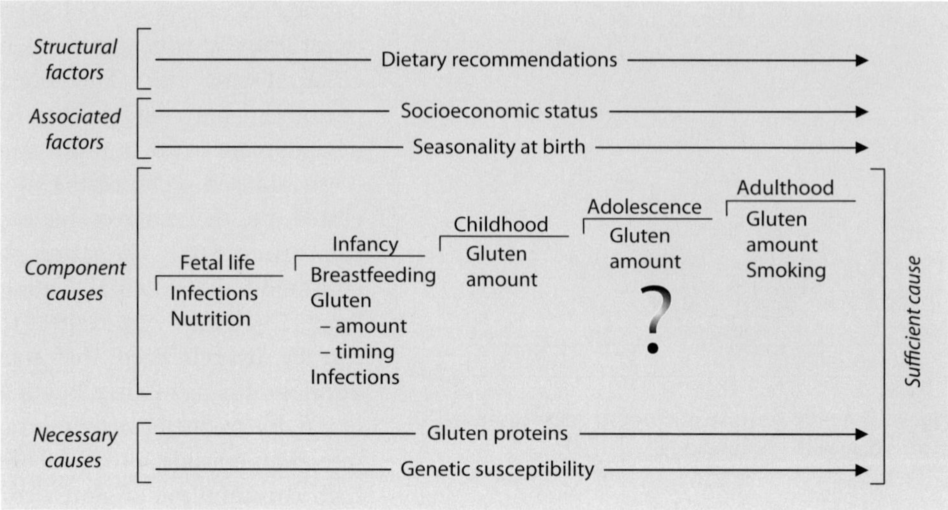

Fig. 3. A life course approach to celiac disease development.

introduced to infants [3]. Structural factors such as dietary recommendations and associated factors, e.g. seasonality in births and socioeconomic conditions [3], are markers for an increased disease risk but are not considered to have a causal effect by themselves.

Environmental and Lifestyle Exposures Affecting Disease Risk

Celiac disease is unique in the sense that the disease process is dependent on exposure to dietary gluten. Some other component causes have been identified, mainly lifestyle-dependent exposures during infancy. However, it is likely that exposures during the whole lifespan, including the fetal period, childhood, adolescence and adulthood, contribute to celiac disease development (fig. 3). This is still, however, a largely unexplored research field.

Fetal Exposures
Fetal exposures are suggested to influence health later in life [23], and may therefore theoretically also influence celiac disease risk. This view is supported by an increased risk being associated with smoking early in pregnancy (OR 1.10, CI 95% 1.01–1.19), being small for gestational age (OR 1.45, 95% CI 1.20–1.75), and neonatal infections (OR 1.52, 95% CI 1.19–1.95); results based on 3,392 celiac disease cases identified through a Hospital Discharge Register and data from the Swedish Birth Register [25]. In a prospective cohort study (ABIS; all babies in southeast Sweden) no association was found with stressful events and parental smoking, based on a cohort of 16,286 newborns but with few cases (n = 50) limiting the value of these findings [26, 27]. Still, it was suggested that mothers who had worked for less than 3 months during pregnancy had offspring with a reduced risk of celiac disease (OR 0.28, 95% CI 0.09–0.92), which remained after adjusting for differences in breastfeeding [28].

Breastfeeding
Evidence is increasing that breastfeeding, besides having short-term beneficial effects, also confers long-term health benefits [29]. Breast milk has

Public Health Impact

Preventive advice should be evidence-based, considering what is practically feasible, and be based on a multidisciplinary evaluation since even obvious advantages might be outweighed by disadvantages. A population strategy is likely to be most effective, i.e. widespread lifestyle changes reducing the average risk in the whole population. The public health impact will be substantial even if the change in risk is small for each individual, provided that the changes are widely spread. A high-risk individual strategy has also been suggested, which would imply focusing on family members of celiacs, or in the future genetic risk assessment at birth to guide lifestyle advice. Recommending that infants be introduced to gluten gradually while being breastfed is of no harm to anyone, and will at the same time benefit the high-risk infants most. Thus, such advice can be given generally without specifically targeting celiac disease families. Changes on a societal level of so-called structural factors, e.g. national recommendations on diet or content of industrially produced foods, are most effective as large groups of people will be influenced, sometimes even without the active choice of the individual. However, as illustrated by the Swedish epidemic, great caution must be taken when giving such general public health advice.

Conclusion

Celiac disease is no longer a rare disease of European children, but a worldwide public health problem. Evidence is accumulating that the etiology is multifactorial. It is likely that throughout life an individual's genes interact with the environment and lifestyle by means of continuous and varying exposures, jointly influencing the complex immunology in humans. These gene–environment interactions determine whether or not, and when in life, celiac disease develops. Importantly, when identified, some environmental and lifestyle factors might be suitable for primary preventive initiatives.

It is urgent to explore any relation between the increased world consumption of wheat and fast foods, and the increase in celiac disease occurrence; as such a relation would have large implications for both food production and dietary advice. However, already today there is reasonable evidence to support a healthy fetal environment, and to suggest infants be introduced to gluten gradually and preferably while still being breastfed. Epidemiology combined with research within other basic and clinical sciences may render possible ways toward preventing celiac disease. If future primary preventive initiatives are widely spread a large public health effect can be expected.

Acknowledgement

This chapter was written within the Centre for Global Health at Umeå University, with support from FAS, the Swedish Council for Working Life and Social Research (2006-1512).

References

1 Green PH, Jabri B: Celiac disease. Annu Rev Med 2006;57:207–221.

2 Rewers M: Epidemiology of celiac disease: what are the prevalence, incidence, and progression of celiac disease? Gastroenterology 2005; 128(suppl 1):S47–S51.

3 Ivarsson A: The Swedish epidemic of coeliac disease explored using an epidemiological approach – some lessons to be learnt. Best Pract Res Clin Gastroenterol 2005;19:425–440.

4 Bonita R, Beaglehole R, Kjellström T: Basic Epidemiology, ed 2. Geneva, World Health Organization, 2006, pp 1–187.

5 Last JM: A Dictionary of Epidemiology, ed 4. Oxford, Oxford University Press; 2001.
6 Dossetor JF, Gibson AA, McNeish AS: Childhood coeliac disease is disappearing. Lancet 1981;1:322–323.
7 Logan RF, Rifkind EA, Busuttil A, Gilmour HM, Ferguson A: Prevalence and 'incidence' of celiac disease in Edinburgh and the Lothian region of Scotland. Gastroenterology 1986;90: 334–342.
8 Gumaa SN, McNicholl B, Egan-Mitchell B, Connolly K, Loftus BG: Coeliac disease in Galway, Ireland 1971–1990. Ir Med J 1997;90:60–61.
9 Greco LMM, Di Donatio F, Visakorpi JK: Epidemiology of coeliac disease in Europe and the Mediterranean area. A summary report on the multicenter study by the European Society of Paediatric Gastroenterology and Nutrition; in Auricchio S, Visakorpi JK (eds): Common Food Intolerances. 1: Epidemiology of Coeliac Disease. Dynamic Nutr Res. Basel, Karger, 1992, vol 2, pp 25–44.
10 Uibo O, Uibo R, Kleimola V, Jogi T, Maki M: Serum IgA anti-gliadin antibodies in an adult population sample. High prevalence without celiac disease. Dig Dis Sci 1993;38: 2034–2037.
11 Catassi C, Ratsch IM, Fabiani E, Rossini M, Bordicchia F, Candela F, Coppa GV, Giorgi PL: Coeliac disease in the year 2000: exploring the iceberg. Lancet 1994;343:200–203.
12 Catassi C, Ratsch IM, Gandolfi L, Pratesi R, Fabiani E, El Asmar R, Frijia M, Bearzi I, Vizzoni L: Why is coeliac disease endemic in the people of the Sahara? Lancet 1999;354: 647–648.
13 Fasano A, Berti I, Gerarduzzi T, Not T, Colletti RB, Drago S, Elitsur Y, Green PH, Guandalini S, Hill ID, Pietzak M, Ventura A, Thorpe M, Kryszak D, Fornaroli F, Wasserman SS, Murray JA, Horvath K: Prevalence of celiac disease in at-risk and not-at-risk groups in the United States: a large multicenter study. Arch Intern Med 2003;163: 286–292.
14 Mäki M, HK, Ascher H, Greco L: Factors affecting clinical presentation of coeliac disease: role of type and amount of gluten-containing cereals in the diet; in Auricchio S, Visakorpi JK (eds): Common Food Intolerances. 1: Epidemiology of Coeliac Disease. Dynamic Nutr Res. Basel, Karger, 1992 vol 2, pp 76–82.
15 Weile B, Cavell B, Nivenius K, Krasilnikoff PA: Striking differences in the incidence of childhood celiac disease between Denmark and Sweden: a plausible explanation. J Pediatr Gastroenterol Nutr 1995;21:64–68.
16 Mitt K, Uibo O: Low cereal intake in Estonian infants: the possible explanation for the low frequency of coeliac disease in Estonia. Eur J Clin Nutr 1998;52:85–88.
17 Ivarsson A, Persson LA, Nystrom L, Ascher H, Cavell B, Danielsson L, Dannaeus A, Lindberg T, Lindquist B, Stenhammar L, Hernell O: Epidemic of coeliac disease in Swedish children. Acta Paediatr 2000;89:165–171.
18 Norris JM, Barriga K, Hoffenberg EJ, Taki I, Miao D, Haas JE, Emery LM, Sokol RJ, Erlich HA, Eisenbarth GS, Rewers M: Risk of celiac disease autoimmunity and timing of gluten introduction in the diet of infants at increased risk of disease. JAMA 2005;293:2343–2351.
19 Ziegler AG, Schmid S, Huber D, Hummel M, Bonifacio E: Early infant feeding and risk of developing type 1 diabetes-associated autoantibodies. JAMA 2003;290:1721–1728.
20 Akobeng AK, Ramanan AV, Buchan I, Heller RF: Effect of breast feeding on risk of coeliac disease: a systematic review and meta-analysis of observational studies. Arch Dis Child 2006;91:39–43.
21 Strobel S, Mowat AM: Oral tolerance and allergic responses to food proteins. Curr Opin Allergy Clin Immunol 2006;6:207–213.
22 Maki M, Holm K: Incidence and prevalence of coeliac disease in Tampere. Coeliac disease is not disappearing. Acta Paediatr Scand 1990;79:980–982.
23 Kuh D, Yoav B-S: A Life Course Approach to Chronic Disease Epidemiology, ed 2. New York, Oxford University Press, 2004.
24 Rothman KJ, Greenland S: Causation and causal inference; in Rothman KJ, Greenland S (eds): Modern Epidemiology, ed 2. Philadelphia, Lippincott-Raven, 1998, pp 7–28.
25 Sandberg-Bennich S, Dahlquist G, Kallen B: Coeliac disease is associated with intrauterine growth and neonatal infections. Acta Paediatr 2002;91: 30–33.
26 Ludvigsson JF, Ludvigsson J: Stressful life events, social support and confidence in the pregnant woman and risk of coeliac disease in the offspring. Scand J Gastroenterol 2003;38: 516–521.
27 Ludvigsson JF, Ludvigsson J: Parental smoking and risk of coeliac disease in offspring. Scand J Gastroenterol 2005;40:336–342.
28 Ludvigsson JF: Socio-economic characteristics in children with coeliac - disease. Acta Paediatr 2005;94: 107–113.
29 Schack-Nielsen L, Michaelsen KF: Breast feeding and future health. Curr Opin Clin Nutr Metab Care 2006;9: 289–296.
30 Troncone R, Scarcella A, Donatiello A, Cannataro P, Tarabuso A, Auricchio S: Passage of gliadin into human breast milk. Acta Paediatr Scand 1987;76: 453–456.
31 Ivarsson A, Hernell O, Stenlund H, Persson LA: Breast-feeding protects against celiac disease. Am J Clin Nutr 2002;75:914–921.
32 Vader W, Stepniak D, Kooy Y, Mearin L, Thompson A, van Rood JJ, Spaenij L, Koning F: The HLA-DQ2 gene dose effect in celiac disease is directly related to the magnitude and breadth of gluten-specific T cell responses. Proc Natl Acad Sci USA 2003;100: 12390–12395.
33 Marsh MN: Gluten, major histocompatibility complex, and the small intestine. A molecular and immunobiologic approach to the spectrum of gluten sensitivity ('celiac sprue'). Gastroenterology 1992;102:330–354.
34 United States Department of Agriculture. Economic Research Service: http:// www.ers.usda.gov/ briefing/wheat/ Accessed May 30, 2007.

35 Food and Agriculture Organization of the United Nations: Cereals and other starch-based staples: are consumption patterns changing?: http://www.fao.org/[CCP:GR-RI/04/4]. Accessed May 30, 2007.
36 Stepniak D, Koning F: Celiac disease – sandwiched between innate and adaptive immunity. Hum Immunol 2006;67:460–468.
37 Forsberg G, Fahlgren A, Horstedt P, Hammarstrom S, Hernell O, Hammarstrom ML: Presence of bacteria and innate immunity of intestinal epithelium in childhood celiac disease. Am J Gastroenterol 2004;99:894–904.
38 Stene LC, Honeyman MC, Hoffenberg EJ, Haas JE, Sokol RJ, Emery L, Taki I, Norris JM, Erlich HA, Eisenbarth GS, Rewers M: Rotavirus infection frequency and risk of celiac disease autoimmunity in early childhood: a longitudinal study. Am J Gastroenterol 2006;101:2333–2340.
39 Austin AS, Logan RF, Thomason K, Holmes GK: Cigarette smoking and adult coeliac disease. Scand J Gastroenterol 2002;37:978–982.
40 Suman S, Williams EJ, Thomas PW, Surgenor SL, Snook JA: Is the risk of adult coeliac disease causally related to cigarette exposure? Eur J Gastroenterol Hepatol 2003;15:995–1000.
41 Carlsson A, Agardh D, Borulf S, Grodzinsky E, Axelsson I, Ivarsson SA: Prevalence of celiac disease: before and after a national change in feeding recommendations. Scand J Gastroenterol 2006;41:553–558.

Anneli Ivarsson, MD, PhD
Epidemiology and Public Health Sciences
Department of Public Health and Clinical Medicine, Umeå University
SE–901 87 Umeå (Sweden)
Tel. +46 90 785 33 44, Fax +46 90 13 89 77, E-Mail Anneli.Ivarsson@epiph.umu.se

Fasano A, Troncone R, Branski D (eds): Frontiers in Celiac Disease.
Pediatr Adolesc Med. Basel, Karger, 2008, vol 12, pp 210–216

Animal Models of Celiac Disease

Eric V. Marietta[a,b] · Joseph A. Murray[c] · Chella S. David[a]

Departments of [a]Immunology, [b]Dermatology and [c]Gastroenterology and Hepatology,
Mayo Clinic College of Medicine, Rochester, Minn., USA

Abstract

Currently no 'true' animal models of celiac disease exist in which all of the elements unique to celiac disease are present. HLA transgenic mice show promise, since these mice have served as good models for other autoimmune diseases, such as diabetes, asthma, arthritis and multiple sclerosis. HLA-DQ8 transgenic mice have been shown to be gluten sensitive and, when placed onto a genetic background that is predisposed to autoimmunity, will develop dermatitis herpetiformis, which is the skin manifestation of celiac disease. Thus, HLA transgenic mice may be valuable in understanding the pathogenesis of celiac disease.

In order to understand the mechanisms involved in the initiation of celiac disease, in vivo (animal) models with significant similarities to human disease need to be generated. The ideal animal model of celiac disease would be one in which both the initiation and disease progression could be studied. With such a model, potential treatments could be administered and their effectiveness determined before clinical trials are conducted with celiac patients [1].

The elements that need to be present in such an animal model are those that are typically associated with celiac disease. These would include: marked villous atrophy, increased numbers of intraepithelial lymphocytes, gluten sensitivity that can be resolved with a gluten-free diet, a tight association with the MHC II and circulating IgA antibodies directed against tissue transglutaminase (tTG). A number of animal models exist today that address some of these elements individually or in certain combinations. These are discussed below and include rabbit, dog and rodent models.

Rabbit Model of Celiac Disease

Rabbits fed a diet enriched in wheat develop high titers of antigliadin IgG antibodies, whereas their 'wild' counterparts raised on a farm do not [2]. Normally rabbits feed on grasses, not grains, and so this study brings up a number of questions about how the intestinal immune system responds to an unusual dietary antigen. Interestingly, the wheat-fed rabbits were not observed to lose weight nor develop any other symptoms related to celiac disease. Most notable though was that the range for the antigliadin IgG in the 18 wheat-fed laboratory rabbits varied greatly and indicated that the intestinal immune response towards an unusual dietary antigen may be under genetic control. Thus, noninbred animals would not serve as good animal models.

Dog Model of Celiac Disease

It has been reported that a certain strain of Irish setter pups fed a standard canine chow that contains gluten develop symptoms similar to that seen in patients with celiac disease [3]. These symptoms included partial villous atrophy and biochemical changes similar to celiac disease [3]. Later studies confirmed that this was a gluten-dependent process and that an abnormal permeability preceded the development of the enteropathy [4, 5]. However, while this canine enteropathy is heritable, there is no association with the canine MHC class II [6].

Mouse Models of Celiac Disease

Nontransgenic Mouse Models of Celiac Disease

The first group to develop a mouse model of celiac disease with intestinal involvement used Balb/c mice [7]. In this model, Balb/c mice were immunized with gliadin in complete Freund's adjuvant, fed a gluten-containing diet, rendered hypersensitive to helminth antigen by infection with the nematode parasite *Nippostrongylus brasiliensis*, and challenged intravenously. This produced an increased intestinal anaphylaxis with an increased crypt cell production rate as compared to controls.

Nonobese diabetic (NOD) mice that are placed on a hydrolyzed-casein-based diet have a reduced incidence of type I diabetes as compared to those placed on a wheat-containing diet [8]. They also have a mild increase in the level of intraepithelial lymphocytes in the small intestine as well as a mild decrease in the height of the villi while on a wheat-based diet [9]. There was also an increase in the level of epithelial expression of MHC II [9]. However, the production of IgA and IgG antibodies specific for tTG was not dependent upon the consumption of gluten [10].

HLA Transgenic Mouse Models of Celiac Disease

The tight association with the MHC II and celiac disease, specifically HLA-DQ2 and HLA-DQ8, is well established and is discussed in the chapter by Zhernakova and Wijmenga [this vol., pp. 32–45]. Therefore an animal model of celiac disease that has such an association with the MHC II would be a significant advance. Thus, transgenic mice that express MHC II alleles directly associated with celiac disease in man (HLA-DQ2 and HLA-DQ8) would be ideal.

Transgenic mice that express human MHC II alleles (HLA-DQ6, -DQ8, -DR2, -DR3 and -DR4) have been generated in our laboratory [11]. Many studies have confirmed that these molecules are expressed at the cell surface of lymphocytes and are recognized by antibodies that specifically bind to these molecules [12–15]. A number of studies have also demonstrated that superantigens are capable of binding to the HLA molecules expressed in transgenic mice [16]. This can lead to cross-linking of MHC II and T-cell receptor and in some cases cause systemic immune activation similar to humans [17, 18]. Interestingly, a number of these superantigens preferentially bind to the HLA molecules and not to the mouse MHC II molecules [16]. Altogether, these studies indicate that the HLA molecules expressed in these transgenic mice are functional.

Of equal importance are the observations that these HLA molecules are capable of presenting peptides to mouse CD4+ T cells [19]. In fact, most of the epitopes that are recognized by T cells derived from the HLA transgenic mice are also recognized by T cells derived from humans that express the same HLA molecules [19–21].

Thus, these HLA transgenic mice can be utilized for understanding the role of HLA class II molecules in the pathogenesis of different diseases. Many groups across the world have utilized

HLA transgenic mice for generating mouse models of autoimmune diseases such as diabetes, arthritis and multiple sclerosis [22, 23]. Collectively, these studies demonstrate the strong role of MHC II molecules in the development of autoimmune diseases. Given the close association between celiac disease and HLA class II genes, HLA class II transgenic mice could serve as an ideal animal model to study the immunological and pathological events that occur in gluten-sensitive enteropathy.

One HLA transgenic mouse that has been well characterized and would be suitable for generating a mouse model of celiac disease is the HLA-DQ8 transgenic mouse, which has been previously used to model polyarthritis [24]. These mice were genetically engineered such that they express a human genomic fragment containing the DQ8 gene [12]. These mice were then mated to mice that lacked endogenous mouse MHC II, resulting in mice in which HLA-DQ8 was the only MHC II molecule that was expressed [25]. Therefore, any presentation of antigen to T cells by MHC II would be via HLA-DQ8.

To determine if the DQ8 transgenic mice could recognize gluten in an MHC-class-II-specific manner, we immunized the transgenic mice with gluten in complete Freund's adjuvant. Spleen cells were isolated and proliferation assays were performed. Using a monoclonal antibody directed against the β-chain of the DQ molecule in inhibition assays, it was determined that these mice can recognize gluten in the context of DQ8 [26]. In addition, the response was dependent upon the specific HLA allele because HLA-DQ6 transgenic mice did not respond as well to gluten as the HLA-DQ8 transgenic mice [26].

With respect to recognition of deamidated gliadin, proliferation assays performed on lymphocytes isolated from the spleen of HLA-DQ8 transgenic mice gave results similar to those using human lymphocytes from celiac patients [26]. ELISA assays performed on sera from gluten-challenged mice also determined that significant levels of gliadin-specific IgG existed within the sera of immunized mice. These results therefore demonstrate that strong DQ8-specific T- and B-cell responses against gliadin are generated in these HLA-DQ8 transgenic mice, lending support for the use of these mice as models for celiac disease.

We have also used these mice to demonstrate that the route of administration affects which epitopes of gliadin are recognized by the DQ8 molecule. Specifically, an oral route of gluten administration led to a strong response against 2 nondeamidated α-gliadin peptides, p13 (amino acids 120–139) and p23 (amino acids 220–239) [27]. As 'native' peptides of α-gliadin, these may have an important role in the initiation of disease.

Surprisingly though, histopathology of the small bowel of these mice revealed a normal bowel architecture with no villous atrophy or crypt hyperplasia despite the different route of administration [26, 27]. They did not produce any IgA antibodies against tTG either [26]. This would indicate that the autoimmune component of celiac disease was lacking in these mice, despite the strong and varied responses against gliadin and deamidated gliadin epitopes. Thus, in these transgenic mice, DQ8 alone conferred gluten sensitivity but not symptomatic autoimmune disease. Therefore, an element of predisposition towards autoimmunity needed to be introduced into the model.

NOD Background

NOD mice spontaneously develop insulin-dependent diabetes and thus have been a useful animal model in the study of this autoimmune disease. As described above, a number of studies have demonstrated that these mice generate a limited immune response towards gluten as well. Based on these data, the NOD background was introduced into the DQ8 transgenic mice under the theory that the introduction of a genetic background associated with autoimmunity may allow symptomatic celiac disease to develop.

Gluten-Sensitive Blistering in NOD AB0 DQ8 Mice

Interestingly, some of the NOD DQ8 transgenic mice that had been sensitized to gluten and later fed gluten developed blistering on the ears [28]. The blisters developed as small white papules which progressed to form erythematous erosions that subsequently scabbed. Hematoxylin and eosin staining of skin biopsies from the ears revealed subepidermal blisters with upper to mid dermal inflammatory infiltrate [28]. The infiltration consisted of neutrophils, eosinophils, histiocytes and lymphocytes. Direct immunofluorescence analysis of the perilesional skin biopsies also showed granular IgA deposition at the basement membrane and the tips of the dermal papillae [28]. No IgA deposits were observed in areas that did not blister, such as the skin on the back of the mice. When these mice were placed onto a gluten-free diet, the blistering resolved in 2–3 weeks. Administration of dapsone resulted in a faster resolution, similar to that observed in dermatitis herpetiformis patients. All of these symptoms are similar to those observed in dermatitis herpetiformis, which is the skin manifestation of celiac disease. Thus, this was characterized as the first animal model of dermatitis herpetiformis [28].

Gluten-Sensitive Enteropathy in NOD AB0 DQ8 Mice

At the same time, some NOD AB0 DQ8 mice, after gluten sensitization and oral challenge with gluten, lost weight and demonstrated an overall appearance of fatigue. These mice produced IgA antibodies to gliadin and also IgA against tTG [29]. When examined histologically, the small intestine had an increased number of lymphocytes and some decrease in the villous height [29]. There was also a direct correlation between the presence of circulating IgA against tTG and the presence of enteropathy. Thus, the addition of the NOD background to the HLA-DQ8 transgenic mouse led to the development of symptomatic disease in these mice.

The results with the NOD AB0 DQ8 mice would demonstrate that genes present in the NOD background are necessary for the development of symptoms similar to celiac disease and dermatitis herpetiformis in DQ8 transgenic mice. Many genes present in the murine diabetes susceptibility loci of the NOD background could be contributing to this phenomenon. The genes most likely to be contributing would be those that predispose the NOD mice towards developing autoimmunity. Supporting this theory is the fact that patients with celiac disease and dermatitis herpetiformis are also predisposed towards they develop other autoimmune diseases such as diabetes and thyroiditis [30, 31].

Generation of DQ2 Transgenic Mice

We have recently generated transgenic mouse lines that express DQ2. Preliminary data demonstrate that the DQ2 molecule in these transgenic mice can present gliadin-derived peptides and activate T cells to proliferate (fig. 1). Both the 33-mer

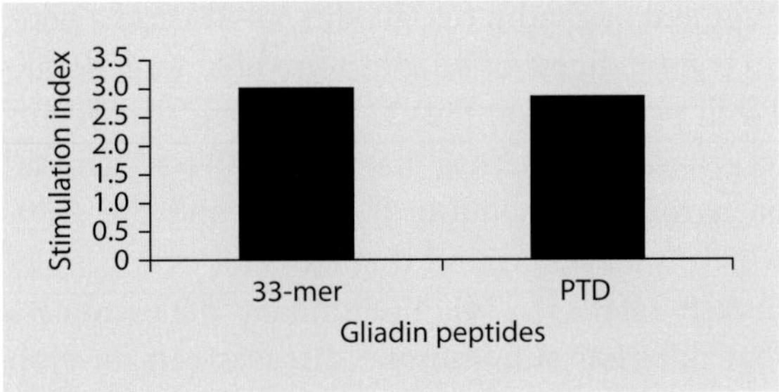

Fig. 1. Recognition of gliadin-derived peptides by DQ2 transgenic mice: mice that express DQ2 were injected subcutaneously with either the 33-mer peptide or a peptic tryptic digest of gliadin (PTD). Draining lymph nodes were extracted and restimulated with the appropriate peptide in vitro, and T-cell proliferation was measured by ^{3}H incorporation.

fragment of gliadin (α_2-gliadin 56–88) and a peptic tryptic digest of gliadin were able to generate T-cell proliferation [32, 33]. We have also begun to generate DQ2 lines that have different genetic backgrounds, including the NOD and the AE0, which is a background that lacks all endogenous mouse MHC II [34]. Preliminary data indicate that different autoimmune diseases can develop in the different DQ2 lines. Some DQ2 mice spontaneously develop a blistering disease with many characteristics similar to dermatitis herpetiformis, including gluten dependency. The DQ2 transgenic mice have therefore a great potential as models for celiac disease.

Use of HLA Transgenic Mice for Testing Novel Therapies

The ultimate goal for generating an animal model of celiac disease is to use them for testing novel therapies. Currently there are a number of proposed therapies, and some have already been tested in some of the aforementioned models.

One proposed therapy is to administer different agents or antigens in order to generate tolerance towards gliadin. This could be done in a number of different ways, and one group using HLA-DQ8 mice used whole gliadin administered intranasally. In those studies, they found that the intranasal administration of α-gliadin before parenteral injection of gliadin decreased the T-cell response towards gliadin in these gluten-sensitive HLA-DQ8 mice [35–37]. They also found that γ-interferon was significantly downregulated in this particular protocol for generating tolerance to gluten. Thus, this approach holds great promise as a therapy for both celiac disease and dermatitis herpetiformis.

Another approach is to inhibit the binding of immunogenic gliadin peptides to HLA-DQ2 and HLA-DQ8 by using 'inhibiting' peptides [38]. These inhibiting peptides would be synthesized with subtle changes in the amino acid sequencing allowing the 'inhibitors' to block the binding of gliadin-derived peptides to the DQ molecules, disrupt the activation of T cells and potentially alter the course of celiac disease [38]. Similar to the tolerance studies, these peptides could also be tested in HLA transgenic mice.

Conclusions

Together these animal models have significantly contributed to our understanding of the pathogenesis of celiac disease. The rabbit and dog models demonstrated that species which did not evolve to have gluten as a main staple of their diet are capable of generating systemic immune responses towards gluten/gliadin. These general immune responses may then result in the development of gluten-dependent enteropathy under the right circumstances. However, since these responses are MHC II independent, the rabbit and dog models may best reflect the 'innate' component of the intestinal immune response to gluten/gliadin. With the generation of HLA transgenic mice, the role of MHC II was able to be evaluated in the development of gluten-dependent enteropathy. These studies demonstrated that MHC II is necessary to develop systemic gluten sensitivity, but not sufficient for a 'true' enteropathy to occur. Furthermore, the addition of the NOD background allowed for the presentation of symptomatic disease, again suggesting that a predisposition towards autoimmunity is needed as well. Thus, it would appear that celiac disease is a complex intertwining of the innate and adaptive immune responses towards gluten in the setting of autoimmunity. HLA transgenic mouse lines, most especially the new DQ2 line, hold great promise as effective tools in characterizing how these adaptive, innate and autoimmune elements of celiac disease interact to result in symptomatic disease.

References

1 Stazi AV, Mantovani A: Possible animal models of endocrine, immune and reproductive complications of celiac disease. Minerva Med 2002;93:457.
2 March JB: High antigliadin IgG titers in laboratory rabbits fed a wheat-containing diet: a model for celiac disease? Dig Dis Sci 2003;48:608.
3 Batt RM, Carter MW, McLean L: Morphological and biochemical studies of a naturally occurring enteropathy in the Irish setter dog: a comparison with coeliac disease in man. Res Vet Sci 1984;37:339.
4 Batt RM, McLean L, Carter MW: Sequential morphologic and biochemical studies of naturally occurring wheat-sensitive enteropathy in Irish setter dogs. Dig Dis Sci 1987;32:184.
5 Hall EJ, Batt RM: Abnormal permeability precedes the development of a gluten sensitive enteropathy in Irish setter dogs. Gut 1991;32:749.
6 Polvi A, Garden OA, Houlston RS, Maki M, Batt RM, Partanen J: Genetic susceptibility to gluten sensitive enteropathy in Irish setter dogs is not linked to the major histocompatibility complex. Tissue Antigens 1998;52:543.
7 Troncone R, Ferguson A: Animal model of gluten induced enteropathy in mice. Gut 1991;32:871.
8 Hoorfar J, Buschard K, Dagnaes-Hansen F: Prophylactic nutritional modification of the incidence of diabetes in autoimmune non-obese diabetic (NOD) mice. Br J Nutr 1993;69:597.
9 Maurano F, Mazzarella G, Luongo D, Stefanile R, D'Arienzo R, Rossi M, Auricchio S, Troncone R: Small intestinal enteropathy in non-obese diabetic mice fed a diet containing wheat. Diabetologia 2005;48:931.
10 Sblattero D, Maurano F, Mazzarella G, Rossi M, Auricchio S, Florian F, Ziberna F, Tommasini A, Not T, Ventura A, Bradbury A, Marzari R, Troncone R: Characterization of the anti-tissue transglutaminase antibody response in nonobese diabetic mice. J Immunol 2005;174:5830.
11 Taneja V, David CS: HLA class II transgenic mice as models of human diseases. Immunol Rev 1999;169:67.
12 Cheng S, Baisch J, Krco C, Savarirayan S, Hanson J, Hodgson K, Smart M, David C: Expression and function of HLA-DQ8 (DQA1*0301/DQB1*0302) genes in transgenic mice. Eur J Immunogenet 1996;23:15.
13 Fugger L, Michie SA, Rulifson I, Lock CB, McDevitt GS: Expression of HLA-DR4 and human CD4 transgenes in mice determines the variable region beta-chain T-cell repertoire and mediates an HLA-DR-restricted immune response. Proc Natl Acad Sci USA 1994;91:6151.
14 Lawrance SK, Karlsson L, Price J, Quaranta V, Ron Y, Sprent J, Peterson PA: Transgenic HLA-DR alpha faithfully reconstitutes IE-controlled immune functions and induces cross-tolerance to E alpha in E alpha 0 mutant mice. Cell 1989;58:583.
15 Zhou P, Anderson GD, Savarirayan S, Inoko H, David CS: Thymic deletion of V beta 11+, V beta 5+ T cells in H-2E negative, HLA-DQ beta+ single transgenic mice. J Immunol 1991;146:854.
16 Rajagopalan G, Smart MK, Marietta EV, David CS: Staphylococcal enterotoxin B-induced activation and concomitant resistance to cell death in CD28-deficient HLA-DQ8 transgenic mice. Int Immunol 2002;14:801.
17 Rajagopalan G, Iijima K, Singh M, Kita H, Patel R, David CS: Intranasal exposure to bacterial superantigens induces airway inflammation in HLA class II transgenic mice. Infect Immun 2006;74:1284.
18 Rajagopalan G, Smart MK, Murali N, Patel R, David CS: Acute systemic immune activation following vaginal exposure to staphylococcal enterotoxin B – implications for menstrual shock. J Reprod Immunol 2007;73:51.
19 Geluk A, Taneja V, van Meijgaarden KE, Zanelli E, Abou-Zeid C, Thole JE, de Vries RR, David CS, Ottenhoff TH: Identification of HLA class II-restricted determinants of *Mycobacterium tuberculosis*-derived proteins by using HLA-transgenic, class II-deficient mice. Proc Natl Acad Sci USA 1998;95:10797.
20 Infante AJ, Baillargeon J, Kraig E, Lott L, Jackson C, Hammerling GJ, Raju R, David C: Evidence of a diverse T cell receptor repertoire for acetylcholine receptor, the autoantigen of myasthenia gravis. J Autoimmun 2003;21:167.
21 Yeung RS, Penninger JM, Kundig TM, Law Y, Yamamoto K, Kamikawaji N, Burkly L, Sasazuki T, Flavell R, Ohashi PS, Mak TW: Human CD4-major histocompatibility complex class II (DQw6) transgenic mice in an endogenous CD4/CD8-deficient background: reconstitution of phenotype and human-restricted function. J Exp Med 1994;180:1911.
22 Sonderstrup G, McDevitt H: Identification of autoantigen epitopes in MHC class II transgenic mice. Immunol Rev 1998;164:129.
23 Taneja V, David CS: HLA transgenic mice as humanized mouse models of disease and immunity. J Clin Invest 1998;101:921.
24 Nabozny GH, Baisch JM, Cheng S, Cosgrove D, Griffiths MM, Luthra HS, David CS: HLA-DQ8 transgenic mice are highly susceptible to collagen-induced arthritis: a novel model for human polyarthritis. J Exp Med 1996;183:27.
25 Neeno T, Krco CJ, Harders J, Baisch J, Cheng S, David CS: HLA-DQ8 transgenic mice lacking endogenous class II molecules respond to house dust allergens: identification of antigenic epitopes. J Immunol 1996;156:3191.
26 Black KE, Murray JA, David CS: HLA-DQ determines the response to exogenous wheat proteins: a model of gluten sensitivity in transgenic knockout mice. J Immunol 2002;169:5595.
27 Senger S, Maurano F, Mazzeo MF, Gaita M, Fierro O, David CS, Troncone R, Auricchio S, Siciliano RA, Rossi M: Identification of immunodominant epitopes of alpha-gliadin in HLA-DQ8 transgenic mice following oral immunization. J Immunol 2005;175:8087.
28 Marietta E, Black K, Camilleri M, Krause P, Rogers RS 3rd, David C, Pittelkow MR, Murray JA: A new model for dermatitis herpetiformis that uses HLA-DQ8 transgenic NOD mice. J Clin Invest 2004;114:1090.
29 Black KE, David CS, Murray JA: Gluten sensitivity in class II transgenic mice. Gastroenterology 2003;124:A26.
30 Schuppan D, Hahn EG: Celiac disease and its link to type 1 diabetes mellitus. J Pediatr Endocrinol Metab 2001;14(suppl 1):597.

31 Reunala T, Collin P: Diseases associated with dermatitis herpetiformis. Br J Dermatol 1997;136:315.

32 Qiao SW, Bergseng E, Molberg O, Xia J, Fleckenstein B, Khosla C, Sollid LM: Antigen presentation to celiac lesion-derived T cells of a 33-mer gliadin peptide naturally formed by gastrointestinal digestion. J Immunol 2004;173:1757.

33 van de Wal Y, Kooy YM, van Veelen PA, Pena SA, Mearin LM, Molberg O, Lundin KE, Sollid LM, Mutis T, Benckhuijsen WE, Drijfhout JW, Koning F: Small intestinal T cells of celiac disease patients recognize a natural pepsin fragment of gliadin. Proc Natl Acad Sci USA 1998;95:10050.

34 Madsen L, Labrecque N, Engberg J, Dierich A, Svejgaard A, Benoist C, Mathis D, Fugger L: Mice lacking all conventional MHC class II genes. Proc Natl Acad Sci USA 1999;96:10338.

35 Maurano F, Siciliano RA, De Giulio B, Luongo D, Mazzeo MF, Troncone R, Auricchio S, Rossi M: Intranasal administration of one alpha gliadin can downregulate the immune response to whole gliadin in mice. Scand J Immunol 2001;53:290.

36 Rossi M, Maurano F, Caputo N, Auricchio S, Sette A, Capparelli R, Troncone R: Intravenous or intranasal administration of gliadin is able to down-regulate the specific immune response in mice. Scand J Immunol 1999;50:177.

37 Senger S, Luongo D, Maurano F, Mazzeo MF, Siciliano RA, Gianfrani C, David C, Troncone R, Auricchio S, Rossi M: Intranasal administration of a recombinant alpha-gliadin down-regulates the immune response to wheat gliadin in DQ8 transgenic mice. Immunol Lett 2003;88:127.

38 Stepniak D, Vader LW, Kooy Y, van Veelen PA, Moustakas A, Papandreou NA, Eliopoulos E, Drijfhout JW, Papadopoulos GK, Koning F: T-cell recognition of HLA-DQ2-bound gluten peptides can be influenced by an N-terminal proline at p-1. Immunogenetics 2005;57:8.

Chella S. David, PhD
Department of Immunology, Mayo Clinic College of Medicine
Rochester, MN 55905 (USA)
Tel. +1 507 284 8180, Fax +1 507 266 0981, E-Mail david.chella@mayo.edu

Author Index

Subject Index